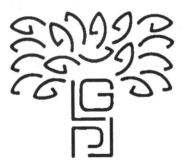

LA GRANGE
PUBLIC LIBRARY

10 West Cossitt Avenue
La Grange, IL 60525
lagrangelibrary.org   708.215.3200

Drugged

Drugged
The Science and Culture Behind Psychotropic Drugs

Richard J. Miller, PhD

Alfred Newton Richards
Professor of Pharmacology
Northwestern University
Medical school
Chicago, IL

OXFORD
UNIVERSITY PRESS

OXFORD
UNIVERSITY PRESS

Oxford University Press is a department of the University of Oxford.
It furthers the University's objective of excellence in research, scholarship,
and education by publishing worldwide.

Oxford   New York
Auckland   Cape Town   Dar es Salaam   Hong Kong   Karachi
Kuala Lumpur   Madrid   Melbourne   Mexico City   Nairobi
New Delhi   Shanghai   Taipei   Toronto

With offices in

Argentina   Austria   Brazil   Chile   Czech Republic   France   Greece
Guatemala   Hungary   Italy   Japan   Poland   Portugal   Singapore
South Korea   Switzerland   Thailand   Turkey   Ukraine   Vietnam

Oxford is a registered trademark of Oxford University Press in the UK and certain other
countries.

Published in the United States of America by
Oxford University Press
198 Madison Avenue, New York, NY 10016

© Oxford University Press 2014

Library of Congress Cataloging-in-Publication Data
Miller, Richard J., 1950- author.
Drugged: the science and culture behind psychotropic drugs / Richard J. Miller.
p. ; cm.
Includes bibliographical references and index.
ISBN 978–0–19–995797–2 (alk. paper)—ISBN 978–0–19–995798–9 (alk. paper)—
ISBN 978–0–19–932196–4 (alk. paper)
I. Title.
[DNLM: 1. Psychotropic Drugs—history. 2. Behavior—drug effects. 3. Brain—drug
effects. 4. Civilization—history. 5. Psychotropic Drugs—pharmacology. QV 77.2]
RM333.5
615.7′88—dc23
2013009308

9 8 7 6 5 4 3 2 1
Printed in the United States of America
on acid-free paper

To Lauren—with all my love for ever and ever.

PREFACE

"I'll have a tall latte with an extra shot."
"Make mine a scotch and soda."
"Excuse me, but do you have a light?"

The chatter of our everyday lives is filled with references to the use of psychotropic drugs. Caffeine, alcohol, nicotine—there can't be many people around today who haven't tried these substances in one form or another. Indeed, many people partake of these things fairly regularly; their use is completely integrated into our society.

But what exactly do we mean by the term "psychotropic drug"? Generally speaking we are talking about chemical substances that enter the brain and change the way it operates. These alterations affect one of the brain's most important outputs: the quality of our conscious experience. In most people's view, consciousness is an expansive property that "emerges" from the complex behavior of the cells that make up the physical substrate of the brain, although exactly how this happens is still a great mystery.

But our consciousness is also limited. Like the prisoners in Plato's cave, our normal experiences may only represent the shadows of a greater reality. Mankind has always been interested in using psychotropic drugs for the purpose of changing or expanding his consciousness so that he might open up new visions of time and space. William Blake, a man whose day-to-day experiences were so mystical and exalted that he didn't really need chemical substances to expand them further, seemed to have this in mind when he wrote, "If the doors of perception were cleansed every thing would appear to man as it is, Infinite. For man has closed himself up, till he sees all things thro' narrow chinks of his cavern." Man has always used psychotropic drugs to enlarge these narrow chinks and unlock the doors of perception.

The use of psychotropic drugs is an ancient practice. Exploration of prehistoric grave sites has frequently yielded evidence suggesting that ancient man was aware of, and presumably used, numerous mind altering substances. These early psychotropic agents were probably employed in the next important therapeutic approaches for psychopharmacology, as the Psychopharmacological Revolution has lost a lot of its momentum in recent years. New drugs and drug targets in the brain are needed. In the final chapter we will talk about the connection between the brain and the immune system and how this may be the key for discovering new treatments for mental illness.

But all that is in the future. The story of psychotropic drugs starts a very long time ago—as early as man himself....

ACKNOWLEDGEMENTS

I am indebted to the many people who helped me in the preparation of this book. Primarily, I would like to thank my wife Lauren, who read the entire thing and helped me type it, edit it, and provided essential critical feedback. Others also provided me with critical reading, including Fletcher White, Jelena Radulovic, Bob Schleimer, Anis Contractor, Phil Hockberger, Anne Marie Malfait, and Brandon Miller.

I would like to thank several people who helped me with preparing the manuscript, including Ghazal Banisadr, Garry Cooper, and Andrew Shum. I would like to thank Wendy Doniger and Bjarke Ebert for their recollections as to significant events described in the book.

Finally, I would like to acknowledge the high level of professional assistance I received from Oxford University Press, particularly from Craig Panner and his team. Thank you all very much!

CONTENTS

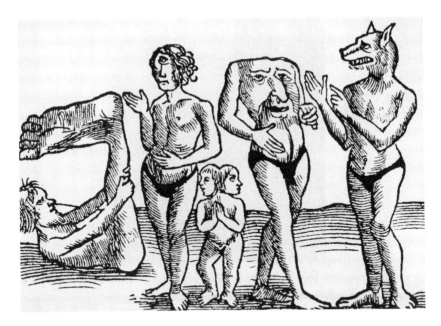

Figure 1.4:
Drawing of "medieval monsters" including the Cyclops, the one-legged man, and the "face in torso" that have been suggested to represent the mushroom *A. muscaria*.[4]
From *Cosmographia* by Sebastien Munster, Basel, 1544 (Corbis Images).

It is true that in some respects, such as their simple symmetry, these mythical creatures could represent the idealized shape of a mushroom. Wasson hypothesized that it was necessary to create these mythical creatures as a way of encoding the existence *Amanita muscaria* because its holy nature made it a taboo to speak of it directly. However, there are clearly other possible explanations. For example, the rare developmental syndrome known as holoprosencephaly[16] is associated with a Cyclops-like appearance (Figure 1.5).

Although very rare, the occasional births of such children in antiquity would surely have received a good deal of attention and could well have become the subject of myths. Indeed, the fact that such things must have occurred intermittently throughout the world would explain the existence of the Cyclops in both Indian and Greek mythology. Moreover, it is quite obvious that the human torso, particularly that of a woman, does bear a close resemblance to a face—something that wasn't lost on the surrealist painter Renee Magritte (Figure 1.6). So there is no real reason to invoke magic mushrooms when thinking about the origins of medieval mythical figures. Thus, when subject to scrutiny, the individual pieces of evidence suggested by Wasson are often not particularly convincing. Scholarly opinion is still divided on these issues. Overall, however, whether or not one is

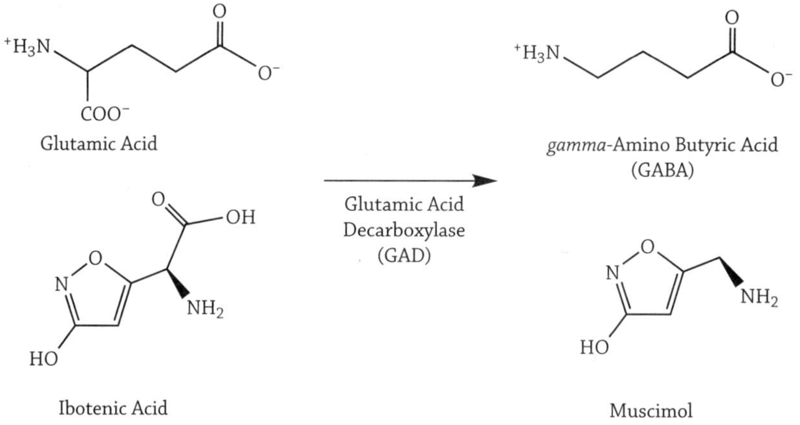

Figure 1.8:
Decarboxylation of glutamic and ibotenic acids by the enzyme glutamate decarboxylase (GAD) produces GABA and muscimol respectively.

decarboxylation and secretion would be repeated.[11] Depending on the initial dose of ibotenic acid ingested, the cycle of decarboxylation and secretion might be repeated several times, and of course this is what is actually observed in practice. It has also been shown that the mushroom's bright red cap contains the highest concentration of ibotenic acid, thus explaining the observation that the mushroom loses its potency when the cap is removed.

HOW DOES MUSCIMOL WORK?

But if muscimol is ultimately responsible for the major psychological effects of *Amanita muscaria,* how exactly does it work? In order to answer this question we must take a step back and consider some of the basic tenets of the science of neuropharmacology. The first and most important of these is the idea that the majority of drugs that produce significant effects on the nervous system do so by either directly or indirectly interfering with the process of chemical neurotransmission—the mechanism through which nerve cells communicate with one another across synapses. According to this model, nerve cells secrete specific chemicals called *neurotransmitters,* which act as messengers that alter the activity of other nerve cells or end organs such as glands and muscle cells. This signaling function is achieved through interaction of the chemical neurotransmitter with a protein receptor molecule expressed by the targeted nerve or muscle cell. This receptor molecule decodes the information imparted by its interaction with the neurotransmitter molecule and "instructs" the targeted nerve to act accordingly—usually by altering its electrical activity and firing "action potentials" more or less frequently. The action potential is an electrical impulse that nerves use to encode information. Groups of action potentials constitute the words and sentences that make up the syntax of nerve cell communication.

These ideas emerged from the research of the great pharmacologists and physiologists of the early twentieth century. The first neurotransmitter molecules to be discovered were acetylcholine and norepinephrine (noradrenaline), which were shown to mediate the effects of nerve stimulation in the peripheral (autonomic) nervous system. However, there was initially considerable resistance to the idea that such molecules might have a similar function in the brain, where it was thought that their actions were too slow to mediate the requirements of the neural circuits responsible for higher brain functions.[24] Nevertheless, it eventually became clear that chemical neurotransmission was the way in which all except a very few nerves functioned. Thus, as the twentieth century proceeded, the hunt was on to identify more molecules that might carry out the functions of neurotransmitters in the brain in particular. In subsequent chapters we shall discuss the properties of several of these substances. Surprisingly, the two most commonly used neurotransmitters in the brain turned out to be simple amino acids, the molecules which we normally think of as being the basic building blocks of proteins.

The detection of novel neurotransmitter molecules in the middle of the twentieth century was aided by the development of new assay systems, frequently derived from the simple nervous systems of invertebrates, which allowed small amounts of these substances to be accurately and conveniently measured. In the mid 1950s Ernst Florey, an Austrian native working in California, had discovered that the brain contained an inhibitory substance which he named "Factor I"—I standing for "inhibition."[25] This substance inhibited the activity of crayfish stretch receptor neurons, the system he was using as an assay. Interestingly, he observed that the effects of Factor I were blocked by picrotoxin, a powerful excitant drug capable of inducing seizures in animals. The mechanism of action of convulsant drugs like picrotoxin, bicuculline, strychnine, and other powerful stimulants that were first identified in the nineteenth and early twentieth centuries were not understood at the molecular level but were part of the developing chemical armamentum available to neuropharmacologists for probing the properties of the nervous system.

Prior to Florey's studies the amino acid GABA (γ-amino butyric acid) had been shown to exist in the brain (Figure 1.8). GABA was not one of the amino acids that were normally used to make protein molecules, and its functions were not understood. However, together with several other colleagues Florey was able to demonstrate that GABA was identical to Factor I. GABA produced inhibition of neuronal activity in his assay preparations, and these inhibitory effects could be reversed by stimulant drugs such as picrotoxin and bicuculline. Subsequent studies confirmed the idea that GABA acted as an inhibitory neurotransmitter and that picrotoxin and bicuculline could block its effects. About this time it was observed that in contrast to the inhibitory effects of GABA, certain other amino acids, particularly glutamate, produced a powerful excitatory effect on neurons. In other words, glutamate produced the opposite effects to GABA. GABA is produced in the brain by decarboxylation of glutamate (Figure 1.8). Thus, the parent molecule, glutamate, and its product, GABA, were observed to have precisely the opposite effects on nerve activity. Further studies suggested that glutamate was a widely used excitatory neurotransmitter in the brain. Subsequently the amino acid glycine was observed to produce neurotransmitter-like inhibitory effects in the spinal cord, and its action was specifically inhibited by the drug strychnine. Thus, by the end of the 1960s a well-defined group of amino acid neurotransmitters had been shown to have widespread inhibitory or excitatory effects on the nervous system.

The idea that glutamate and GABA have important neurotransmitter roles in the brain is key to understanding how *Amanita muscaria* produces its effects. It is easy to see from a brief inspection of their chemical structures that ibotenic acid and muscimol represent slightly modified versions of the two amino acid neurotransmitters glutamate and GABA (Figure 1.8). The inclusion of chemical ring systems in ibotenic acid and muscimol means that they represent "conformationally restricted" versions of the two amino acid neurotransmitters—that is, the movement of the atoms in muscimol and ibotenic acid is more restricted than in GABA and glutamate. Nevertheless, the pharmacological properties of the two mushroom molecules are similar to those of the two neurotransmitters they resemble, muscimol being inhibitory like GABA and ibotenic acid being excitatory like glutamate.

Indeed, it can be shown that the ibotenic acid activates receptors for glutamate and muscimol activates receptors for GABA. Thus, ibotenic acid and its decarboxylation product muscimol mimic the effects of glutamate and its decarboxylation product GABA. Given the model discussed above, which suggests that it is muscimol that is the ultimate determinant of the effects of ingested ibotenic acid, it would be interesting for us to know exactly how GABA produces its effects on nerve cells, how these can be mimicked by muscimol, and how these lead to the observed psychotropic effects of mushroom ingestion.

As we have discussed, receptor proteins are the molecules which are activated by neurotransmitters in order to produce their effects. Drugs that mimic the effects of neurotransmitters and activate receptors are known as *agonists,* and drugs that inhibit the activation of receptors are known as *antagonists*. Receptors for the neurotransmitter actions of GABA represent the predominant inhibitory receptors in the central nervous system. That is to say that their activation usually leads to an inhibition of nerve cell activity. Two major types of GABA receptors, known as GABA-A and GABA-B receptors, have been identified and they typify the two major molecular classes of receptors for virtually all neurotransmitters. GABA-A receptors are ion channels, meaning that they are protein molecules that allow the movement of electrically charged ions across the nerve cell membrane. The opening and closing ("gating") of this kind of receptor is regulated by the binding of the neurotransmitter GABA.

The second type of receptor (GABA-B) generates cellular messages by a variety of means, including the activation of intracellular protein molecules such as G proteins, the molecule β–arrestin, and numerous other biochemical pathways. Generally speaking these latter receptor molecules are known as *G protein coupled receptors* (GPCRs), being so named after their first identified function, the activation of G proteins. Because the activation of GPCRs and subsequent generation of biochemical messenger molecules normally involves several molecular steps, the information they transduce is relatively slow. On the other hand, receptors such as GABA-A receptors that are ion channels produce extremely rapid changes in the distribution of ions across the nerve cell membrane. This movement of ions across the nerve cell membrane changes its electrical properties, and this acts as a very rapid signal (<1 sec) responsible for mediating synaptic transmission in the brain. The receptors for both glutamate and GABA, which mediate fast excitatory and inhibitory synaptic responses respectively, are ion channels. In technical parlance the molecule activating the receptor, glutamate or GABA in this instance, is called a *ligand* and so these receptors are known as *ligand gated ion channels.*

GABA-A receptors have turned out to be of central importance for understanding rapid synaptic inhibition in the brain and are also the sites of action of many important classes of drugs such as sedatives, hypnotics, anesthetics, and anxiolytics—including benzodiazepines, barbiturates, and alcohol (Chapter 6). It is these GABA-A receptors that are also activated by muscimol. In the 1980s it became clear that the GABA-A receptors were related in structure to those of previously well-studied ligand gated ion channel receptors known as *nicotinic acetylcholine receptors*. Like GABA receptors, the receptors for the neurotransmitter acetylcholine can also be separated into two families, represented by ligand gated ion channels and GPCRs. The former types of receptors can be activated by the drug nicotine (Chapter 8) and, as we have discussed, the latter class can be activated by muscarine. Thus, just as we speak of GABA-A and GABA-B receptors for GABA, we speak of nicotinic and muscarinic receptors for acetylcholine.

Nicotinic receptors were shown to mediate the fast synaptic actions of the neurotransmitter acetylcholine in sympathetic ganglia and at the motor neuron synapses innervating skeletal muscle. When GABA-A receptors arrived on the scene, a great deal of information had already been obtained about the structure of nicotinic receptors and so this was very helpful in understanding the structure and functions of GABA-A receptors. Like nicotinic receptors, the structure of GABA-A receptors consists of 5 protein subunits arranged in a pentameric array. Each protein subunit snakes its way across the cell membrane four times, so that both its beginning and end, known as the N- and C-termini, are outside the cell. The 5 protein subunits are arranged so that the second membrane-spanning region from each subunit surrounds a pore or ion channel that crosses the membrane. The subunits resemble the staves of a barrel surrounding a central pathway that allows the flow of ions across the cell membrane when the receptor is activated. Normally the GABA-A receptor channel is closed. However, when agonist molecules like GABA or muscimol bind to the receptor they cause a conformational change in its structure so that the channel opens, allowing the flow of Cl ions until the channel closes once again. One could imagine that GABA or muscimol are the "keys" that open the GABA-A receptor "door."[26-28] The flow of negatively charged Cl ions into the neuron has an inhibitory effect, making it harder for the cell to fire action potentials.

MUSCIMOL BECOMES GABOXADOL

Something that is frequently the case in neuropharmacology is that the development of a useful drug begins with a natural product, and the story of muscimol is an excellent example of this. When we consider the effects of *Amanita muscaria*, certain things might suggest to us that muscimol is actually an attractive candidate for modern drug development. After all, drugs like benzodiazepines and barbiturates that also activate GABA-A receptors have found widespread utility in treating epilepsy and as hypnotics (that is, drugs that help people sleep)—so why shouldn't muscimol be developed in the same way?

This seems a perfectly reasonable idea. Indeed, it is an idea that has been given considerable attention. We might predict that muscimol itself is unlikely to make a useful drug—the evidence resulting from its use over many thousands of years suggests that it is likely to produce too many unwanted psychotropic and other effects to be useful. Moreover, it would not be possible to patent muscimol and so it would not be an attractive target for a drug company to develop. However, medicinal chemists and pharmaceutical companies may also think about muscimol in an entirely different light. The currently used GABA-A receptor activating drugs all have certain problems associated with them. For example, benzodiazepines certainly work very well for many purposes but they are associated with some undesirable side effects such as causing a drug dependency syndrome. Moreover, the sleep pattern they produce in patients is not exactly like normal sleep (Chapter 6). Hence, one might suppose that they could be improved upon. Muscimol represents a completely different type of chemical structure than previously developed GABA-A receptor activating drugs. So the idea is that perhaps if one plays around with its chemistry enough, a new compound will emerge that will have improved properties in comparison to all the preceding GABA-A receptor activating drugs. For example, perhaps it will have fewer side effects or do something that is completely unique.

It was with this in mind that Dr. Povl Krogsgaard-Larsen and his colleagues in Denmark started to explore the properties of the muscimol molecule in the 1970s, with a view to making changes to its chemical structure and examining the effects this had on its properties. Over the years they produced hundreds of GABA and muscimol analogues and have invented some very interesting substances.[29]

To understand what they achieved, let us begin with GABA itself and think about how we might alter its structure to make an effective drug. One of the first things to note is that GABA is a very flexible molecule; that is to say, its atoms can take up a large number of positions in space relative to one another (Figure 1.9). GABA is rapidly metabolized by the body and doesn't get into the brain at all easily if ingested or injected, so it wouldn't make a useful drug. Now let us consider the properties of muscimol, which *Amanita muscaria* has already made for us. The carboxyl acid group (-COOH) of GABA has been replaced by a 3-isoxazolol group, thereby restricting the conformation of this part of the molecule (Figure 1.9). As we have seen, this substitution allows the molecule to cross the blood–brain barrier fairly well while maintaining its ability to activate GABA-A

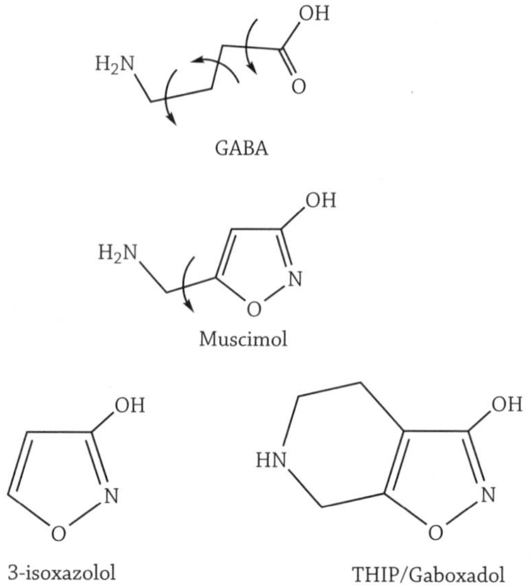

GABA

Muscimol

3-isoxazolol   THIP/Gaboxadol

Figure 1.9:
Restricted conformation of the carboxyl terminal of GABA in muscimol and of the carboxyl and amino termini in gaboxadol/THIP.

receptors. In technical parlance one says that the 3-isoxazalol group is a very efficient "bioisostere" for the carboxyl group in GABA.

Now muscimol activates GABA-A receptors very nicely, and also gets into the brain relatively easily, but are there any further things one can do to improve its effects by increasing its stability and access to the nervous system? How about incorporating the other end of the GABA molecule—that is, the amino function—into something like a piperidine ring system to restrict its conformation even further? When this is done, relatively stable molecules are produced that also retain their ability to activate GABA receptors. So now, how about incorporating these same changes into muscimol to produce a GABA analogue with conformationally restricted carboxyl and amino functions (Figure 1.9)? The resulting molecule is THIP (or in chemical language: 4,5,6,7-tetrahydroisoxazolo[3,4-c]pyridine-3-ol). When Krogsgaard-Larsen and his colleagues made this molecule they found that they had produced a very potent GABA-A agonist, which was metabolically very stable and entered the brain even more easily than muscimol—excellent progress!

But was THIP just another version of muscimol or was it different in some way? Did it have any novel and interesting properties when administered to animals indicating that it might be a lead for future drug development? Initial animal studies were promising and encouraged the view that

be used clinically. Gaboxadol did turn out to produce side effects at these high doses when tested in a population of known drug abusers. The side effects included visual hallucinations, but more importantly restlessness and anxiety reminiscent of an abrupt benzodiazepine withdrawal syndrome. A retrospective analysis of previous data also revealed that a few patients in the clinical trials who had taken higher than the recommended dose of gaboxadol also displayed similar behavioral effects. When this data was presented to Merck, one of their top executives commented, "Looks like LSD to me!" This was not meant to be a compliment and that just about did it. Merck pulled out and it was decided that Lundbeck would not go forward alone and make an NDA to the FDA.

At the time when they made their decision, Lundbeck didn't know much about the mechanisms underlying these side effects, which were never seen in insomniacs or even in drug abusers at normal therapeutic doses, but they didn't dare to use the compound in the general population just in case. Since that time Lundbeck and others have performed a series of rodent studies and published data demonstrating that drug abusers do get a bizarre response to GABA-A agonists even months after abusing drugs like amphetamine or cocaine. Indeed, it seems as though longterm drug abuse produces similarly long-lasting changes in the properties of neurons in the brain which underlie the rewarding effects of abused drugs. Published research demonstrates that drugs like muscimol and gaboxadol produce a response on these nerves in addicted animals that is actually the opposite of the response they produce normally.[31] Instead of inhibiting these neurons, they activate them.

The story of gaboxadol is a good illustration of the drug development process in general. Gaboxadol certainly did deliver. It produced unique, potentially highly beneficial effects on sleep, no tolerance or dependence, and no abuse potential, thereby distinguishing itself from drugs like benzodiazepines that are already on the market. And yet it failed. It didn't perform well in US clinical trials and it showed some bizarre effects in the drug abuse population. Lundbeck's chosen partner Merck was suffering from post-traumatic stress disorder as a result of its Vioxx fiasco and were not in any mood to invest in anything that wasn't a 100% conservative bet. Should Lundbeck have seen any of this coming? They could be forgiven for not anticipating the effect of the typical US diet on their clinical trials. However, given the history of muscimol it isn't too surprising that some type of bizarre psychiatric side effects had turned up eventually, even if they were outside the intended dose regimen. In addition, it is possible that the company didn't approach the FDA correctly and didn't stress the unique character of their drug appropriately.

So, what does the future hold in store for gaboxadol? The original patent obtained by Krogsgaard-Larsen has expired at this point—one of the consequences of being well ahead of your time. Nevertheless, Bjarke Ebert is excited about new possibilities. It seems as though gaboxadol has beneficial effects in tinnitus (ringing in the ears), one of the up and coming iPod-induced diseases of the twenty-first century, and there are some other possibilities as well.

Thus, thousands of years after our distant ancestors began consuming *Amanita muscaria,* the mushroom is finally giving up its secrets and pointing the way to the future. It is certainly not hard to believe that the inhabitants of Gobekli Tepe used entheogenic plants like *Amanita muscaria* as part of their religious life. Perhaps it is also true, as believed by many archeologists, that the vast array of giant monoliths they constructed look quite humanoid in certain respects. But then again, maybe they just look like giant mushrooms (Figure 1.10).

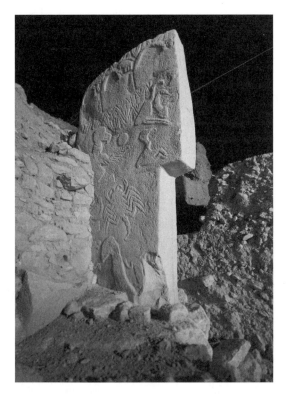

Figure 1.10:
Man or mushroom?
(National Geographic Image Collection / Alamy)

NOTES

1. Sir Thomas Browne (1605–1682) was one of the greatest writers on science and related topics. The *Hydriotaphia, Urn Burial, or a Discourse of the Sepulchral Urns lately found in Norfolk,* was published in 1658 and discusses the discovery of a buried trove of Roman urns in Norfolk. Browne was an incredibly erudite person and a marvelously eloquent writer. See *The Major Works* by Sir Thomas Browne, Penguin Books, 1977.

2. National Geographic (June 2011) contains a detailed description and discussion about the excavations at Gobekli Tepe.

3. Henderson GL. Designer drugs: Past history and future prospects. *J Forensic Sci,* 1988, 33:569–575.

4. Wasson RG, Kramrisch SK, Ott J, Ruck CAP. *Persephone's Quest.* Yale University Press. 1992.

5. Louis Lewin. *Phantastica.* Park Street Press. 1931.

6. Ibid., p. 84.

7. Discussed in *Acid Dreams* by Martin A Lee and Bruce Shlain. Grove Press. 1985.

8. Griffiths R, Richards W, Johnson M, McCann U, Jesse R. Mystical-type experiences occasioned by psilocybin mediate the attribution of personal meaning and spiritual significance 14 months later. *J Psychopharmacol.* 2008, 22:621–632.

9. *The Rigveda: Complete.* Translated by Ralph TH Griffiths. Forgotten Books. 2008.

10. Gordon R Wasson. *Soma: divine mushroom of immortality.* Harcourt Brace Jovanovich, Inc. 1972.

11. Discussed in two very useful and interesting books: *Shroom* by Letcher A, Harper-Collins, and *Pharmacotheon* by Ott J, Natural Products Co. The latter book is a very detailed source of information concerning the chemistry and biology of psychoactive drugs.

12. Oliver Goldsmith (1730–1774) wrote a novel entitled *Citizen of the World* which described, among other things, the possible effects of urine-drinking in British society (see Letcher A, p. 122–123).

13. See Letcher A (ref 11) p. 125 for a discussion of Mordecai Cubitt Cooke.

14. Wasson wrote many books and articles on this topic, particularly his *magnum opus* (ref 10). "Persephone's Quest" (ref 4) represents a good summary of his diverse work.

15. Prester John was a legendary monarch of a lost Christian kingdom said to be situated somewhere in the Orient, possibly India. Stories relating to Prester John and his kingdom were popular between the twelfth and seventeenth centuries in Europe. His kingdom was said to be the domain of many wonders and mythical creatures.

16. Holoprosencephaly is a condition in which the two hemispheres of the brain fail to separate properly. It is associated with deformation of midline structures along the face and head (lips, eyes, nose) so that they tend to fuse together. The disease can range from being very mild, such as the fusion of a single central incisor, to moderate, as in cleft palate syndrome, to very serious as in cyclopia. Serious forms of the disease are usually fatal *in utero* or early in life. The condition also exists in other species, such as cats, or may result from cattle or sheep eating plants such as the corn lily that contain the alkaloid cyclopamine.

17. John M Allegro. *The Sacred Mushroom and the Cross.* Gnostic Media Research & Publishing. 2009.

18. In his short story "*Tlon, Uqbar, Orbis Tertius*" Jorge Luis Borges describes how the fictional culture of Tlon, invented in the Middle Ages by a group of seventeenth-century intellectuals including Bishop Berkley, eventually takes over the real physical world.

19. This conclusion is very controversial. Many other authors, such as Wasson, have concluded that the tree in the fresco is a stylized representation of a pine tree rather than an *A. muscaria*.

20. For example see *Magic Mushrooms in Religion and Alchemy* by Clark Heinrich. Park Street Press. 2002.

21. Michelot D, Melendez-Howell LM. *Amanita muscaria*: chemistry, biology, toxicology, and ethnomycology. *Mycol Res*. 2003, 107(Pt 2):131–146.

22. Existence. "Infinite Nothingness. An experience with Amanita Muscaria (var. formosa)". *Erowid Extracts*. 2011, 20:p20.

23. Hanus LD, Rezanka T, Spizek J, Dembitsky VM. Substances isolated from Mandragora species. *Phytochemistry*. 2005, 66:2408–2417.

24. Elliot S Valenstein. *The War of the Soups and the Sparks*. Columbia University Press. 2005.

25. Bowery NG, Smart TG. GABA and glycine as neurotransmitters: a brief history. *Br J Pharmacol*. 2006, 147 (Suppl 1):S109–119.

26. D'Hulst C, Atack JR, Kooy RF. The complexity of the GABA-A receptor shapes unique pharmacological profiles. *Drug Discov Today*. 2009, 14:866–875.

27. Nutt D. GABA-A receptors: subtypes, regional distribution, and function. *J Clin Sleep Med*. 2006, 2:S7–11.

28. Orser BA. Extrasynaptic GABA-A receptors are critical targets for sedative-hypnotic drugs. *J Clin Sleep Med*. 2006, 2:S12–18.

29. Krogsgaard-Larsen P, Brehm L, Schaumburg K. Muscimol, a psychoactive constituent of Amanita muscaria, as a medicinal chemical model structure. *Acta Chem Scand B*. 1981, 35:311–324.

30. Lancel M. Role of GABAA receptors in the regulation of sleep: initial sleep responses to peripherally administered modulators and agonists. *Sleep*. 1999, 22:33–42.

31. Vargas-Perez H, Ting-A Kee R, Walton CH, Hansen DM, Razavi R, Clarke L, Bufalino MR, Allison DW, Steffensen SC, van der Kooy D. Ventral tegmental area BDNF induces an opiate-dependent-like reward state in naive rats. *Science*. 2009, 324:1732–1734.

32. Nikolai Nikolaevich Dikov. *Mysteries in the Rocks of Ancient Chukotka*. Moscow, Nauka. 1971.

33. Roessler E, Belloni E, Gaudenz K, Jay P, Berta P, Scherer SW, Tsui LC, Muenke M. Mutations in the human Sonic Hedgehog gene cause holoprosencephaly. *Nature Genetics*. 1996, 14:357–360.

CHAPTER 2

✧

Bicycle Day

"Sandoz, Sandoz who taught me love,

Sandoz, Sandoz, heavens above,

They could all learn something from your mind

Yeah baby!"

Eric Burdon and the Animals, "A Girl Named Sandoz" (1967)

If you were going to predict which country would jumpstart the counter-culture movement of the 1960s, it wouldn't be Switzerland. In Switzerland nothing seems out of place. Sitting in the Lindenhof overlooking the river Limmat, the capital of Zurich looks like the perfect Mittel-European small city. It is the essence of picturesqueness—that is, of course, if you ignore the heroin addicts strewn all over the Spitzplatz behind the Hauptbahnhof. The worthy citizens of Switzerland have a well earned reputation for being no-nonsense folk, hardworking and sensible. But perhaps there is another Switzerland percolating just below the surface? If we consider the life of the religious revolutionary Ulrich Zwingli, the work of the great alchemist Philippus Aureolus Theophrastus Bombastus von Hohenheim (aka Paracelsus), or the brooding canvases of the painter Arnold Böcklin, then we may realize that there is a very different Swiss personality strain that emerges every so often if the opportunity arises. Perhaps that is the best way of understanding the career of Albert Hoffman—the man who discovered LSD.

Basel is the center of the Swiss pharmaceutical industry, with its many drug and chemical companies arrayed along the banks of the river Rhine.

These companies are tucked into a corner of Europe where the borders of three countries—Switzerland, Germany, and France—all meet. I remember visiting the Sandoz company in the 1980s and being surprised that if I parked my car near the main research building I was in Switzerland, but if I parked at some distance across the parking lot I was actually in Germany!

The chemical company of Kern & Sandoz was founded by Alfred Kern and Edouard Sandoz in 1886. As can be seen from the names of the two founders, German and French, this was a typically Swiss mixture. As with many successful pharmaceutical companies, Kern and Sandoz began by making dyestuffs. Subsequently, the company became known solely as Sandoz and began making pharmaceuticals, the analgesic and antipyretic antipyrine being its first major product of this type.

In 1917 Sandoz created a pharmaceutical department headed by Professor Arthur Stoll (1887–1971) and started a pharmaceutical research group to search for novel drugs. It was this department that the young Albert Hoffman joined following the completion of his PhD at the University of Zurich in 1929. Just as we have described in the case of gaboxadol (Chapter 1), the Sandoz research department was interested in following up therapeutic leads based on natural products. Indeed, they had already had some success with this approach, having succeeded in the isolation and marketing of ergotamine, a leading drug for the treatment of migraine. After a period of time in which the young Albert Hoffmann was concerned with attempts to isolate substances known as cardiac glycosides from the Mediterranean Squill (a small hyacinth-like plant), he shifted his attention to making semisynthetic derivatives of lysergic acid—an intermediate in the biosynthesis of all the ergot alkaloids including ergotamine. In 1938 he synthesized lysergic acid diethylamide (LSD) or LSD-25, as it was the 25th substance he had made. Hoffmann had predicted that LSD might possess "analeptic" actions; that is to say, it would act as a respiratory stimulant. He thought this because its structure was similar to nikethamide (nicotinic acid diethylamide), a drug that was known to have this kind of effect. Unfortunately, when LSD was tested on animals, analeptic activity was not observed. Hoffmann did observe that the animals became somewhat restless during the experiments, but this was not considered to be very interesting and the compound was shelved.

However, there was something of the genius about Hoffmann. He had "insights" and "hunches" that normal people just don't have. Science is supposed to be an entirely logical enterprise. However, every scientist knows this is not entirely true. Really good scientists have an instinct about how things work. Where it comes from, nobody knows. As Hoffmann recounts in his memoirs, for no real reason he couldn't get LSD-25 out of his mind and had a hunch that there was more to the compound than had been observed. But he was very busy with his project and didn't get round to making it again until 1943. What happened next was detailed in a report he sent to his superior, Prof. Stoll:[1]

"Last Friday, April 16, 1943, I was forced to interrupt my work in the laboratory in the middle of the afternoon and proceed home, being affected by a remarkable restlessness, combined with a slight dizziness. At home I lay down and sank into a not unpleasant intoxicated-like condition, characterized by an extremely stimulated imagination. In a dreamlike state, with eyes closed (I found the daylight to be unpleasantly glaring), I perceived an uninterrupted stream of fantastic pictures, extraordinary shapes with intense, kaleidoscopic play of colors. After some two hours this condition faded away."

Hoffmann realized that his experiences were likely due to the substance he had been preparing in the laboratory and that it seemed possible that he might have absorbed some of it through his skin. Because Hoffmann was very meticulous he knew that if this was the case the amount must have been very small indeed. A few days later he tested this hypothesis by self–experimentation, taking some LSD tartrate orally at a dose (0.25 mg) which would have been appropriate if he were taking one of the other Sandoz ergot-based drugs such as ergotamine. Of course he didn't realize that he had synthesized one of the most potent drugs known to man and that the dose he took was about 10 times greater than the actual minimum amount of LSD required to produce an effect. Here are his laboratory notes.

"4/19/43 16:20: 0.5 cc of 1/2 promil aqueous solution of diethylamide tartrate orally = 0.25 mg tartrate. Taken diluted with about 10 cc water. Tasteless.

17:00: Beginning dizziness, feeling of anxiety, visual distortions, symptoms of paralysis, desire to laugh.

Supplement of 4/21: Home by bicycle. From 18:00 – ca. 20:00 most severe crisis."[1]

His journey home was by bicycle owing to the fact that it was wartime and travel by car was restricted. Hoffmann was accompanied by one of his laboratory assistants. Here are some comments on his journey.

"On the way home, my condition began to assume threatening forms. Everything in my field of vision wavered and was distorted as if seen in a curved mirror. I also had the sensation of being unable to move from the spot. Nevertheless, my assistant later told me that we had traveled very rapidly. Finally, we arrived at home safe and sound, and I was just barely capable of asking my companion to summon our family doctor and request milk from the neighbors."

Once at home, Hoffmann lay on his bed as he found himself quite unable to carry on normally. The requested milk did arrive, although his neighbor had been transformed into "a malevolent insidious witch with a colored mask."[1] Hoffmann worried about his sanity. A doctor was called and arrived but was quite baffled as to what was going on, as Hoffmann displayed few external symptoms apart from mydriasis (dilated pupils). Hoffmann recounts that eventually he got somewhat used to the situation and that he began to enjoy the wonderful "kaleidoscope" of shifting shapes and colors that presented itself when he closed his eyes. Hoffmann's wife returned from a trip to Lucerne—she had been contacted by phone—and eventually he went to sleep. He woke the next day with no hangover or any ill effects. In fact he recalls that he had never felt better and that the drug made him see everything "in a new light."

Hoffmann reported his experiences to his superiors, Prof. Stoll and Dr. Rothlin. They were extremely skeptical about the entire thing. So Hoffmann suggested that if they didn't believe him, they should also try the new substance. This they did, taking one-third the dose he had taken. Hoffmann relates that as a result, "all doubts about the statements in my report were eliminated." Thus, the first people ever to "trip out" on LSD were a number of Swiss drug company executives! LSD aficionados around the world now celebrate April 19th every year as "Bicycle Day."

ERGOT AND ITS ALKALOIDS

Ergot (*Claviceps purpura*), the ultimate source of the major molecular components of LSD, is a fungus of the *Claviceps* family that attacks grasses and related crops.[2,3] Rye is the most susceptible to attack, whereas some other crops including barley, oats, and wheat are less so. The word *ergot* comes from the French word *argot* meaning a "spur" (Figure 2.1).

This is a description of the dark brown or black peg-like protuberances which the fungus forms on ears of rye when they are ripe. As we shall see, this humble fungus is arguably the most amazing source of natural products that affect the nervous system known to man. It is truly a treasure trove of extremely active molecules (generally known as alkaloids, Chapter 5), that produce a very wide range of effects. Some references to ergot are very ancient, dating back to around 1000 BC where it is mentioned in the context of its use in obstetrics, which is still one of its major medical

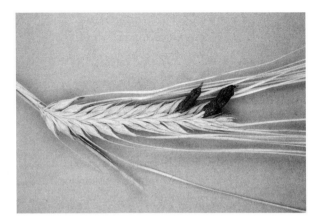

Figure 2.1:
Example of ergot growing on barley.
(Reproduced with permission of Prof. Carl Bradley, University of Illinois, Urbana).

applications. It also enters human history in association with "ergotism," a disease associated with eating ergot-contaminated rye whose symptoms include convulsions, gangrene, and hallucinations. Given the large number of powerful substances contained in the fungus, it is hardly surprising that the effect of consuming all of them simultaneously produces such a remarkable syndrome.

The occurrence of ergotism became particularly associated with the cultivation of rye, which in the Middle Ages became the major grain consumed by the lower classes in parts of the European mainland including Germany, Austria, Czechoslovakia, Poland, and Russia. The successful attack of the rye crop by ergot depends on the appropriate climatic conditions. These would usually begin with a period of wet weather, which would encourage the fungus to germinate, and then a dry period during which the fungal spores would be distributed by the winds. The first accurate modern description of the fungus was published in 1582 by Adam Lonitzer who described it growing on rye—"There are long, black, hard, narrow pegs on the ears, internally white, often protruding like long nails from between the grains in the ear."

However, a complete understanding of ergot's fungal nature and a complete description of its life cycle was not forthcoming until 1853. The ergot life cycle starts when the wind distributes fungal spores which land on plants such as rye that can act as susceptible hosts. Filaments of the fungus, which are called "hyphae," colonize the host plant's ovaries resulting in the production of a large number of fungal spores packed into a thick liquid known as "honeydew." The honeydew can then be spread to other plants in the vicinity, particularly by insects. After about 5 weeks the formation of honeydew ceases and hard pegs (sclerotia) appear on the plant. In the autumn, the ripe pigmented sclerotia fall to the ground where they lie dormant until activated by warmer temperatures the following spring, thereby completing the cycle.

As we have discussed, the consumption of ergot-tainted rye results in ergotism, a syndrome that can take on two different forms—gangrenous and convulsive. Presumably this difference results from the precise alkaloid composition in the particular ergot sample involved, as this may be expected to be quite variable depending on the environmental conditions prevailing at the time. The gangrenous form of ergotism results from extreme constriction of the peripheral blood vessels in the extremities. The lack of blood flow produces swelling and intense burning pains. In the end, atrophied hands and feet will actually fall off. In some patients all four limbs may become detached in this way! The convulsive form of ergotism involves excruciating muscle spasms and diarrhea accompanied by delirium and hallucinations.

As can be imagined, outbreaks of this disease—the result of eating batches of contaminated flour—could involve large numbers of people and numerous deaths. For example, some 20,000 deaths were reported to have occurred from an outbreak of ergotism in Aquitaine in 944 AD. The burning sensation associated with the gangrenous form of ergotism became known as St. Anthony's fire or Sacred Fire (Sacer Ignis) in the Middle Ages. Indeed, the symptoms were so common that an order of monks, known as the Hospital Order of St. Anthony, was established in 1095 and specialized in the treatment of patients with this form of ergotism. The name "St. Anthony's fire" is derived from this holy order. The association of St. Anthony and ergotism was most spectacularly realized in Matthias Grunewald's great altarpiece commissioned by the Antonite monks of the monastery at Isenheim in the Alsace in the early sixteenth century. It is certainly worth a 15-mile detour to the south to visit the charming old town of Colmar and view this great masterpiece in the Unterlinden Museum. In the altarpiece, the figure of the suffering Christ appears to involve the symptoms of gangrenous ergotism, and other figures in the tryptich also bear reminders of the symptoms of the disease[4] (Figure 2.2).

As we have discussed in Chapter 1, the powerful effects of natural products such as Amanita muscaria or ergot suggest that they contain important chemical substances that, if isolated and understood from the structural point of view, might provide us with new insights into disease mechanisms or potential therapeutic opportunities for treating diseases. As the science of natural products gained momentum in the nineteenth and twentieth centuries, it was inevitable that ergot should become the subject of serious

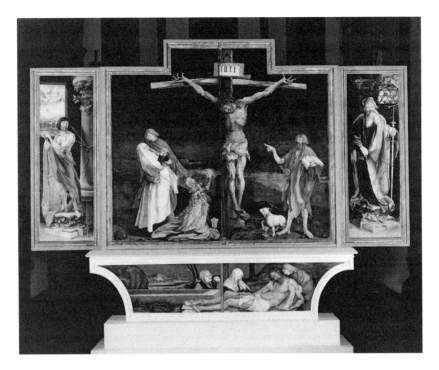

Figure 2.2:
Initial portion of the Isenheim altarpiece.
(Grunewald, Matthias (Mathis Nithart Gothart) c.1480–1528) / Musee d'Unterlinden, Colmar, France / Giraudon / The Bridgeman Art Library)

investigation. Prior to the isolation of its active chemical principles preparations of ergot were already widely used for a number of medical purposes. For example, ergot preparations have powerful effects on the uterus, and there is evidence that it has been used for hundreds if not thousands of years as an aid to parturition. In 1808 John Stearns, a doctor in New York, described the use of ergot preparations to stimulate labor. It was also used early in pregnancy to induce abortion. Nevertheless, the use of crude ergot was found to be rather an inexact science which could be accompanied by serious side effects, not least of which was the occurrence of ergotism if the dose used was too high. Hence, it was clear that if ergot was to be truly useful, its active constituents would have to be identified.

The first major steps in this direction were made early in the twentieth century. In 1904 the 29-year-old Henry Dale joined the Burroughs Wellcome research labs in London.[5] Dale was later to emerge as one of the twentieth century's greatest scientists and would receive the Nobel prize for his work on identifying neurotransmitters and their receptors. When he first joined Burroughs Wellcome, it was suggested that he might attempt to identify the active principle in ergot. Together with George Barger he identified the effects of different ergot extracts on blood pressure and even crystallized what he thought to be a pure substance which he named "ergotoxine." However, this ultimately proved to be a mistake as ergotoxine was actually a mixture of three different ergot alkaloids. In the end, the real progress in identifying ergot's secrets came with work conducted at Sandoz.

Arthur Stoll, who became Albert Hoffman's immediate superior at Sandoz, was the head of the company's research laboratory. In 1917 he began trying to identify the active principles in ergot and isolated the first pure ergot alkaloid naming it "ergotamine" (Figure 2.3). The chemical structure of the alkaloid was not actually determined until 1951, and its synthesis achieved in 1961; a collaboration, appropriately enough, between Stoll and Hoffmann. Ergotamine proved to have extremely powerful vasoconstricting (i.e., blood vessel–constricting) effects and rapidly found an important medical use as a treatment for migraine. Not surprisingly the drug is known to produce side effects in some people that are reminiscent of the symptoms of gangrenous ergotism. Indeed, it is probably ergotamine that is mostly responsible for the gangrenous aspect of ergot toxicity, but clearly at doses that are much greater than those used in the treatment of migraine. As we shall discuss, the effects of all ergot alkaloids are produced through their interactions with the receptor molecules for

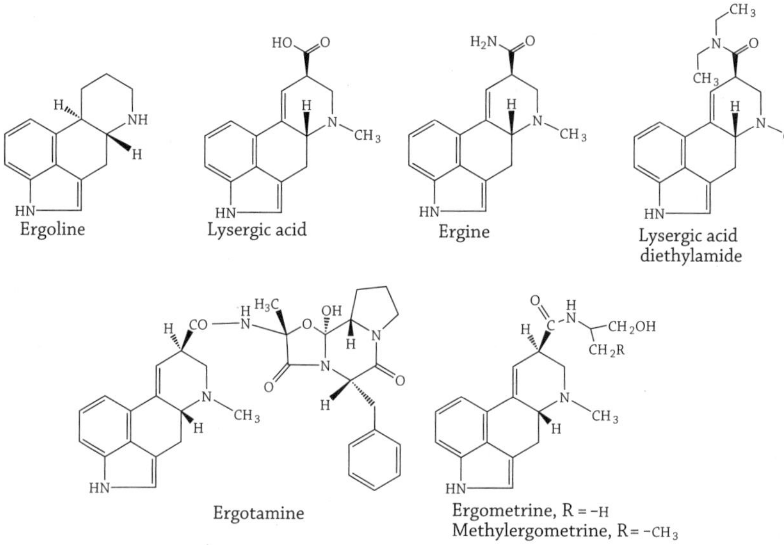

Figure 2.3:
Structures of lysergic acid, lysergic acid diethylamide (LSD), and other important ergot alkaloids.

the biogenic amine neurotransmitters epinephrine, norepinephrine, dopamine, and 5-hydroxytryptamine (serotonin). Remarkably, however, there is a great deal of variability in terms of which receptors are targeted by a particular ergot alkaloid, resulting in unique effects of different members of the chemical family.

The structure of ergotamine typifies all the major features of the ergot alkaloids in general (Figure 2.3). Ergot alkaloids are all biosynthetically derived from the amino acid L-tryptophan and actually constitute the largest group of fungal alkaloids known to man. There are three basic classes of molecules: the water-soluble lysergic acid amides, the water-insoluble peptide derivatives (ergopeptines), and the clavine group. The sclerotia contain somewhere in the region of 0.15%–0.5% pure alkaloid material, of which about 20% are water-soluble derivatives.

The structure of ergotamine contains both an ergoline/lysergic acid alkaloid portion (Figure 2.3), which is central to the structure of all ergot alkaloids, and an L-proline-containing complex tripeptide (three amino acids) moiety. Although there are a huge number of naturally occurring ergopeptines, ergotamine is the only one to be currently used in medicine. However, small chemical modifications made in the laboratory to some of the other ergopeptines have yielded useful semisynthetic drugs. For example, the original "ergotoxine" described by Dale and Barger ultimately proved to consist of a mixture of three closely related ergot alkaloids: ergocornine, ergocristine, and ergocriptine. A slight chemical modification to the latter yields bromocriptine, a substance that has unique dopamine receptor activating properties and is used in the treatment of hyperprolactinemia and pituitary prolactinoma. The lysergic acid amides have also yielded important drugs. Here ergonovine (aka ergometrine) is the most prominent example and is the alkaloid primarily responsible for the ability of ergot to stimulate the uterus, increasing the rate of uterine contractions. The drug is also used to facilitate the delivery of the placenta and to produce constriction of the blood vessels, helping to prevent bleeding after childbirth[6] (Figure 2.3).

As can be seen from this brief discussion, the ergoline/lysergic acid structure has clearly been a fertile chemical starting point for the development of new therapeutic agents which might have diverse interesting effects.[7] One can therefore see why the further modification of this molecule would have interested Albert Hoffmann and his colleagues at Sandoz. However, in 1943 with the synthesis of LSD (Figure 2.3) and the discovery of its unique and completely unexpected properties, the genie was really out of the bottle. Sandoz quickly went to work trying to understand the structural and mechanistic basis for its unique effects and, perhaps more importantly from their point of view, to try to find a therapeutic niche for their new superstar molecule.

One thing to note is that although ergot contains numerous chemical substances which produce extremely potent biological effects, none of them is particularly hallucinogenic in the same way as LSD. LSD, a semi-synthetic molecule made in a laboratory which does not exist in nature, has a unique profile in this regard. One question therefore is whether there are also naturally occurring substances that act like LSD and whether they have entheogenic properties as defined in the previous chapter. As we shall see, powerful naturally occurring hallucinogenic molecules that have properties that are similar to LSD have been identified, and these have certainly been used for entheogenic purposes. However, before proceeding with that discussion we must first turn to another of Albert Hoffmann's remarkable discoveries.

THE "LITTLE ROUND THINGS"

Following the conquest of Mexico by the Spanish in 1521, the Spanish clergy began to settle in the New World with a view to taking care of the religious well-being (that is, forced conversion) of the indigenous Indian population. Some of these men were considerable scholars. Bernardo de Sahagun was actually a Marrano Jew who had become a Franciscan missionary and then moved to Mexico. He lived near Mexico City, where he became fluent in the local Nahuatl language. He also taught Spanish and Latin to several of the local people who, like Sahagun, were then trilingual (Spanish, Latin, and Nahuatl). Working with his students he compiled a vast compendium of the Nahuatl language and its grammar and recorded facts about the local culture in Mexico prior to the Spanish conquest. This compendium became known as the *Florentine Codex* and is one of the richest sources of information about the habits of the original Aztec society. It was clear that the indigenous population used numerous plants and fungi for entheogenic purposes and that such practices were extremely ancient.

The seeds of one plant in particular were known as *Ololiuhqui* ("little round things").[8] Many of these ancient entheogenic practices were still in use in Mexico well into the twentieth century when anthropologists began to take an interest in them. Compelling evidence was collected that Ololiuhqui corresponded to the seeds of the morning glory plant, a common type of climbing vine with bright flowers of many different colors (Figure 2.4). In particular it was suggested that they corresponded to the seeds of a variety called *Turbina* (also known as *Rivea*) *corymbosa*. Further

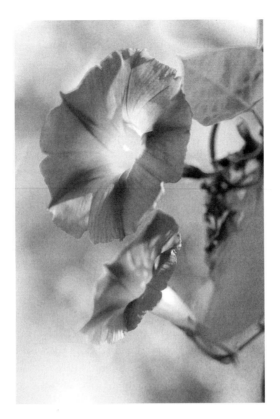

Figure 2.4:
The morning glory plant.
(Wei-Chieh Wu © Photoscom)

investigations with different populations of Indians also revealed the use of other morning glories such as *Ipomoea violacea*. In 1959 Gordon Wasson, who was carrying out his own investigations in Mexico, sent a supply of morning glory seeds to Albert Hoffmann in Switzerland in an effort to isolate their entheogenic principles. To everybody's surprise, including Hoffmann's, he demonstrated that the seeds contained ergot alkaloids. In particular they contained ergine (Figure 2.3) and also isoergine, which had been originally synthesized and tested by Hoffmann around the time he first made LSD. Hoffmann originally reported that ergine and isoergine were only weakly hallucinogenic at best, although they did give him a feeling of "unreality" and made him feel "life was completely meaningless." Other authors have also reported being somewhat underwhelmed by the hallucinogenic nature of these ergot alkaloids, although it is generally agreed that they do have some type of psychotropic effect and so may explain the psychoactive effects of Ololiuhqui. In contemporary Mexican Indian culture the morning glory seeds are ground up (by a virgin, naturally) and then an aqueous extract is made and drunk, sometimes in combination with other plant-derived drugs.

However, the fact that ergot alkaloids of any type are found in morning glory seeds is itself a remarkable observation, as these plants are not closely related to *Claviceps purpurea* and presumably indicate an unusual instance of convergent evolution, although the reason for the selective advantage that is associated with the biosynthesis of these substances is unknown. We now know that ergot alkaloids are widely represented in diverse morning glories and are found in all parts of the plant in addition to their seeds. Just for the record, the most highly ergot-endowed species is known as the "Hawaiian Baby Woodrose," whose seeds weigh in at 0.3% ergot alkaloid content. At any rate, the possible use of ergine as an entheogenic substance has implications for another interesting debate associated with ergot and its alkaloids. This time it concerns the myths of ancient Greece and one of the greatest mysteries of the ancient world.

MYSTERIOUS MYSTERIES

The Greek goddess Demeter was the deity who ruled the harvest and so controlled the fertility of the earth in general, as well as the regular occurrence of the seasons. Demeter had several children including a daughter by Zeus, whose name was Persephone (she was also known as Proserpine; see Figure 2.5 for Dante Gabriel Rossetti's gorgeous painting). One day Persephone was out collecting wildflowers with her two friends Athena and Artemis when an enormous chasm opened up and a fellow riding a chariot appeared. It was Hades, Lord of the Underworld! He abducted Persephone and took her down to his subterranean realm, where she became his queen. Demeter and Persephone were very close, and Demeter was devastated by the loss of her daughter. She spent all of her time wandering about searching for her. During her search Demeter neglected her other duties such as the harvest. All the plants died and people had nothing to eat.

Eventually Helios, the all-seeing Sun, told Demeter what had actually happened to her daughter. Moreover, Zeus was perturbed at the state of things in the world and persuaded Hades to let Persephone return to her mother. Unfortunately there was a rule that anybody who ate anything while they were in the underworld had to stay there *for ever,* and it seems that Persephone had eaten a pomegranate while she was there (Figure 2.5). Well, not an entire pomegranate—actually just a few seeds. Olympian realpolitik demanded a compromise. Persephone could return to her mother,

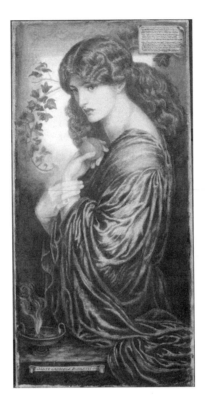

Figure 2.5:
Rossetti, Dante Charles Gabriel (1828–1882), Proserpine (oil on canvas).
Birmingham Museums and Art Gallery / The Bridgeman Art Library

but she had to return to Hades and the underworld for 4 months each year, during which time Demeter would predictably get depressed again and all of the plants would die, only to come to life once more next spring when Persephone returned to her again.

According to the "Homeric Hymn to Demeter," at one point in her wanderings Demeter initiated a temple and cult at the town of Eleusis near Athens, and it is well known that an ancient fertility cult that worshiped Demeter and Persephone did really exist there. Initiates into this cult had numerous duties; however, the most famous of these was to take part in a ceremony known as the *Eleusinian mysteries*. This ceremony took place at the temple of Demeter in Eleusis each year over a period of 9 days in the month of September and was open to all Greeks. The ceremonies were very ancient and may have started as early as 1500 BC, possibly representing the continuation of a truly ancient fertility rite. The ceremonies were eventually phased out in Roman times following the ascendancy of Christianity. The Eleusinian mysteries were very elaborate and involved all kinds of acts such as fasting, speaking special words, and drinking a special drink called the *kykeon,* which the Homeric Hymn tells us consisted of barley and mint mixed in water. The participants entered a special inner sanctum called the *Telesterion,* where a ceremony took place involving the revelation of some type of esoteric knowledge.

However, exactly what went on in the Telesterion and exactly what was in the kykeon, as well as other details of the ceremony, are unknown. Initiates were sworn to secrecy under pain of death, so almost no information is available. Nevertheless, there has been much speculation that following their entry into the Telesterion the initiates were subject to visions provoked by a secret psychoactive ingredient in the kykeon. For example, Hoffmann and Wasson speculated that the barley in the kykeon was specially selected by the Hierophant who led the ceremony to be infected with ergot.[9] However, as we have discussed, ergot itself is not particularly psychoactive in the hallucinogenic sense. So it has been further speculated by several authors that chemical treatment of the ergot in the preparation of the kykeon may have yielded an increase in its psychoactive ingredients.[10] In this way it is possible that ergot could be treated to yield ergine, which as we have seen from discussion of Ololiuhqui, may well be active as an entheogen. Moreover, there are things about the mysteries that may have enhanced the effects of the compound. First of all there was the fact that the participants were mentally prepared to have mystical experiences, something that certainly helps. One of the other stipulations for initiates was that they had to fast prior to imbibing the kykeon, and it is also likely that this might encourage a psychotropic experience. It has to be said that, just as with the theory equating soma with muscimol, there are many objections that can be raised to the hypothesis that ergot alkaloids were responsible for the effects of the kykeon. Nevertheless, it is an intriguing idea. Whatever the truth of the matter, it is absolutely the case that other substances related in structure to LSD are widely found in nature and have clearly been used as entheogens throughout history. To understand this we must revisit both mushrooms and Gordon Wasson.

MAYAN MUSHROOMS

As we have seen, it is clear that ergot alkaloids in the form of Ololiuhqui were used from ancient times as entheogens in Central America. Ancient texts from the same part of the world also attest to the use of mushrooms for similar purposes. Mushrooms used for religious purposes are mentioned in the Popol Vuh, the great epic poem of the ancient Mayan Quiche civilization from the highlands of Guatemala.[11] Sahagun and other writers at the time of the Spanish conquest also refer to the use of mushrooms by the Indians to intoxicate themselves in ceremonies where they communicated with their gods. Of particular interest, as we shall see, was Sahagun's observation that the mushrooms in question were frequently found growing in animal waste or dung. The mushrooms were known as teonanácatl, or "God's flesh" in the Nahuatl language. As with the petroglyphs of Siberia that may illustrate *Amanita muscaria,* there are also pictures, murals, and sculptures from ancient Mexico that display human/mushroom hybrid figures and other images suggestive of their religious importance (Figure 2.6).

The Spanish were definitely not enthusiastic about the use of mushrooms in religious ceremonies or, for that matter, in anything else that they thought distracted from strict Catholic practice. The use of teonanácatl was specifically outlawed and anybody found to be using it was tortured. Hence, the practice soon went underground. However, it never entirely disappeared and, as with many of these things, it reemerged in the twentieth century with the arrival of anthropologists who were interested in such topics. Just as we have seen in the previous chapter that anthropologists were interested in the question "what was soma?", they were also interested in the question "what was teonanácatl?" The first real breakthroughs in answering this question came around 1940 when an Austrian/Mexican anthropologist named Blas Pablo Reko, and an ethnobotanist at Harvard named Richard Schultes, obtained samples of what appeared to be teonanácatl. Reko had determined that it was still being used by Mexican Indians in secret ceremonies in many inaccessible parts of the country. Their initial

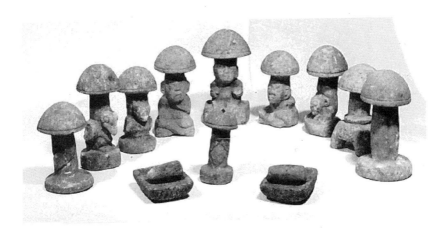

Figure 2.6:
Hybrid human/mushroom sculptures from Guatemala (1000–500 BC).
(Picture reproduced courtesy of Prof. Carl de Borhegyi.)

attempts at identification pointed toward the mushrooms being of the genus *Psilocybe*. Interestingly, scattered reports concerning the psychotropic effects of accidently ingested liberty cap (*Psilocybe semilanceata*) mushrooms (Figure 2.7) growing in the wild had appeared in the US and British press over the years.[12] At the same time that Reko and Schultes were collecting and identifying teonanácatl mushrooms, Jean Johnson, another anthropologist, actually sought out and observed a ceremony in the Indian town of Huautla in which mushrooms were used by a shaman or "curandero" to intoxicate himself in efforts to engage spirits who could aid in healing a sick patient. Hence by the middle of the twentieth century there was good evidence that mushrooms were still being used in Central America for entheogenic and related purposes.

In 1952 Gordon Wasson received a letter from the poet Robert Graves providing him with details concerning reports about the apparent entheogenic use of mushrooms in Mexico. Without further ado he set off with his wife and made a series of visits to isolated villages in Mexico where he not only observed mushroom ceremonies but also became the first modern non-Mexican to actually participate in one. He collected his experiences in a lengthy article he wrote for *Life Magazine* in 1957 entitled " Seeking the magic mushroom: a New York banker goes to Mexico's mountains to participate in the age old rituals of Indians who chew strange growths that produce visions." The article proved quite sensational and was read by millions of people. It is reasonable to state that Wasson almost singlehandedly brought hallucinogenic mushrooms into the consciousness of the modern

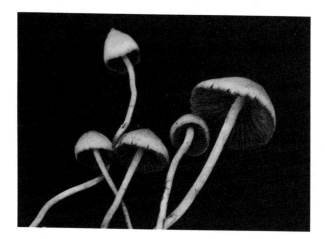

Figure 2.7:
Liberty cap mushrooms (*Psilocybe semilanceata*).
(Ivan Mikhaylov © Photoscom)

public, and did much to encourage interest in them in the United States and Europe. As Wasson describes, he became friendly with an important curandera named Maria Sabina who was active as a healer in the region of Huautla. She provided Wasson and his wife with mushrooms so that they could participate in a "velada," the name for the nighttime ceremonies that involved mushroom intoxication. Wasson made films of Maria Sabina, recorded her singing and chanting, and basically turned her into a celebrity. This was something that wasn't necessarily appreciated by other curanderos who had always taken the view that their ceremonies should be closely guarded secrets. Nevertheless, following Wasson's investigations the mushroom was well and truly out of the bag and Mexican mushroom veladas became a *de rigeur* tourist destination for many hippies in the 1960s.

In addition to his anthropological interests, Gordon Wasson was also active in establishing the ethnobotanical and ethnopharmacological aspects of his discoveries. Here he allied himself with two excellent investigators. The first of these was Roger Heim, a very well known French mycologist who helped with identifying and cultivating the different species of Psilocybe mushrooms used in veladas. He also needed the collaboration of a chemist/pharmacologist who was experienced in the isolation of the hallucinogenic principles from natural products. Here there was only one clear choice, and that was Albert Hoffmann. Heim was able to cultivate *Psilocybe mexicana* mushrooms in his laboratory and sent samples of these to Hoffmann. The Sandoz company also began cultivating these mushrooms in large quantities. In 1958 Hoffmann announced in a publication in the journal *Experientia* that he had successfully isolated the two major substances that appeared to be responsible for the activity of *Pilocybe Mexicana,* as determined by self experimentation—clearly the best bioassay for hallucinogenic activity, as Hoffmann had realized when he discovered LSD.[1] He named the two substances *psilocybin* and *psilocin,* or 4-phosphoryloxy-N, N-dimethyltryptamine and 4-hydroxy-N,N-dimethyltryptamine respectively (Figure 2.8). Hoffmann also quickly established synthetic schemes for making both of these substances. Ten years later two other potentially psychoactive compounds with related structures named *baeocystin* and *norbaeocystin* were isolated from the mushroom *Psilocybe baeocystis.* Psilocybin, psilocycin, baeocystine, and norbaeocystine have now been isolated from numerous types of psilocybin mushrooms.

Hoffmann performed a classic experiment for establishing the veracity of psilocybin's identity as the entheogenic component of psilocybin mushrooms. He returned to Mexico and gave Maria Sabina a sample of the powdered synthetic product made in his laboratory and asked her if she could distinguish it from using wild mushrooms. Basically the answer was

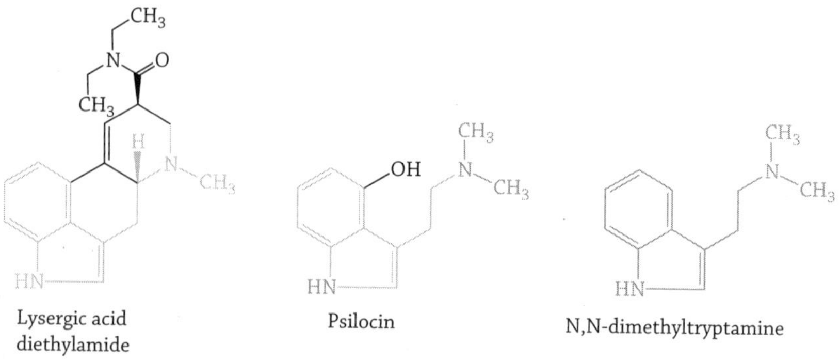

Figure 2.8:
Psilocybin and related structures.

that she couldn't. Now Maria's subjective "experience" as a user of mush-rooms was certainly the most sensitive assay available for testing these compounds, so this can be considered the best possible proof. Indeed, as we shall discuss, similar assays called "drug discrimination tasks" are used in animals if one wants to know if a new substance that has been isolated corresponds in its psychoactive properties to a previously known molecule.

HALLUCINOGENIC TRYPTAMINES

It has subsequently been determined that upon ingestion psilocybin is dephosphorylated to form psilocin (Figure 2.8), which is actually the species responsible for the production of psychotropic effects. This is somewhat analogous to the situation with ibotenic acid and muscimol (Chapter 1), where the precursor molecule (ibotenic acid) is metabolized to produce the ultimately active species (muscimol). Interestingly, psilocybin is not the only substance of this chemical type that exists in nature. The skin of toads such as *Bufo marinus* contain a very similar compound called bufotenine which is just a positional isomer of psilocin—in other words, the hydroxyl group is in a different ring position (Figure 2.8). Historically there are many stories of "toad licking" and the smoking of dried toad skins to engender psychotropic effects, so it seems the witches in Macbeth must have known a thing or two when they were cooking up their spells. Interestingly, research on bufotenine both in animals and humans has demonstrated that it doesn't produce very potent classic hallucinogenic effects, more a feeling of profound discomfort.

Psilocybin-containing mushrooms are saprophytic; that is to say, they grow on dead plant material. Like *Amanita muscaria*, psilocybin mushrooms are not rare. Indeed there are many varieties that grow in virtually all parts of the world. Many of the mushrooms are members of the genus *Psilocybe*, which has more than 80 species, but others also belong to separate genera including *Panaeolus* and *Inocybe*. It is thought that the widespread nature of the occurrence of psilocybin-containing mushrooms is partly the result of human development, because many of these mushrooms like to grow on wood chips, refuse, or other types of human detritus resulting from the clearing of woodlands. Other types, such as the liberty cap, *Psilocybe semilanceata*, grow well on animal dung and so parallel the spread of domestic animals. As might be expected, the different species also vary a great deal in their content of hallucinogenic alkaloids. For example the super-potent *Psilocybe azurescens* contains an average of 1.78% psilocybin, 0.38% psilocin, and 0.35% baeocystin. *Psilocybe semilanceata,* on the other hand, contains 0.98%, 0.02% and 0.36%; *Psilocybe cubensis* 0.63%, 0.60%, and 0.025%; and *Psilocybe stunzii* 0.36%, 0.12%, and 0.02% respectively. The great popularity of these mushrooms has given rise to a "shroom" industry throughout the world catering to psilocybin gourmets. Detailed field guides now describe how to identify the appropriate mushrooms in the wild through different tests, such as the fact that they tend to show blue bruising when damaged, and how to avoid picking a deadly α-amanita-containing Galerina mushroom by mistake.[12,13] Although the attraction of a sunny day trekking though woods and pastures collecting psilocybin mushrooms is clear, it is certainly safer to use mushrooms that have been artificially cultivated, something that has now been widely achieved.

It is instructive to examine the structure of psilocin and to compare it to LSD (Figure 2.9). The similarities will be obvious. Psilocybin and related substances all contain tryptamine built around the indole nucleus, as also found in the amino acid tryptophan. The tryptamine outline is clearly present within the LSD structure as well. Overall, however, psilocin is a much simpler structure than LSD. Nevertheless, it has been demonstrated that the hallucinogenic experience obtained from taking psilocin/psilocybin is really qualitatively very similar to that of taking LSD—so it is likely that the two compounds ultimately share the same biological mechanism of action. Hence, we can conclude that the basic chemical structure required to obtain this type of hallucinogenic activity is contained within the substituted tryptamine moiety. Now compared to ergot alkaloids, substituted tryptamines are relatively easy to synthesize and so there has been a great deal of experimentation with their structures and this has yielded many insights into their mechanisms. Moreover, it is also the case that hallucinogenic mushrooms are not the only tryptamine-containing plants that have been used for their hallucinogenic entheogenic effects. To understand this we must now leave Mexico and travel to South America.

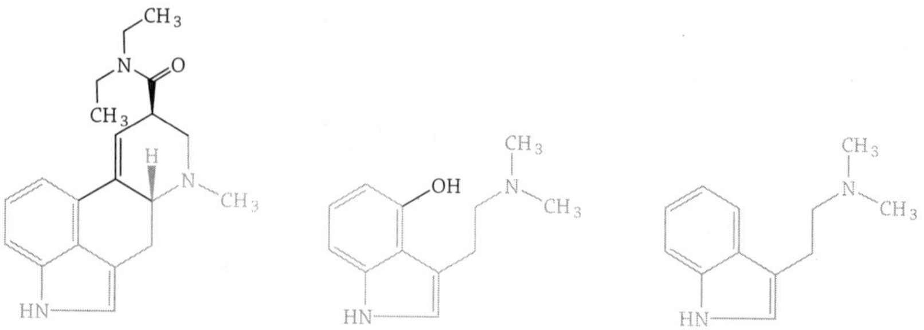

Figure 2.9:
Common features (grey) in the structures of LSD, psilocin and N,N-dimethyltryptamine.

THE AYAHUASCA OF THE INDIANS

In the latter part of the nineteenth century, reports started to emerge from travelers to Brazil, Ecuador, and Peru of intoxicating drinks and potions prepared by the local Indian tribes. A general feature of these reports were that the potions were based on decoctions or extracts of the vine *Banisteriopsis caapi* and called "yage" or "ayahuasca" in the local languages. Indeed, these potions are referred to by Louis Lewin in his *Phantastica* where he describes the hallucinogenic effects they produce. The quality of the visions and hallucinations provoked by ayahuasca prompted him to write that they were "like those evoked by *Anhalonium Lewinii* (aka mescaline) in a perfect form." Here he was very perceptive, as we shall see, because it seems clear that like LSD and psilocin all of these substances are capable of inducing what we might call a classic "hallucinogenic syndrome," which is typified by all of the symptoms originally reported by Albert Hoffmann. This would indicate that they all ultimately produce their effects by the same cellular and molecular mechanisms. The active principle of *Banisteriopsis caapi* was isolated in the 1920s by Lewin and by others and named "banisterine" or "telepathine," and was subsequently identified as the β-carboline alkaloid, harmine. Interestingly, harmine, harmaline (a related alkaloid), and several other similar substances had been previously isolated from the Syrian rue, *Peganum harmala* (Figure 2.10). Lewin tested harmine on human subjects and by self-experimentation and deemed it to be psychotropic. But psychotropic in what fashion? Subsequent authors such as Ott and Shulgin[14,15] have reported that the effects of β-carboline alkaloids are not at all similar to compounds like psilocybin or LSD. Ott reported that they made him feel like he was taking diazepam (Valium).[15] So, generally speaking, they do not seem to recapitulate the experience of drinking ayahuasca.

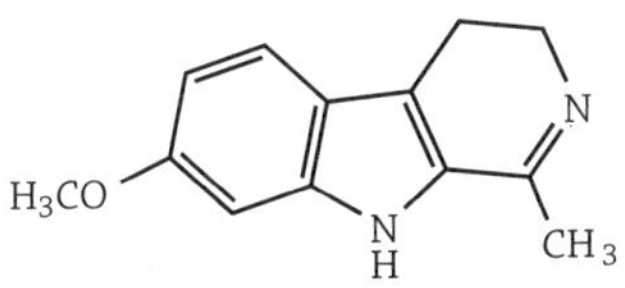

Harmaline

Figure 2.10:
The alkaloid harmaline, derived from the vine *Banisteriopsis caapi*. Harmaline is an inhibitor of the enzyme monoamine oxidase.

The mystery of how ayahuasca produces its effects can be solved by considering three key observations. The first of these is that *Banisteriopsis caapi* is usually not the only ingredient in ayahuasca. Typically the drink also contains the leaves of a second plant. This is often leaves of the coffee-like shrub *Psychotria viridis*, but in actuality could be hundreds of different things. When these extracts are added together, the true effects of ayahuasca are observed. The second observation is that the indole alkaloid NN,dimethyl tryptamine (DMT) (Figure 2.9) and also the related substance 5-MeO-DMT are found in all of the secondary plant ingredients of ayahuasca. Indeed, as the famous hallucinogen researcher Alexander Shulgin has pointed out, "DMT is everywhere"[14]—it is extremely widely distributed throughout the plant and animal kingdoms. If one looks at the chemical structure of DMT, one can see that it is closely related to substances like psilocin and LSD (Figure 2.9).

So, is DMT hallucinogenic in the same way as these other compounds? Some reports have demonstrated that it can produce hallucinogenic effects if administered in a way so that it gains access to the brain very easily, for example intranasally (it is found in psychoactive snuffs) or by smoking. However, its effects are gone in a matter of minutes, presumably due to the fact that it is easily metabolized. Indeed, we know that DMT is a substrate for the enzyme monoamine oxidase (MAO), which metabolizes most biogenic amines including the neurotransmitters 5-hydroxytryptamine and norepinephrine, as well as substances such as psilocin. The other key observation to consider is the fact that in the 1950s substances like harmine and harmaline were found to be very effective MAO inhibitors. So, here we have an excellent example of the discovery of an important biochemical principle purely by empirical observation, a biochemical problem being solved even prior to understanding the precise nature of the problem. *Psychotria viridis* leaves or the leaves of another plant provide the DMT, and *Banisteriopsis caapi* provides the MAO inhibitor—when put together in ayahuasca, the psychotropic effects of DMT are clearly apparent as its metabolism by MAO is inhibited. The veracity of these ideas have been demonstrated by self-experimentation studies in which pure DMT is taken with a modern synthetic MAO inhibitor such as isocarboxazid (Chapter 4), following which an ayahuasca-like hallucinogenic experience is obtained.[15]

Exactly what events led to the understanding that an MAO inhibitor in *Banisteriopsis caapi* was necessary to bring out the psychoactive properties of DMT found in numerous plant sources is unknown, but it is a fascinating development that presumably reflects both years of informal experimentation and the ancient nature of these practices. In summary, therefore, substances like LSD, psilocin, and DMT, under the appropriate circumstances, can all produce classical hallucinogenic experiences that are qualitatively indistinguishable from one another. DMT appears to be the simplest naturally occurring indole-containing structure that is capable of producing these effects. Nevertheless, there are also other, even simpler, chemical structures that can produce the same types of hallucinations. To understand this we will stay in Central and South America and switch our attention from mushrooms and vines to cacti.

PEYOTE: THE CACTUS HALLUCINOGEN

As we have seen, the early Spanish conquerors of Mesoamerica included men such as Bernadino de Sahagun who described the use of entheogenic drugs by the local population. In addition to teonanácatl, Sahagun also described other types of drugs such as one obtained from a particular cactus:

> "There is another herb called peiotl. It is found in the north country. Those who eat or drink it see visions either frightful or laughable; this inebriation lasts two or three days and then ceases. It is a sort of delicacy of the Chichimecas, it sustains them and gives them courage to fight and not feel fear, nor hunger nor thirst, and they say it protects them from danger."

As with other drugs, the Spaniards actively discouraged the use of peiotl or peyotl but, as with the use of mushrooms, the practice continued and survived up to the present day. In fact it eventually spread to the Southwest of the United States. Ultimately the American Indians that use it founded their own church and, after diverse legal battles, won the right to use it legally in the United States. The peyotl or peyote cactus mentioned here by Sahagun is a slow-growing variety found in the north of Mexico and into Texas and Oklahoma (Figure 2.11). The "crown" of the cactus can be cut

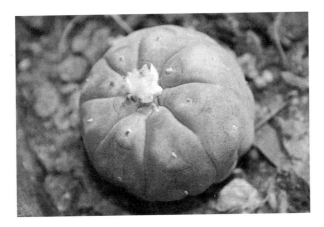

Figure 2.11:
Lophophora williamsii, the peyote cactus.
(Charlie Edward © Shutterstock)

into pieces and dried to produce "peyote buttons," which can be extracted or chewed directly to release the psychoactive principles of the cactus.

The story of mescaline, which is the name used these days for the psychoactive principle of the peyote cactus, is just as fascinating as the parallel story of psilocybin and its discovery. It is certainly the case that the cultures of pre-Columbian Mesoamerica were probably the most sophisticated we know of when it comes to the integration of entheogenic substances into their daily lives. Again it was Louis Lewin who was the first to study the peyote cactus in the modern era. Following a trip to the United States at the end of the nineteenth century, Lewin had been given samples of dried peyote from the Parke Davis drug company. Back in Germany he isolated a substance he called *anhalonium* which he considered to be the active principle. Detailed descriptions of the psychological effects of anhalonium are provided by Lewin in his book *Phantastica* (16). The visions, hallucinations, synesthesia, and profound introspection produced by the drug are clearly very similar to descriptions that others such as Hoffmann have provided concerning the effects of LSD or psilocybin, indicating a common mechanism of action. Subsequent work by Arthur Heffter and by Spath further characterized the different alkaloids obtainable from peyote. Heffter used self-experimentation to demonstrate that one of the substances he had isolated and named mescaline produced psychoactive activity that was indistinguishable from the native cactus, which is now known as *Lophophora Williamsii.*

In 1919 Spath determined the structure of mescaline as being 3,4, 5-trimethoxy-β-phenethylamine (Figure 2.12). The psychological effects of

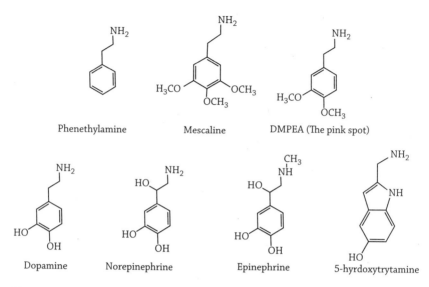

Figure 2.12:
Structures of important phenethylamines and 5-hydroxytryptamine.

mescaline are very similar to those of DMT, LSD, and psilocybin, which are all tryptamine derivatives. However, mescaline is related in structure to phenethylamine and the catecholamine neurotransmitters norepinephrine, epinephrine, and dopamine (Figure 2.12).This observation tells us that it is not possible to make the simple equation tryptamine = classical hallucinogen, as we can now see that other types of chemical structures can also produce the same effects. One thing to note is that mescaline is very much less potent than either LSD or psilocybin. Mescaline requires hundreds of milligrams of material to produce effects in humans, whereas psilocybin is effective using tens of milligrams and LSD in the ten to hundreds of microgram range. This is not to say, however, that the phenethylamine structure is incapable of yielding potent hallucinogens. As we shall discuss, several of the synthetic derivatives of mescaline are very potent indeed, rivaling the effects of LSD.

The fact that mescaline has a phenethylamine-related structure is of critical importance when we consider some of the influential theories of mental illness in the 1950s and 1960s. Around the time that Lewin was working on the isolation of Anhalonium/mescaline, the effects of peyote were becoming widely known in medical and artistic circles in Europe and the United States. The influential US and British physicians, S. Weir Mitchell and Havelock Ellis, tried it and wrote about it. It was even taken up by the famed occultist Aleister Crowley ("the wickedest man in the world"),[17] who recommended it to his acquaintances including, if the story is to be believed, the young Aldous Huxley who was later to play a prominent role in the popularization of hallucinogenic drugs and mescaline in particular. Physicians and psychologists throughout Europe began experimenting with peyote or pure mescaline. Two ideas started to circulate. First, the close structural similarity was noted between mescaline and the known catecholamine neurotransmitters such as norepinephrine. Second, it was also noted that some of the effects of taking mescaline "resembled" the positive symptoms of schizophrenia; particularly hallucinations, alternative perceptions of reality, and so on. In other words, the effects of mescaline were in some way "psychotomimetic"; that is, it produced a model of psychosis. It wasn't long before people started to put these ideas together. Perhaps schizophrenics actually metabolized substances like norepinephrine by inappropriately transmethylating them, yielding endogenous mescaline like substances that were then responsible for their aberrant behaviors? Were they producing an endogenous "psychotogen?"

THE MOLECULES OF MADNESS

In 1952 the British psychiatrists Humphrey Osmond and John Smythies proposed that in schizophrenia a compound might be formed which resembled both epinephrine and mescaline and which had the hallucinogenic properties of mescaline,[18] Harley-Mason (1952) suggested that such a compound might arise during the methylation reaction that occurs in the final stage of the biogenesis of epinephrine.[18] This hypothesis was extended in 1963 by Smythies, who postulated that a more generalized disturbance of methylation might occur in schizophrenia, resulting in the formation of abnormally methylated metabolites of catechol or indoleamines which were related to known psychoactive compounds. Indeed, following a move to Canada, Osmond and his colleague Hoffer began clinical trials giving patients nicotinic acid, which they postulated would be transmethylated and, if given in excess, would "mop up" any abnormal transmethylating reactions preventing the formation of any endogenous psychotogen.

Then something extremely exciting happened. In 1962 Friedhoff & Van Winkle reported the presence of 3,4-dimethoxyphenylethylamine (DMPEA), detected chromatographically as a "Pink Spot" in the urine of schizophrenics but not in the normal control population[18] (Figure 2.12). Obviously DMPEA is very closely related to mescaline in terms of its structure,—but that did not prove to be the case in terms of its biological activity, as DMPEA proved to be completely inactive as a hallucinogen.[19]

Nevertheless, the fact that it was present was deemed to be a sign or "bio-marker" of abnormal transmethylation reactions existing in schizophren-ics that could in principle yield an endogenous psychotomimetic substance. Whether the source of the abnormal methylation was based on the endog-enous biochemistry of the patient, their diet, or combinations of these two things was not really understood. Reports as to the existence of the Pink Spot now flooded the scientific literature, some pro, some con.[18,19] In the end it was shown by Alexander Shulgin that the Pink Spot was just a metab-olite of the antipsychotic drug chlorpromazine, which was being routinely given to schizophrenic patients but not to normal controls. Shulgin and some of his colleagues actually took chlorpromazine and "Hey Presto," the Pink Spot appeared in their urine.[19] So, the endogenous psychotomimetic theory of schizophrenia, at least in its simplest "one compound = one dis-ease" form, gradually died out.

In 1969 I read a small announcement on the front page of the venerable *Times of London* newspaper. In those days the front page of the *Times* was completely given over to small ads and announcements covering a wide variety of topics. The announcement called to my attention a meeting that was going to take place in a church in London to discuss the implications of the Pink Spot, the overall concept of "Orthomolecular Psychiatry," and to found a society for the investigation of schizophrenia from a biochemical point of view. I was about to go to the university to study biochemistry and had recently finished Huxley's *Doors of Perception*. I had also read the lit-erature as to the existence of the Pink Spot. The whole thing made perfect sense to me: this had to be the source of mental illness! These patients were constantly high because they were manufacturing their own hallucinogens.

One should remember that at that time, everybody was very infatuated with hallucinogenic drugs and the society they represented. We were all rev-olutionaries. We thought revolutionary thoughts, listened to the Jefferson Airplane, and ingested psychedelic drugs (a term actually first introduced in 1956 by Humphrey Osmond to mean mind-altering or mind-expanding or something of the sort). So, the idea and importance of psychedelic sub-stances was very much in the air. The application of such ideas to psychia-try therefore only seemed reasonable and was very much in tune with the ideas of orthomolecular psychiatry. *Orthomolecular medicine* was a term that originated with Linus Pauling and concerned the treatment of disease by using vitamins, nutrients, and other natural substances to rectify imbal-ances in the internal biochemical milieu of individuals. An example of such an approach would be the attempt discussed above by Osmond to "correct" the supposed aberrant methylation reactions in schizophrenics by giving them nicotinic acid. These imbalances could give rise to phenomena like the Pink Spot and its associated effects.

When I went to the meeting at the church, I found that it was being run by a Mrs. Gwynneth Hemmings. She was a passionate believer in the concept that things like schizophrenia, depression, and addiction were real diseases with real physical causes (e.g., things like the Pink Spot) whose symptoms could be cured by interventions of the orthomolecular type. She was greatly opposed to the views of people like R. D. Laing and Thomas Szasz, who didn't believe that there was really such a thing as mental illness that could be rectified by pharmacological or other types of intervention. It turned out that Mrs. Hemmings' husband had been diagnosed with schizophrenia and she hoped to organize people with common interests in understanding and battling the disease. So it was that the British Association for Schizophrenia was founded and I was one of the founding members. I had it in mind that I should carry out research to identify the endogenous psychotogen made by schizophrenics. If it wasn't DMPEA then it must be something else. But how should one go about this?

By a strange quirk of fate, the answer was rapidly forthcoming. At that time I also regularly visited the H. K. Lewis medical bookstore on Gower Street near University College in London. They would always have the latest issue of the journal *Nature*. In February of 1969 I went into the bookstore to browse through the journal and read one of the most amazing papers I had ever seen. It was authored by Alexander Shulgin and two colleagues. In a tour de force of medicinal chemistry and psychopharmacology, Shulgin and his colleagues had prepared more than 40 structural analogues of mescaline and tested them all by experimentation on human subjects. The identity of the human subjects is never made clear. However, the experiments were apparently conducted at the University of Chile and it has subsequently become known that the "subjects" were most likely Shulgin and his two collaborators. As a result of his investigations, Shulgin provided key information suggesting which mescaline-like molecules might act as endogenous psychotogens, if indeed they existed. DMPEA, for example, was found to be inactive, but numerous other mescaline analogues were as active as mescaline or even more so.[20] This paper seemed to me to be the epitome of courageous scientific investigation. There were also some odd things about it; for example, Shulgin's address on the author line was not given as Dept. of X at Prestigious University Y or as the Dept. of Discovery Research at Big Pharmaceutical company Z. All that was listed was 1483 Shulgin Rd., Lafayette, California—and thereby hangs a tale.

DR. SHULGIN'S COOKBOOKS

Dr. Alexander Shulgin has had anything but a normal career path, and yet he is certainly one of the most influential scientists of the twentieth century. While Albert Hoffmann has been the great pioneer of hallucinogenic tryptamine development, Alexander Shulgin has played a similar role in the development of hallucinogenic phenethylamines. Initially their career paths were similar. Hoffmann started as a researcher at Sandoz, and Shulgin at Dow Chemicals in the United States. However, after that their career paths diverged: Hoffmann remained with the same company all of his life, whereas Shulgin's career turned out to be extremely unconventional. He received his PhD in biochemistry from the University of California Berkeley and did postdoctoral work in psychiatry and pharmacology at University of California San Francisco. He then began work at Dow Chemical Company, where he developed a highly profitable biodegradable insecticide called *Zectran*. Because of this Dow gave Shulgin a lot of freedom to pursue his own research interests, which by that time were concerned with the psychopharmacology of mescaline in particular. Eventually Shulgin and Dow went their separate ways, and Shulgin set up his own research lab at his home. His status has been consistently controversial. On the one hand, because of his unique expertise in the area he has acted as an advisor to the Drug Enforcement Administration. On the other hand he has also been an *agent provocateur,* constantly expanding the horizons of hallucinogenic drug chemistry and development and taking a libertarian position on individuals' right to use whatever chemical agents they please.

Over the years Shulgin has embarked on an incredible series of investigations that have uncovered the seemingly infinite psychoactive potential of the phenethylamine nucleus as a chemical starting point for drug development. Consider the chemical structures of mescaline, amphetamine, and norepinephrine (Figures 2.12 and 2.13). One doesn't need a sophisticated background in chemistry to see that they are all closely related molecules, all containing the phenethylamine nucleus. However, the biological properties of these molecules are vastly different. Mescaline has the properties of a classical hallucinogen, amphetamine is a psychostimulant (see Chapter 8), and norepinephrine is a neurotransmitter that activates adrenergic receptors. Shulgin has systematically explored what happens when one makes small chemical changes to these structures. Importantly, one should note that there are still further classes of psychoactive substances that can be obtained in this manner. For example consider the compound methylenedioxymethamphetamine (MDMA). This substance was actually first synthesized in 1912 but was not really developed further until Shulgin

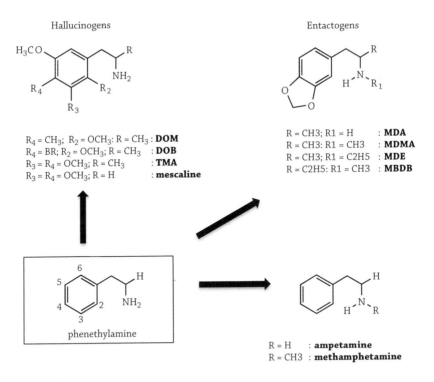

Hallucinogens

$R_4 = CH_3$; $R_2 = OCH_3$: $R = CH_3$: **DOM**
$R_4 = BR$; $R_2 = OCH_3$; $R = CH_3$: **DOB**
$R_3 = R_4 = OCH_3$; $R = CH_3$: **TMA**
$R_3 = R_4 = OCH_3$; $R = H$: **mescaline**

Entactogens

R = CH3; R1 = H : **MDA**
R = CH3; R1 = CH3 : **MDMA**
R = CH3; R1 = C2H5 : **MDE**
R = C2H5; R1 = CH3 : **MBDB**

phenethylamine

R = H : **ampetamine**
R = CH3 : **methamphetamine**

Figure 2.13:
Different classes of psychoactive compounds derived from the phenethylamine structure. MDMA is also known as Ecstasy (see Chapter 8).[7]

and his colleague David Nicholls resynthesized it and tested it in the 1970s. It can be seen that the structure of MDMA, which is also known by its street name XTC or Ecstasy, is related to both amphetamine and mescaline. However, its psychotropic actions proved somewhat unique and in fact it represents a prototype of a entirely separate family of drugs that have been named *entactogens* by David Nichols (see Chapter 8).

The numerous synthetic chemical riffs on the mescaline/phenethylamine theme that Shulgin has prepared are described in his book *PiHKAL*, or "Phenethylamines I Have Known And Loved." Here he describes many chemical analogues of mescaline that are actually much more potent that the parent molecule. For example, the series of substituted amphetamine-like structures DOI, DOB, DOC, and DOM all have profound classical hallucinogenic activity (Figure 2.13). Many of these molecules approach the potency of LSD. Some, like DOM (also known as STP or "Serenity, Tranquility, Peace") have had an independent street life. The numerous small modifications in structure that can be easily produced have enabled the creation of "designer drugs," new structures that could potentially be used for recreational purposes but which are not specifically covered by the drug laws. This is a cat and mouse game in which the producers of drugs attempt to stay one step ahead of the Drug Enforcement Administration (DEA).

For example, the compound 2C-B (4-bromo-2,5-dimethoxyphene-thylamine) is clearly related to the potent hallucinogen DOB and can be further modified in numerous fanciful ways. Addition of dihydrofuran rings (or in this case wings) yields 2C-B-FLY, or if only one ring is added, 2C-B-hemiFLY. With such compounds the fanciful chemical structure of the molecule has become a metaphor for the effects that it produces (Figure 2.14). Many of these compounds possess structural determinants of hallucinogens, amphetamines, and entactogens all combined in different ways, and the subjective experience obtained with many of them is hard to categorize, as it may have components of more than one drug type. Hence in *PiHKAL* (or the corresponding work *TiHKAL*, which covers adventures in tryptamine synthesis and psychopharmacology), Shulgin, who has tested every drug on himself, is careful to describe each experience as accurately as possible including all the little idiosyncrasies associated with each substance.

LSD HITS THE STREETS

Following its original discovery, the news about the amazing effects of LSD was rapidly disseminated. Sandoz supposed that the drug, marketed under

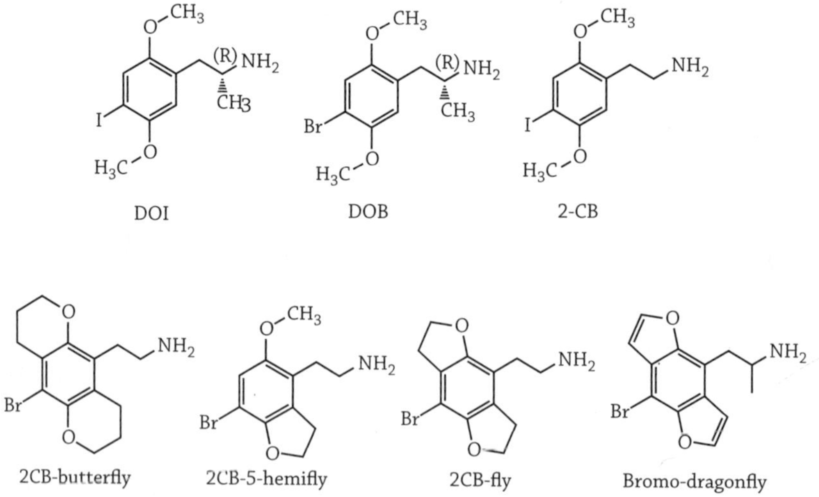

Figure 2.14:
Structures of hallucinogenic phenethylamines including insect like fly structures.

the name Delysid, might find a useful niche in the psychiatric market. But what exactly should it be used for? In order to understand its potential, the drug would need to be tested by psychiatrists "in the field." The original report on the effects of LSD were published by the psychiatrist Werner Stoll—none other than the son of Dr. Arthur Stoll, Albert Hoffmann's superior at Sandoz. Thereafter, Sandoz made samples of their new drug widely available to those who wanted to test it under the appropriate clinical conditions. However, the cat was very much out of the bag at that point and the first major group to examine the potential use of LSD was, of course, the CIA. In the 1950s and '60s the CIA had several top secret initiatives under the names BLUEBIRD, ARTICHOKE and MK-ULTRA, which sought to develop mind control techniques or "brainwashing" a la Manchurian Candidate[21] as an aid to the interrogation of subjects as part of their Cold War activities. These programs had been inspired by, among other things, documents that the CIA had obtained after World War II describing experiments with mescaline performed by Nazi doctors on the inmates of the Dachau concentration camp. LSD was first brought to the United States in 1949 by Dr. Max Rinkel, who carried out research using the drug on a population of 100 volunteers. Together with his colleague Dr. Paul Hoch they noted that LSD produced effects that mimicked schizophrenic psychosis. Indeed, they postulated that LSD produced a model psychosis—that is, it was "psychotomimetic." As we have seen, similar ideas circulated about the properties of mescaline. Such ideas were very influential and stimulated a great deal of subsequent research, which ultimately fell out of favor but has recently been revived.

The idea that LSD could produce mental disorganization encouraged the CIA to start using it in experiments similar to those carried out by the Nazi doctors. CIA operatives began administering the drug in secret to different subject populations (or indeed to each other). Like the Nazis, the CIA used different populations of helpless individuals such as prisoners, drug addicts, and mental patients in their experiments, often with appalling results. The CIA not only performed experiments on individuals but also came up with schemes for contaminating the water supply of potential enemies with LSD so as to incapacitate entire hostile populations. For this they would need large amounts of the drug, at one point ordering the equivalent of 100 million doses from Sandoz. When they found out that obtaining such a large amount as this might be somewhat problematic they turned to Eli Lilly and Company, whose capable chemists broke the secret Sandoz patent and assured the CIA that they could produce LSD in tons or similar amounts. Thankfully for the future of humanity, this eventuality never came to pass. In the end the CIA concluded that the effects of hallucinogenic drugs like

LSD were just too unpredictable for general use in the Cold War, and should just be reserved for very specific circumstances. Nevertheless, in the atmosphere of general paranoia that pervaded the postwar era, the CIA maintained an important role in manipulating the developing drug culture. CIA operatives acted as drug suppliers if they were interested in observing drug effects under particular circumstances, and infiltrated different drug-using groups with political points of view deemed to be of "interest" so as to relay information back to Washington.

However, it was not just the CIA who started the nascent drug culture simmering in the United States. As we have seen, Gordon Wasson had published his article on the use of psychedelic mushrooms in Mexico in *Life Magazine* in 1957, and this was very widely read and discussed. Aldous Huxley was another individual who greatly enhanced the awareness of the potential of psychedelic drug use. His interest in this subject clearly preceded the drug revolution of the 1960s as his famous book *Brave New World,* which had described the use of psychotropic drugs to control an entire society, had been published in 1931. Of course, much of the research on hallucinogenic drugs at the time was not just being performed at the behest of the CIA. There was enormous excitement in the psychiatric community about the possible uses of hallucinogens in psychiatry. Not only was there the idea that these drugs could be psychotomimetic and represented models of psychosis, but simultaneously other theories were being proposed suggesting the potential use of these same drugs in the treatment of mental disorders. Hence, LSD was simultaneously viewed as being psychotomimetic and a treatment for psychosis, reflecting the ferment in the psychiatric research community that the arrival of such a powerful drug had stirred up. LSD-mediated psychotherapy became highly popular and film stars such as Cary Grant were treated in this way, becoming propagandists for the drug.[22]

In the vanguard of LSD research in psychiatry was Humphrey Osmond, whom we have already encountered as the man who introduced the word *psychedelic* and who, along with John Smythies, suggested the endogenous psychotogen theory of schizophrenia. Osmond attempted to use LSD as a treatment for a variety of disorders such as alcoholism, and claimed to have had considerable success. Aldous Huxley became aware of Osmond's writings and volunteered to be a subject in one of his experiments. So, in May 1953 Osmond agreed and travelled to Huxley's home in California to supervise his drug experience. Huxley was duly impressed and continued experimenting with the drug on subsequent occasions. Huxley's final novel *Island,* published in 1960, summarized his views on the use of hallucinogens (called *moksha* in this novel) as an integral part of an ideal society.

When he died in 1963 Huxley had his wife administer LSD to him on his deathbed as he slid into the hereafter. Other writers such as the "Beats," including Allan Ginsberg and William Burroughs, also experimented with hallucinogens. Their book "*The Yage Letters*" (1963) details their sojourn in South America experimenting with ayahuasca.

It can therefore be seen that in the 1950s hallucinogenic drugs including mescaline, psilocybin, and LSD had become a widely discussed topic in medical, political, and artistic circles. However, in order for the use of hallucinogens to really take off in society in general, something else was needed. Proselytizing leaders were required, and one was soon at hand.

In 1960 Timothy Leary was a 39-year-old psychology lecturer at Harvard. He clearly had a bright career ahead of him, having carried out important basic research in behavioral psychology. Leary read Wasson's article in *Life Magazine* and, like many others, was intrigued. That summer he traveled down to Cuernavaca in Mexico with friends and obtained some samples of psilocybin mushrooms. Leary was profoundly impressed with his experience. Basically, he was bored with the kind of life he was leading as a faculty member at Harvard and saw that hallucinogens represented an entirely new path for the exploration of the psyche. Soon after returning to Boston he was sharing psilocybin with students and faculty alike and, together with his colleague Richard Alpert, set up an entire psilocybin-based research project which included "experiments" such as the Marsh Chapel religious event discussed in the previous chapter. Eventually Leary was also introduced to LSD, and this became his experimental drug of choice. However, the authorities at Harvard had soon had enough of Leary's antics, self-promotion, and his entire *modus operandi*. In 1963 both Leary and Alpert were dismissed from their faculty positions.

However, Leary was not deterred in the slightest. Initially he and Alpert started their own organization, the International Federation for Internal Freedom (IFIF) for the further study of the religious and psychological potential of hallucinogenic drug use.[22] The IFIF was headquartered in a Mexican resort town. However, the reports of wild orgies and other unseemly behavior caused the Mexican authorities to evict the group, and Leary was back in the United States once again. By this time experimenting with LSD had developed a cachet that was attracting the attention of many high rollers throughout the country. Eventually Leary encountered the fabulously wealthy William Mellon Hitchcock (aka "Mr. Billy"), the grandson of the founder of Gulf Oil. Mr. Billy took to LSD and to Timothy Leary and offered him and his acolytes the use of his 64-room country estate. Here at the Millbrook estate Leary established the Castalia Foundation, named after the priestly sect in Hesse's novel *The Glass Bead Game*,[23] which was dedicated to the scholarly study of LSD and its spiritual applications. Apparently Leary saw himself as a latter-day Joseph Knecht[23] and proceeded to hold court with anybody who cared to visit, partake of the LSD experience, and discuss the matter with him. As a guide to the direction and understanding of LSD-induced psychedelic experience, Leary used the Tibetan Book of the Dead which deals explicitly with different states of consciousness. Leary reinterpreted this so that it ended up as a sort of mixture of Buddhist wisdom and Scientology. Clearly at this point Leary had become the high priest of an LSD-fueled religion complete with its own bible. Millbrook was visited by a wide variety of high-profile individuals from the arts and politics, and its place in the general public's consciousness rapidly increased.

However, it was not only Leary who catalyzed the popularity of LSD. In 1960 Ken Kesey, who had graduated from Stanford's creative writing workshop, answered an advertisement for human guinea pigs to take part in one of the CIA-sponsored research studies on psychedelic drugs at a local hospital and ended up working there in the psychiatric ward. Here the ample availability of both psychedelic drugs and mental patients inspired him to write his first novel, *One Flew Over the Cuckoos Nest*—a considerable critical and popular success. The money that he earned from the book allowed Kesey, like Leary on the East Coast, a certain degree of freedom. While continuing to write, a group of like-minded and frequently stoned associates began to form a loose association with him.

Kesey's take on the use of the LSD experience, however, was very different from Leary's. He saw himself as a sort of *agent provocateur* whose role was to shake up the entire bourgeois establishment. In1964, together with his band of "Merry Pranksters," he purchased a bus, painted it in bright Day-Glo colors and, with the Pranksters attired in outrageous garb, traveled across the country handing out LSD—or "acid" as it was becoming known—to anybody who wanted to try it. In this way Kesey began to democratize the use of LSD, and things began to take on the characteristics of the drug counterculture movement of the 1960s. While in New York, Kesey and the Pranksters visited Leary at Millbrook in what clearly could have been an interesting meeting. However, the presence of two egos as large as theirs was too much even for the 64 rooms of Millbrook. Indeed, Leary did not deign to meet personally with Kesey, and the latter was not impressed with the priestly atmosphere pervading the upper class Millbrook estate where, in spite of everything else, attempts were made to study the effects of LSD on behavior in a conventional sense. So, the result was a culture clash—East coast versus West Coast, upper class versus working class, exclusivity versus egalitarianism. Kesey wanted to popularize the entire "acid trip" in a way that was fundamentally different from what Leary was doing. Following his return to California, Kesey began to mount a series of "Acid Tests," basically the precursors to hippie happenings where acid-laced "Electric Kool-Aid" was readily available accompanied by the latest music played by Kesey's favorite rock group, The Warlocks, soon to reemerge as The Grateful Dead.

In 1965, when large amounts of easily available acid hit the streets of US cities, American society was a powder keg ready to explode. The combination of the Vietnam war, the assassination of Malcolm X, the race riots in Watts and other cities, and the volatile mood on US college campuses, all contributed to the general ferment. Society was becoming increasingly radicalized and many young people felt completely disillusioned with their government and society in general. They sought to distance themselves from the status quo and to distinguish themselves as revolutionaries in as many ways as possible. Hallucinogenic drugs were the perfect things to help to define their defiant and alternative life style. As Leary had declared, it was time to "Turn on, tune in, and drop out." Drop out was what young people wanted to do; they certainly didn't want to actively participate in the society in which they found themselves. The Haight-Ashbury area of San Francisco became the crucible where all these elements came together, and the mass drug culture movement really got going. Owsley Stanley and Tim Scully began the local large-scale manufacture of ultrapure LSD dispensed at low cost as different batches of tablets, each one manufactured in a different psychedelic color. Stanley and Scully continued in their role as the local "alchemists" of Haight-Ashbury for several years and not only distributed LSD but other agents such as DOM/STP as well.

The mass use of acid by elements of the counterculture now spread incredibly rapidly, and by 1966 the US government realized it would have to step in. The government and their allies in the press mounted a smear campaign blaming LSD for everything from psychotic behavior in young people to chromosomal damage, and whipped the general public into a frenzy. Eventually, Sandoz stopped supplying the drug to scientists in the United States and the government placed strict legal controls on its possession and use. To understand the tenor of the times, it is very revealing to watch the 1967 "Blue Boy" episode of the crime drama *Dragnet*,[24] a very popular television series in the 1960s and 1970s. In this episode Sgt. Joe Friday, veteran of the LA police force, and his sidekick set out to rid the Los Angeles area of the LSD menace that is stalking Southern California. Using a semidocumentary style, the drama made it clear that LSD was destroying the lives of young people in the area by making them permanently psychotic and inducing them to behave in a generally lewd manner. This was the type of information that middle-class America was exposed to at the time, and so it was hardly surprising that drug use polarized society in the way it did.

By 1967 the situation at Millbrook had started to deteriorate and Mr. Billy decided to move to the West Coast. Here he joined forces with Owsley Stanley's colleague Tim Scully (Stanley being in jail at this point) and another chemist called Nick Sand to bankroll the production of large quantities of LSD for general distribution. This they achieved and by 1969 had manufactured over 10 million doses of acid, most of which was in the form of pills known as "Orange Sunshine" (OS). In order to distribute their product they joined forces with a group of ex-bikers from Anaheim who had started experimenting with LSD and had transformed themselves into a hippie church dedicated to bringing people closer to God through the use of acid. The group was known as the Brotherhood of Eternal Love and its leader was "Farmer" John Griggs. Initially giving vast quantities of OS away for free and then setting up an international LSD trading cartel, the Brotherhood was extremely successful in spreading the LSD message and within a year OS was turning up all over the world including with US troops in Vietnam. When Scully's original supply finally ran out, the Brotherhood teamed up with a remarkable character named Ronald Stark who turned up on their doorstep with a kilogram of pure LSD for the Brothers to do business with. Stark's actual identity and the source of all of his acid (eventually mounting up to over 50 million hits) have always been something of a matter for speculation—even to suggestions that he was actually a CIA operative.

In 1967 Timothy Leary found his way down to Southern California, where he hung out with the Brothers and became a Hollywood-style celebrity. However, by this time he had already started running afoul of the law and was eventually sentenced to a long prison term for drug possession. The story of what happened after that is so incredible that in truth it is much stranger than fiction. Leary was sent to a low security prison and was "sprung" from there by the notorious Weather Underground, who made great political capital out of the publicity they obtained from freeing a "political prisoner of the capitalist pigs." The Weathermen then smuggled the disguised Leary out of the country to sojourn with Eldridge Cleaver and his Black Panther government in exile in Algeria. However, Cleaver and Leary did not get on and the Panthers put him under local house arrest. Eventually the Brothers ransomed him for $25,000, and Leary and his wife fled to Switzerland. Leary always found wealthy patrons to support him, and this was true in Switzerland where he eventually settled down to a comfortable existence for the next 18 months and, in what must surely be one of the more interesting meetings of the century, dined with none other than Albert Hoffmann. Naturally they discussed matters pertaining to LSD and its potential uses.[1,22] In the end, however, the Swiss denied Leary political asylum and the US government started to press for Leary's extradition, so he decided to move on. In 1973 he flew to Kabul, possibly intending to journey on to Southeast Asia. This proved to be a big mistake. He and his latest wife (another possible CIA operative) were immediately arrested and deported back to the United States where the man labeled by president Nixon as "the most dangerous man in America" was sent back to jail until finally released by California Governor Jerry Brown in 1976. The use of LSD in the United States peaked in the late 1960s around the time of the great "love-in" rock concert at Woodstock in 1969. However, the use of hallucinogens has not gone away, and mushrooms in particular have recently undergone a new surge of popularity.

HALLUCINOGENIC MECHANISMS

The drugs discussed in this chapter, including LSD, psilocybin, DMT, and mescaline, are those which produce similar types of effects and are generally considered to be the "classical" hallucinogens. However, today the term *hallucinogen* has come to be rather widely employed in the context of psychoactive drug use. The word *hallucination* was originally a neologism introduced by Sir Thomas Browne in his great compendium the *Pseudodoxia Epidemica,* in a chapter in which he examined the truth of the widely held notion that moles are blind.[25] He thought not. Today what we really mean by the word *hallucination* is a conscious sensory experience devoid of any real stimulus. Numerous categories of drugs appear to be able to provoke this type of effect, including muscimol, as we have seen (Chapter 1), as well as others including antimuscarinic (anticholinergic) drugs, PCP (phencyclidine), cannabinoids, and opiates.

However, there is a particular quality to the experiences produced by LSD, psilocybin, mescaline, and DMT that indicate that they share a similar mechanism of action. This is indicated by drug discrimination studies performed in rodents. In such experiments animals are trained to receive a reward by pushing a lever if they distinguish between a particular type of drug—say LSD and saline. If an animal trained in this way is given a drug that produces the same type of effects, in this case mescaline or psilocybin for example, it will be fooled and press the same lever as it would when given LSD. In other words, the animal is saying to the experimenter: "You just gave me some LSD, thank you very much indeed!" On the other hand, if the animal was given a different type of psychoactive drug, such as an opiate or cocaine that produced a different type of effect, it would not push the LSD lever. These studies indicate that the animals cannot distinguish between the effects of drugs like LSD, mescaline, and psilocybin, but can clearly distinguish them from other drugs such as cocaine or opiates, thereby supporting the hypothesis that the classical hallucinogenic compounds all share the same mechanism of action. Of course we cannot know what kind of effects the animals are using for a cue, as it is certainly unlikely that they are experiencing the same type of subjective effects as a human being. Nevertheless, there is clearly something that all these drugs do to an animal which causes them to be recognized as a group.[7]

Now if we are satisfied that LSD, psilocybin, mescaline, and DMT all have the same mechanism of action, what might that be? We can obtain a clue by examining the structures of these compounds. As we have discussed, they resemble certain neurotransmitters, and we might imagine that interfering with the way that such neurotransmitters carry out their functions in the brain is the key to understanding their mechanism of action. In particular we have noted that LSD, psilocybin, and DMT resemble the neurotransmitter 5-hydroxytryptamine (5-HT), whereas mescaline and the hallucinogenic amphetamines resemble the catecholamine neurotransmitters such as dopamine and norepinephrine (Figure 2.12). As we shall see, it appears to be the 5-HT neurotransmitter system that is the important one in this instance. What then do we know about the functions of 5-HT? The existence of such a substance was actually first indicated by observations made well over a century ago. In 1868 Ludwig and Schmidt observed that defibrinogenated blood could contract blood vessels in perfused dog muscle. However, the identification of the substance responsible for this activity did not take place until much later, when in 1949 Maurice Rapport in Cleveland identified the mysterious substance as the indolealkylamine, 5-hydroxytryptamine. As we have indicated, 5-HT is also known as *serotonin* and the two terms are used interchangeably.

The modern classification of the receptors for 5-HT, including those in the brain, had to await the development of novel approaches for identifying receptor molecules that were pioneered in the 1970s by Solomon Snyder and his colleagues. Snyder's incredibly fruitful approach to the study of all neurotransmitter receptors was very direct, and we shall refer to it several times in subsequent chapters. He took the neurotransmitter molecule itself, or drugs thought to interact with the neurotransmitter receptor, and made them as radioactive as possible. Then, because radioactivity can be readily measured, one could examine the ability of these radioactive molecules to interact directly with tissue preparations from the brain or elsewhere. The idea was that if the radioactive molecules stuck tightly to the tissue and could not be easily washed off, it was more than likely that the entity they were sticking to was their receptor—just as an address tag can readily identify a suitcase. Snyder's innovative approach led the way to the modern identification of 5-HT receptors. By performing studies with radioactive drugs, Snyder and Peroutka[26] concluded that there must be more than one kind of 5-HT receptor in the brain and that LSD could clearly interact with some of these receptor classes. Some 10 years later (1988) the emerging tools of molecular biology were brought to bear on the problem and the first 5-HT receptor molecule was cloned, and as a result its entire sequence of amino acids was precisely identified.[27]

If you are a pharmacologist and you are interested in 5-HT, you have really hit the proverbial jackpot because it turns out that there are more receptors for 5-HT than any other neurotransmitter we know of. Currently there appear to be 7 families of 5-HT receptors named 5-HT1, 5-HT2, and so on up to 5-HT7. Many of these families contain subtypes, and so there are a total of 14 5-HT receptors altogether.[28] Each of these receptors has a unique pattern of expression throughout the body, including the brain, allowing 5-HT to regulate the functions of many different tissues. Indeed, 5-HT is synthesized and stored by many kinds of cells including neurons in the brain, platelets in the blood, and in specialized cells of the gut called *enterochromaffin* cells. It can be released from all of these sources to act upon its many widely distributed receptors. Investigations have shown that the major type of 5-HT receptor that LSD interacts with is known as the *5-HT2A receptor,* and it is particularly widely distributed in the brain. Moreover, other potent hallucinogens like DOI, which as we have seen has a completely different kind of chemical structure, also strongly activate 5-HT2A receptors, further implicating them as the major conduit for these types of effects.

What then is the molecular structure of a 5-HT receptor? One receptor type, the 5-HT3 receptor family, closely resembles the GABA-A receptors discussed in the previous chapter. Like the GABA-A receptors, the 5-HT3 receptors consist of a series of protein subunits that define an ion channel. Also, like GABA-A receptors, this ion channel is normally closed. However, when 5-HT binds to 5-HT3 receptors, the ion channel opens and cations like Na and K redistribute themselves across the membrane. Thus, as opposed to GABA-A receptors which are anion-specific channels, 5-HT3 receptors are cation channels. 5-HT3 receptors have been found to play a key role in the nausea and vomiting response to chemotherapeutic agents, and so drugs that block this receptor have found an important use as anti-emetic drugs in cancer chemotherapy.

However, all of the other known receptors for 5-HT have a completely different structure. These receptors all resemble the GABA-B receptors briefly mentioned in the previous chapter and are members of the superfamily of molecules known as the *Gprotein coupled receptors* (GPCRs). GPCRs are the major types of receptors used by cells all over the body and they make up more than 1% of the human genome—and that's a lot. GPCRs act as the receptors for numerous substances, including many neurotransmitters and hormones. Furthermore, many important drugs act by either activating or inhibiting GPCRs. The structure of a GPCR is quite different from that of the ligand gated ion channel. However, the job of these receptor proteins is still to issue a set of instructions to the interior of the cell as a consequence of the binding of an agonist. Structurally, the chain of amino acids that makes up a GPCR is characterized by an extracellular N-terminus, followed by seven transmembrane α-helices connected by three intracellular and three extracellular loops, and finally an intracellular C-terminus. In effect, the sequence of amino acids threads its way back and forward across the cell membrane like a snake or possibly the Loch Ness Monster. Because of this, GPCRs are sometimes referred to as "serpentine" receptors. When an agonist binds to a GPCR on the outside of the cell it produces a change in the shape of the protein, which then acts as a signal to elements within the cell and changes their activity. The first of these intracellular signaling elements to be discovered is known as a *Gprotein,* so called because it possesses intrinsic enzymatic activity and can degrade the molecule GTP which is found within all cells.

GPCRs have turned out to be extremely fascinating and versatile molecules. Nowadays we know that activation of GPCRs can not only lead to the activation of Gproteins but also to other intracellular signaling proteins as well, including an important protein known as β-arrestin. We also know that different types of agonists can cause a GPCR to assume a number of slightly different conformations, and that each of these may activate different intracellular signaling pathways which can involve the activation of different Gproteins or other signaling molecules. Hence a given GPCR may act in different ways depending on the specific agonist employed. Thus, depending on the exact nature of the GPCR there may be a large number of potential signaling consequences for the cell once it is activated.

We also know that some agents are better than others at activating receptors. If one substance works at lower concentrations than another we say it is more "potent." If another substance can make the receptor attain a higher maximal activity, we say it is more "efficacious." If a substance occupies the receptor but does not activate it at all (that is, it has zero efficacy), we say it is an "antagonist." Such considerations turn out to be important if we wish to understand the current hypothesis as to how hallucinogens like LSD produce their effects.

The subjective effects of LSD and other classical hallucinogens on human conscious experience are truly remarkable. A complete understanding of the way these drugs produce their effects would entail a comparable understanding of the neurobiology of consciousness, something that we don't really possess. Consequently we are unable to say precisely how activation of a particular group of nerve cells allows us to perceive our internal and external environments. However, we can make some attempts at defining those components of the brain which might be important in this process. It is interesting to note that although there are so many types of 5-HT receptors in the body, and we know 5-HT has many important roles to play, the actual source of 5-HT in the brain is extremely restricted. This can be compared to the numerous neurons that synthesize and release the neurotransmitters GABA and glutamate, for example. Only one group of nerve cells in the brain can synthesize and release 5-HT. These are neurons of the raphe nuclei, which are localized in pairs along the entire length of the brainstem. Although the number of raphe neurons is small, their axons spread out very widely to reach nearly every part of the central nervous system, including the higher regions of the brain such as the cortex, thought to be responsible for higher cognitive functions. Thus one raphe neuron may release 5-HT that influences hundreds of thousands of other neurons. These neurons will respond to 5-HT because they express 5-HT receptors. In particular, 5-HT2A receptors are also widely expressed in the brain particularly, as one might expect, near most of the 5-HT nerve terminal–rich areas of the cerebral cortex. This includes the prefrontal, parietal, and somatosensory areas. This kind of information suggests that cortical 5-HT2A receptors could act as an important target for hallucinogens in the higher cognitive centers of the brain.

One problem in trying to elucidate the mechanism of action of psychotropic drugs using animals like rats and mice is trying to establish what types of effects to measure in such animals. If we want to measure something that mimics a disease like Parkinson's disease (PD), we might be able to come up with something reasonable. In PD, patients have a problem with movement owing to the destruction of specific nerves that utilize the neurotransmitter dopamine. So, if we selectively destroy such neurons in a mouse, we find that the mouse then has movement problems which at least have a passing resemblance to those seen in human PD. Hence we can use such a mouse model for doing things like testing new drugs that might help in the disease—if they help the mouse, they might well help humans.

But this is not the case when trying to make a mouse model of a complex human cognitive phenomenon like the disease schizophrenia, or in this case the highly subjective effects of hallucinogenic drugs. Recall that when the doctor was called to visit Albert Hoffmann at his home while he was experiencing the world's first LSD trip, all the doctor could observe was the fact that Hoffmann had dilated pupils. He needed Hoffmann to actually tell him about the things he was experiencing. Also recall that when Sandoz first tested LSD in mice, they found its effects quite unremarkable. This for one of the most remarkable drugs the world has ever discovered! It is unlikely that mice are experiencing the same kind of thing that a human experiences—and anyway, even if they were, they can't tell us about it. We know from drug discrimination studies that rats and mice all "think" that LSD, mescaline, psilocybin, and DMT do the same thing—but what that thing actually is we cannot say.

So, how do we know that LSD is having any type of effect on the brain of a mouse? Is there some kind of behavior that we can observe that would suggest this is the case? The answer is that they twitch their heads! That's it! In lieu of all the spectacular and interesting effects hallucinogenic drugs produce in humans, in mice this is reduced to a mere twitch of the head. It turns out that only hallucinogenic drugs like LSD, mescaline, psilocybin, and DOI induce mice to twitch their heads in a specifically recognizable fashion, and nonhallucinogenic drugs with similar chemical structures do not. Hence neuropharmacologists tend to believe that the "head twitch" response in mice, unlikely though this might seem, is actually a measure that at least correlates with hallucinogenic activity in humans.

Once we cross this particular Rubicon and subscribe to this view, several things follow. First, we have noted that 5-HT2A receptors are very widely expressed in the brain. Which 5-HT2A receptors are the important ones that mediate the effects of hallucinogens? We might hypothesize that the receptors in higher cortical structures are important. To test this possibility, neuropharmacologists have performed a remarkable experiment.[29] First they have used the techniques of mouse genetic engineering to produce mice that lack 5-HT2A receptors. These mice seem "normal"; that is, they do not exhibit any obvious behavioral abnormalities. Giving LSD or DOI to such mice no longer results in head twitching, thereby "proving" the importance of 5-HT2A receptors in producing this behavior. It was noted that a particular type of neuron called a *pyramidal neuron* located in layer V of the cortex normally expresses lots of 5-HT2A receptors. Using a sophisticated genetic engineering procedure, investigators took mice that had no 5-HT2A receptors and put them back again—but only into the cortical layer 5 pyramidal cells and nowhere else. Now, when LSD or DOI were given to these mice, they twitched their heads again just like ordinary mice. So this experiment leads us to conclude that the 5HT2A receptors expressed by cortical layer 5 pyramidal cells are the ones that mediate the head twitch response and, in so far as this head twitch response represents hallucinogenic activity in man, then such receptors are also the important ones for producing the hallucinogenic effects in humans. This is the type of logic that neuropharmacologists employ when they are investigating questions like this one.

Recently it has also been possible to examine the patterns of brain activity produced by hallucinogenic drugs by using modern brain imaging techniques. An important observation is that some of the patterns of cortical activity produced by drugs like LSD are also produced by other types of "hallucinogenic" compounds, particularly drugs known as dissociative anesthetics which include phencyclidine (PCP, aka Angel Dust) and ketamine.[30] Although the effects produced by such drugs are clearly distinct from those produced by the classical hallucinogens, they do produce effects in humans which are thought by some to mimic aspects of schizophrenia (Chapter 3). Interestingly, the mechanism of action of drugs like PCP is quite different from that of LSD. Rather than being agonists at 5-HT2A receptors, these drugs act as antagonists at the receptors for the excitatory neurotransmitter glutamate. Therefore, at present a research area of great interest is to try and understand how the 5-HT and glutamate systems interact with one another in the prefrontal cortex and related structures in the brain. Indeed, there have been recent attempts to develop novel antipsychotic drugs that work by activating glutamate receptors and simultaneously inhibiting 5-HT2A receptors. We will discuss these interactions further when we consider the pharmacology of antipsychotic drugs in detail in the next chapter. The fact is, however, that over 50 years after Albert Hoffmann first synthesized LSD and suggested it might lead to insights into the pathology of psychiatric disease, his predictions may now be coming true. Like many great men he was just ahead of his time.

NOTES

1. Albert Hoffmann. *LSD: My Problem Child*. MAPS (Multidisciplinary association for psychedelic studies) contains a detailed description of how LSD was discovered.
2. Schiff PL. Ergot and its alkaloids. *Am J Pharm Educ*. 2006, 70(5):1–10.
3. Lee MR. The history of ergot of rye (*Claviceps purpurea*) I: from antiquity to 1900. *J R Coll Physicians Edinb*. 2009, 39(2):179–184.

4. The Isenheim altarpiece was painted by Matthias Grunewald between 1506 and 1515 and is surely one of the greatest works of art ever produced. The altarpiece has two wings and a predella. The precise scenes depicted depend on which parts of the altarpiece are opened. Scenes of the annunciation and resurrection are portrayed. Other scenes show St. Anthony in the desert being tormented by demons. All the pieces of the work can be seen on display at the Museum Unterlinden in Colmar. The altarpiece was the inspiration for Paul Hindemith's opera "Mathis der Maler" (Matthius the Painter).

5. Lee MR. The history of ergot of rye (*Claviceps purpurea*) II: 1900–1940. *J R Coll Physicians Edinb.* 2009, 39(4):365–369.

6. Lee MR. The history of ergot of rye (*Claviceps purpurea*) III: 1940–80. *J R Coll Physicians Edinb.* 2010, 40(1):77–80.

7. Nichols DE. Hallucinogens. *Pharmacol Ther.* 2004, 101(2):131–181.

8. Jonathan Ott. *Pharmacotheon.* Natural Products Co. Pp. 119–162 discusses Ololiuhqui and its alkaloids.

9. Wasson RG, Hofmann AA, Ruck CAP. *The road to Eleusis: Unveiling the secrets of the mysteries.* North Atlantic Books. 2008.

10. Peter Webster, Daniel M. Perrine, Carl A. P. Ruck. "Mixing the Kykeon" in *Eleusis: Journal of Psychoactive Plants and Compounds.* New Series 4. 2000.

11. Popol Vuh and Chilam Balam are classic works describing aspects of Mesoamerican cultures. The earlier Popol Vuh describes several pre-Columbian histories of the Mayan K'iche' (Quiche) people of Western Guatemala whose kingdom existed from the thirteenth century until the arrival of the Spaniards in the sixteenth century.

12. Andy Lechter. *Shroom: A Cultural History of the Magic Mushroom.* HarperCollins, publisher. This informative book contains many examples of the inadvertent consumption of hallucinogenic mushrooms in the nineteenth and twentieth centuries.

13. Paul Stamets. *Psilocybin Mushrooms of the World: An Identification Guide.* Ten Speed Press 1996.

14. Alexander and Anne Shulgin. *TiHKAL: The continuation.* Transform Press. 1997. (Chapter 15—DMT is everywhere). TIHKAL is an acronym for "Tryptamines I Have Known And Loved." Together with PIHKAL ("Phenethylamines I Have Known And Loved"), these two volumes contain a huge amount of information concerning the chemistry and pharmacology of hallucinogenic drugs. This includes instructions of how to synthesize hundreds of them and the effect of every one of these on the author(s).

15. Jonathan Ott. *Pharmacotheon.* Natural Products. Co. Pp. 163–197 and 199–273 contains detailed discussions of DMT and ayahuasca.
Alexander Shulgin. *TIHKAL: the continuation.* Pp. 285–310 contains a discussion of the chemical constituents of ayahuasca.

16. Louis Lewin. *Phantastica.* Park Street Press. Pp. 80–90 contains a description of "Anhalonium," Lewin's name for mescaline.

17. John Symonds. *The Great Beast: The life and magick of Aliester Crowley.* Macdonald and Co. 1971.

18. Harley-Mason J. The Pink Spot: The Lancet. *J ment Sci.* 1952, 98:313.
Friedhoff AJ, Van Winkle E. *Nature.* 1962a, 194:897.
Friedhoff AJ, Van Winkle E. *J Nerv Ment Dis.* 1962b, 135:550.
Friedhoff AJ, Van Winkle E. *J Chromatog.* 1963, 11:272.
Osmond H, Smythies JR. *J Ment Sci.* 1952, 98:309.
Smythies JR. *Postgrad Med J.* 1963, 39:26.

19. Alexander Shulgin. *PiHKAL: a chemical love story.* 614–616: Shulgin describes how he took a large dose of chlorpromazine and observed the pink spot appearing in his urine. It went away when he stopped taking the drug.
Ridges PA, Bourdillon PE. The Pink Spot. *Proc Royal Soc Med.* 1967, 60:29–31.
Pink spot in schizophrenia. *Br Med J.* 1966, 1(5480): 119.

20. Shulgin AT, Sargent T, Naranjo C. Structure–activity relationships of one-ring psychotomimetics. *Nature.* 1969, 221(5180):537–541.

21. *The Manchurian Candidate.* John Frankenheimer's 1962 movie in which Laurence Harvey plays a US serviceman who is brainwashed by the Communists as a prisoner in the Korean war and trained to assassinate a presidential candidate.

22. Martin A. Lee, Bruce Shlain. *Acid Dreams.* Grove Press 1992.

23. *The Glass Bead Game* by Herman Hesse takes place in the fictional country of Castalia and tells the story of Joseph Knecht, who becomes the head of the priestly order described in the book.

24. This is available on YouTube: http://www.youtube.com/watch?v=P0zgIzqgxFU.

25. Sir Thomas Browne. *Pseudodoxia Epidemica.* "of moles, or molls" (chapter 18).
Browne is perhaps the greatest of all writers on science. In the *Pseudodoxia Epidemica* or *Vulgar Errors* he examines different opinions that are generally held and presents arguments showing that they are incorrect. For example, in this case he examines the opinion that all moles are blind and concludes that this cannot be the case.

26. Peroutka SJ, Snyder SH. Multiple serotonin receptors: differential binding of [3H]5-hydroxytryptamine, [3H]lysergic acid diethylamide and [3H]spiroperidol. *Mol Pharmacol.* 1979, 16(3):687–699.

27. Leysen JE. 5-HT2 receptors. *Curr Drug Targets CNS Neurol Disord.* 2004, 3(1):11–26.

28. Hannon J, Hoyer D. Molecular biology of 5-HT receptors. *Behav Brain Res.* 2008, 195(1):198–213.

29. González-Maeso J, Weisstaub NV, Zhou M, Chan P, Ivic L, Ang R, Lira A, Bradley-Moore M, Ge Y, Zhou Q, Sealfon SC, Gingrich JA. Hallucinogens recruit specific cortical 5-HT(2A) receptor-mediated signaling pathways to affect behavior. *Neuron.* 2007, 53(3):439–435.

30. Vollenweider FX, Kometer M. The neurobiology of psychedelic drugs: implications for the treatment of mood disorders. *Nat Rev Neurosci.* 2010, 11(9):642–651.

CHAPTER 3

Purple Haze

"Purple haze all in my brain. Lately things just don't seem the same. Actin' funny, but I don't know why, 'Scuse me while I kiss the sky."

Jimi Hendrix (1966)

How does science progress? This is a subject that has been discussed in great detail over the years. One influential book on this topic is *The Structure of Scientific Revolutions* by the philosopher of science Thomas Kuhn.[1] One of Kuhn's major ideas was that science does not always progress in a gradual manner but is driven by seismic events, which he named "paradigm shifts." For example, sometimes the discovery of a new drug produces revolutionary changes in the practice of medicine. The introduction of this new type of drug may not only improve the lives of many patients who had previously not been effectively treated, but might also tell us a great deal about the underlying causes of the disease in question.

In the middle of the twentieth century there were two revolutions of this type. The first of these was the discovery and development of antibacterial agents, such as the sulfonamide drugs and the antibiotic penicillin. These discoveries completely revolutionized the treatment of many infectious diseases that had previously been untreatable. The second, equally revolutionary change concerned the way we treat different types of psychiatric disorders. Although there are numerous reasons why these changes took place, one of the most important was the appearance of new classes of drugs in the 1950s that could effectively alleviate the symptoms of mental disorders such as clinical depression, schizophrenia, bipolar disorder, and anxiety. Drugs such as the antipsychotic "major tranquilizers," the anti-depressants, and anxiolytic "minor tranquilizers" have subsequently been given to billions of people throughout the world. One might well describe these events as the "Psychopharmacological Revolution" in psychiatric medicine. Exactly how successful this revolution has been has also been widely discussed. While there is general agreement that these drugs have brought considerable relief to numerous patients, and dramatic changes in the way psychiatry is practiced, some critics have raised questions about the social forces that have engineered these changes. Nevertheless, it is undeniable that the revolution did take place, and its importance is not in question.

Consider the situation of mental patients prior to the 1950s. Montague Lomax, a retired general practitioner, wrote the following in his *Experiences of an Asylum Doctor* in 1921, describing the "lunatics in the refractory ward of our public asylums. Beastialised, apathetic, mutinous, greedy, malevolent . . . their habits quarrelsome and filthy, their persons dirty and malodorous."[2] Following the introduction in the early 1950s of chlorpromazine, the first antipsychotic drug, and the subsequent introduction of haloperidol in the early 1960s, the situation changed rapidly. This change can be illustrated by statistics on the number of psychiatric inpatients over this time period. In 1950 more than half the hospital beds in the United States were occupied by psychiatric patients, whose numbers had risen from around 150,000 in 1900 to 500,000 in 1955. However, after the start of routine antipsychotic drug use the number of patients fell rapidly and by 1975 it was down to 200,000. Indeed, between 1954 and 1996 numbers fell by approximately 90%.[3]

Although it would be an oversimplification to state that these changes were entirely due to the introduction of antipsychotic drugs rather than fiscal and administrative factors, it is clear that antipsychotics played a major role. The development of chlorpromazine was the result of an extremely long and convoluted series of events that is as old as the pharmaceutical industry itself. In fact, its story begins with a consideration of something that could not have been further from the treatment of psychiatric disease nor a seemingly more unpromising starting point—a sticky, gooey substance called coal tar.

MAUVE MADNESS

Coal tar is formed during the distillation of bituminous coal—that is, coal that results from the compression of peat bogs. Coal tar is obtained from the coking of this coal, which produces coke for many industries and coal gas for numerous processes including the lighting of streets in many cities in the nineteenth century. During the coking process, coal is heated to very high temperatures in an airless furnace, which drives off volatile constituents like coal gas and coal tar, leaving behind a fused carbon residue.

Coal tar is a thick dark liquid which smells like naphthalene (as in moth balls) and produces a burning sensation on the tongue. It is a highly complex mixture of many organic substances. This chemical richness has ultimately been exploited in numerous ways. The use of coal tar in topical applications such as soaps and shampoo will be familiar to many people. In the 1820s Charles Macintosh invented a method for using coal tar for waterproofing cloth, and so developed the raincoat. However, coal tar also played an enormously important role in the development of chemistry in the nineteenth century, particularly as a source of many important organic molecules that acted as the starting points for the subsequent synthesis of many other, more complex substances. For example, naphthalene was isolated from coal tar in 1820, aniline in 1841, and benzene in 1845. Substances such as these were the building blocks of the burgeoning science of organic chemistry and ultimately played a critical role in the development of the entire chemical and pharmaceutical industries (Figure 3.1).

Some of the most important events that led to these developments took place in England, although the fact that this was the case is surprising. In the early nineteenth century the science of chemistry was not taken particularly seriously in England. There were chemists, of course, but the subject was generally the provenance of dilettantes rather than professionals. Chemistry courses, of a sort, were taught at Oxford and Cambridge but they certainly didn't include anything as practical as work in a laboratory. It was widely believed that the study of pure chemistry was unlikely to lead to anything "useful." On the other hand, attitudes in Germany were completely different. Here, professors such as Justus von Liebig at the University of Giessen taught laboratory-based courses on synthetic chemistry and so trained large numbers of skilled chemistry students.

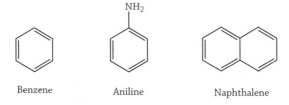

Figure 3.1:
Important organic chemicals isolated from coal tar.

This tradition was to put Germany at the forefront of research in the latter part of the nineteenth century when the need ultimately arose for skilled chemists to work in the chemical and pharmaceutical industries. Apart from being an important chemist, Justus von Liebig was also a wonderful teacher and speaker. In 1830s and '40s he made lecture tours of England and excoriated the English as to the state of chemistry in their country. His words sunk in and persuaded a group of influential individuals, which included the Prince Consort, the Prime Minister Mr. Gladstone, and the great chemist and physicist Michael Faraday, to open a Royal College of Chemistry, which found a permanent home in Oxford Street in 1845.

The fact that the school was a success was mainly due to the inspired choice of its initial director. August Wilhelm von Hofmann had been a student of Liebig's at Giessen and was extremely well qualified. His recruitment even involved the personal intervention of Queen Victoria and Prince Albert. Following his appointment Hofmann kept the "Royals" up to date with the latest results in chemical research by giving private lectures on the subject at Windsor Castle. He also lectured widely at venues like the Royal Institution, spreading the news of new breakthroughs in the subject. Like Liebig, Hofmann was an energetic and inspirational teacher who had an enormous influence on his students. Among these was an 18-year-old from London by the name of William Perkin.

William Perkin was born in the East End of London in 1838, the son of a fairly well to do carpenter.[4] A clever boy and a good student, Perkin had many early hobbies and enthusiasms including photography, music, art, and engineering. However, when at the age of 13 a friend demonstrated some basic chemistry experiments to him, he was hooked. He attended the City of London school and persuaded his father to pay a small extra fee for chemistry lessons, which were taught as an addition to the basic courses that naturally included Latin, Greek, Divinity, and suchlike.

Once he started attending chemistry lessons, Perkin's enthusiasm continued unabated. His teacher was impressed with him and at some point suggested that Perkin set up his own small laboratory at home to conduct simple experiments. This is surely the way that most budding chemists start out even today. (I well remember my own laboratory in the garage of my boyhood home in North London). He also suggested that Perkin write to Michael Faraday asking if he could attend Faraday's lecture series at the Royal Institution. Faraday sent him a personal reply giving him permission. Hence, at the age of 14 Perkin was already privy to the latest developments in cutting-edge chemistry.

Naturally Perkin wanted to enroll in the new Royal College of Chemistry, but this was equally naturally opposed by his father who wanted to do something "useful" like architecture. Nevertheless, following several meetings with Hofmann, Perkin's father relented and in 1853, at the age of 15, Perkin enrolled at the Royal College.

At this time one of the major goals of the young science of organic chemistry was to attempt to provide chemical syntheses for natural products. Some of these substances were extremely important but very hard to come by. It was thought that success in such ventures would help to demonstrate that chemistry was not just an academic or gentlemanly pursuit, but could actually provide useful answers to important practical questions. Two such substances of great interest were the drug quinine and the dye indigo. Hofmann was particularly interested in the former question but, as we shall see, came to play a major role in the answering the latter.

South American Indians had been using the bark of the cinchona tree to treat "ague" (malaria) for many centuries. The Spanish conquistadors learned about quinine following their conquest of Peru around 1532, and the drug was brought back to Europe for the first time by the Jesuits. The active drug was isolated in 1820 by two French doctors, Pierre Joseph Pelletier and Joseph Bienaimé Caventou, who named it "quinine" from the Amerindian word for the cinchona tree, *quinaquina,* meaning "bark of barks."[5] In the nineteenth century the British Empire had spread to all parts of the world and included many areas where malaria was a particularly serious problem. Hence, the availability of quinine at a reasonable price was a considerable concern. As it turned out, a chemical synthesis for quinine proved to be an extremely difficult problem and it was only ultimately achieved in 1944. Even now, synthetic quinine is not really an economical alternative to the natural product. However, in the 1850s all of this was unknown. August Hofmann had considered the problem of synthesizing quinine and gave this project to Perkin, suggesting that he might use coal tar–derived bases as a starting point for his investigations.

Perkin decided to perform some of these studies in his home laboratory and began experiments with several substances including aniline. One reaction he performed, in which he attempted to oxidize aniline with potassium dichromate, resulted in the production of a black sludge. Perkin extracted this product with alcohol and found to his surprise that it gave a beautiful purple lilac colour. Now, it should be remembered that Perkin had always been interested in the arts, and the vibrant color he had produced certainly caught his attention. He was intrigued, and instead of discarding it as a curiosity he decided to investigate further. In particular he attempted to dye a piece of silk cloth, and observed that not only did the material turn a beautiful purple but that the color did not wash out after several attempts. Perkin wondered whether he might be able to commercialize the production of his newly discovered dyestuff, and spoke to several dye manufacturers for their opinions and advice.

At the time all dyes were produced from natural sources. For example, blue was produced from the indigo plant, red from the root of the madder plant, yellow from saffron, purple from the rare mollusk *Murex,* and so on. Not only were these colors usually expensive to produce but they were also complicated, requiring numerous steps in their preparation. Purple in particular was an extremely expensive product, and Perkin was advised by the dyers he consulted that a reliable synthetic form of the dye would in fact be extremely valuable. Although it caused something of a rift with Hofmann, Perkin decided that he would indeed try to turn his new discovery into a commercial product and left the Royal College to follow this path. Amazingly, this decision would ultimately lead all the way to the development of chlorpromazine, the first antipsychotic drug.

To begin with, he found it difficult to secure financing for his new business and eventually his father had to step in with the money. Perkin built a small factory at Greenford near Harrow in London and started to make his new purple dye in larger quantities. He named the new dye *mauveine,* or "mauve," after the French for the mallow flower which is precisely this color (Figure 3.2). As it turns out, the chemical reaction Perkin had created involved the formation of a mixture of isomers of the mauveine molecule such as the structure in Figure 3.2. It should be noted that this contains a tricyclic ring system; that is, three ring structures fused together at its center. This is something which, as we shall see, would yield numerous substances of great importance to the field of psychopharmacology.

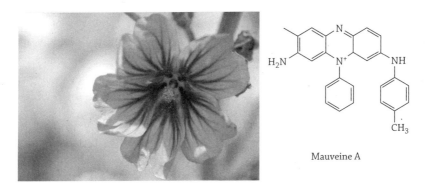

Mauveine A

Figure 3.2:
The mallow flower from which the word "mauve" was derived by William Perkin.
(Bojidar Beremski © Photoscom)
The chemical structure of mauveine, the chemical basis of synthetic mauve dyes.

The fact that Perkin had come up with a French name for the dye was appropriate because it was the French who ensured the success of his new venture. Paris was the center of the fashion world then as it is now. In particular, the Empress Eugenie, wife of Napoleon III, was the undoubted tastemaker supreme, perhaps the Paris Hilton or Lady Gaga of her day. With infinite sources of money and a great sense of style and pomp, the empress was the person all women looked to as a fashion icon. This not only included the *hoi polloi* but also other aristocrats such as her friend across the channel, Queen Victoria of Great Britain.

Soon after her marriage Eugenie decided that mauve was the very color that showed her eyes off to their best advantage, and started to wear elaborate gowns in this shade. At this point in time, fashion magazines for women were just starting to make their appearance and so the Empress's new look was rapidly disseminated throughout Europe and the rest of the world. Unfortunately Perkin hadn't acted quickly enough to obtain the patent for synthetic mauve in France. However, another stroke of luck was to set him on his way. In 1858 Queen Victoria's daughter, the Princess Royal, was married—quite the social event of the season. And guess what color the Queen wore for the occasion? Perhaps influenced by Eugenie, she was described in the illustrated *London News* in the following way ([4]):

> "The train and body of her Majesty's dress was composed of rich mauve velvet, trimmed with three rows of lace; the corsage ornamented with diamonds and the celebrated Koh-i-noor brooch; the petticoat, mauve and silver moiré antique, trimmed with a deep flounce of Honiton lace; the head dress, a Royal diadem of diamonds and pearls."

Moreover, both Eugenie and Victoria continued to favor mauve in their wardrobe for some time. This was enough to ignite "mauve madness" and it became all the rage. Of course in order to fulfill the wishes of the great masses of women who wanted crinolines and other items of this color, it was important to have a way of making a reliable mauve dye relatively cheaply that did not involve mashing up millions of hard-to-come-by mollusks, beetles, or other creatures. So, William Perkin's invention was just the right thing at just the right time (Figure 3.3).

THE RISE OF THE CHEMICAL INDUSTRY

Of course fads in fashion do not last, and after about half a dozen years mauve was out of favor. However, now the genie was out of the bottle.

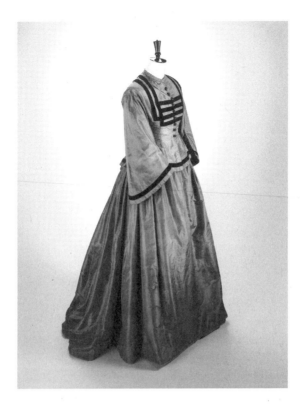

Figure 3.3:
Classic Victorian mauve dyed ladies gown.
(Reproduced with permission of the Science Museum, London).

Following Perkin's discovery, an enormous amount of experimentation began with a view to making new and fashionable synthetic dyes or synthetic versions of older natural dyes. The next big success to hit the market was a magenta dye (fuchsine) invented in France. Over the next few years this was followed by new dyes of every conceivable shade—Hofmann's violet, Bismarck Brown, aniline black, malachite green, Congo red, and so on. Together with the synthesis of these new dyes came a more sophisticated appreciation of the chemical reactions that were involved in their creation. So, gradually, the synthesis of new compounds became more rational and less serendipitous.

Originally, many of the new compounds were made in the United Kingdom or France. But there was a big change just around the corner. As we have discussed, it was in Germany, or at least in the collection of states that were soon to become Germany, where the science of chemistry received the most respect. Many great chemists such as Adolf von Baeyer, Bunson, and Kekule were German, and a large number of energetic and well trained young students were being produced by German universities. Many of these students made their way to the United Kingdom to gain knowledge about the new advances in the dye-making industry being pioneered by the likes of Perkin and others. Following this training, most of them returned to Germany ready to make use of their new knowledge in the service of the German chemical industry. Even August Hofmann returned to Germany in 1865, having tired of the unenlightened attitude of the British toward chemistry and with the promise of a professorship in Berlin.

Coal tar dyestuff companies began to appear in Germany in great numbers. By 1876, for example, there were 6 in the United Kingdom, 5 in France, and 17 in Germany. Many of these were established along the Rhine river, which provided an excellent water supply and was an ideal conduit for the transport of materials. Around 1860 Badische Anilin und Soda Fabrik (BASF) was established in Ludwigshafen. Other new companies that were to make their mark included Hoechst, Bayer, Kalle, and Cassella. Aktiengesellschaft für Anilinfabrikation (Corporation for Aniline Production), which became known as Agfa, was founded in Berlin by Carl Martius, who had studied with Hofmann in England, together with Paul Mendelssohn-Bartholdy, the son of the composer.

It was in companies such as these that the industrial research laboratory as we now know it first developed.[6] These research laboratories became the engines that drove the developing chemical industry. The German dye companies actively recruited professional chemists to develop new products and attempted to collaborate as closely as possible with the leading chemists in academia. Indeed, a battle broke out between the various companies to recruit the most prominent university professors as collaborators, each company forging associations with particular universities in an effort to exclude their rivals. For example, Hochst and Bayer used Adolf von Baeyer as a consultant and had first choice in attempting to recruit some of his most prominent students, such as Ludwig Knorr and Emil and Otto Fischer. On the other hand, Agfa established a close collaboration between Hofmann and his students. These collaborations with the finest minds in organic chemistry at the time gave the German pharmaceutical industry a huge advantage. Indeed, it was two of von Baeyer's students who were responsible for the next giant step forward in the story of dyes and medicine.

Following the decline in the popularity of mauve, Perkin needed another big hit to keep his company profitable. Alizarin, the red dye traditionally prepared from the root of the madder plant, seemed an excellent target, as its popularity was something that was not subject to the ups and downs of fashion (Figure 3.4).

Around the same time, von Baeyer's students Graebe and Liebermann at BASF were also working on this problem and were able to make considerable

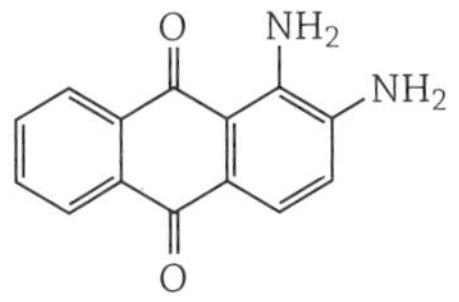

Alizarin

Figure 3.4:
The chemical structure of the red dye alizarin.

progress on the actual chemical structure of the dye. Consequently the desired structure was mostly known, so they could attempt to devise a rational chemical synthesis for it. Graebe and Liebermann were able to do this, although the synthesis they came up with was not really economically practical on an industrial scale. Nevertheless, this was a significant chemical milestone as it was the first time a known natural product dye of great importance had been successfully synthesized in the laboratory. Heinrich Caro, who actually knew Perkin very well because he had been one of the German scientists trained in the United Kingdom, and who was now head of research at BASF, began to work with Graebe and Liebermann and soon a more reasonable synthetic route was devised. However, Perkin and his brother had come up with a virtually identical synthesis at the same time, and the two groups filed their rival patent claims within 24 hours of each other. In the end it was declared a tie, and Perkin and Caro met to divide up the synthetic alizarin territory between Perkin and BASF. Needless to say, both companies profited greatly. However, the writing was on the wall and in the future, more and more of the great successes in the chemical industry were the product of the highly organized and professional German industrial research laboratories rather than those in Britain or France.[4]

An example of this was the synthesis of indigo. Indigo is the striking blue dye used for many thousands of years for numerous purposes including the dyeing of ancient Egyptian mummy coverings. Indigo retains its importance today and is used in the dyeing of blue jeans. Throughout the years its use has never ceased to be popular. However, the preparation of natural indigo from the tropical plant *Indigofera tinctoria*, like many other natural dyes, was an expensive and time consuming affair. Traditionally, the indigo business was virtually a British monopoly involving dye production from plantations in India, Jamaica, and South Carolina. The artificial synthesis of indigo was considered to be one of the great prizes of organic chemistry in the nineteenth century. As with many other things, the prize went to the great German chemist Adolph von Baeyer, who was involved in many important discoveries including the original synthesis of the precursor for barbiturate sedative drugs (Chapter 6). Indeed, von Baeyer won the Nobel

Prize in 1905 for his work on the synthesis of organic dyes. Von Baeyer first achieved the synthesis of indigo in 1880 after many years devoted to this project, with the help of many colleagues in the German chemical industry.[6] In the end the synthesis devised by von Baeyer, which is now known as the Baeyer-Drewson procedure, did not prove to be very efficient and wasn't able to provide the large amounts of dye required by the chemical industry. However, a few years later in 1890 a Swiss scientist named Karl Heumann devised a more efficient synthesis for indigo. BASF started to produce the dye using this procedure, resulting in enormous profits.[6]

And so by the end of the nineteenth century the chemical industry was well established, particularly in Germany. Aniline and other coal tar derivatives had been used by Perkin and others as the building blocks for the synthesis of increasingly more complex and novel structures. Although originally these were usually dyes, the stage was now set for employing this expertise in the production of chemicals with many diverse uses. In particular, many of the dye companies turned to pharmaceuticals.

FROM CHEMICALS TO DRUGS

In the 1880s several companies in Germany observed that fairly simple aniline derivatives had excellent antipyretic (fever reducing) properties. Antipyrine was synthesized by Ludwig Knorr in 1884 while, like Perkin before him, he was actually trying to produce quinine. Originally antipyrine and a related molecule, antifebrin, were marketed for these purposes. They were not entirely successful owing to side effects they produced, such as pronounced gastric irritation. However, the Bayer company then produced a further compound of this type that they marketed under the name *phenacetin*. This was very effective and much easier to take. It became a blockbuster drug and put Bayer firmly on its way. Now it wasn't just a dye-making company, it was a "pharmaceutical" company (Figure 3.5).[7]

Following these early successes it became a common strategy to start testing dyes for any potential therapeutic activities they might possess.

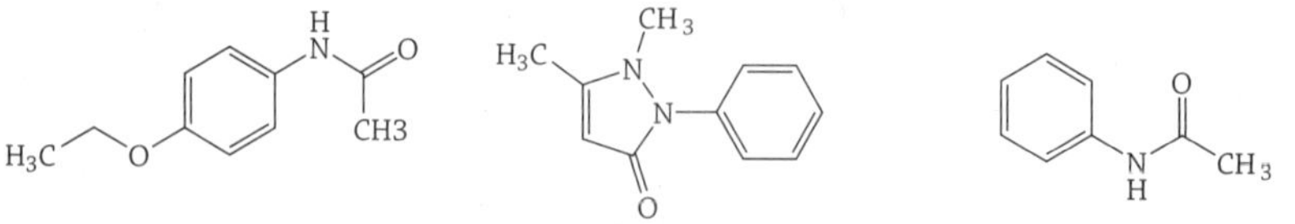

Phenacetin   Antipyrine (Phenazone)   Antifebrine (acetanilide)

Figure 3.5:
Chemical structures of some of the earliest aniline-derived antipyretic drugs.

There are many interesting stories of how substances that started life as dyes eventually became, or led to the discovery of, useful medicines. For example, in the 1930s a red azo dye called sulfamidochrysoidine, known commercially as "Prontosil Red," was shown by Gerhard Domagk and his colleagues, also working at Bayer, to protect mice from normally fatal streptococcal infection. It ultimately proved to be the case that Prontosil Red was actually acting as a "pro-drug." This means that it was metabolized *in vivo* to produce something else, in this case the active antimicrobial agent sulfanilamide. In this manner the entire field of antimicrobial sulfa drugs was born (Figure 3.6).[8]

From the point of view of the present discussion, however, we should concentrate on two other dyes. In 1876 Lauth synthesized a deep purple dye, which he named "Lauth's violet." In the same year Perkin's friend Heinrich Caro at BASF synthesized the dye methylene blue. Bernthsen then investigated the structure of methylene blue and related dyes. He suspected the presence of the then unknown phenothiazine structure in these substances and went on to prepare phenothiazine. As can be seen, the phenothiazine structure is another tricyclic molecule such as had been found at the center of many other dye molecules—including mauve (Figure 3.7).

MAGIC BULLETS

During the latter part of the nineteenth century another idea was also developing. This idea was pioneered by scientists like Paul Ehrlich, one of the fathers of modern pharmacology. It was well known that in addition to staining textiles, dyes could also stain biological tissues and microorganisms. Indeed, the Danish biologist Gram had developed a precise staining system for microbes based on their abilities to be stained by different types of dyes. Thus, dyes didn't stain biological materials in a completely

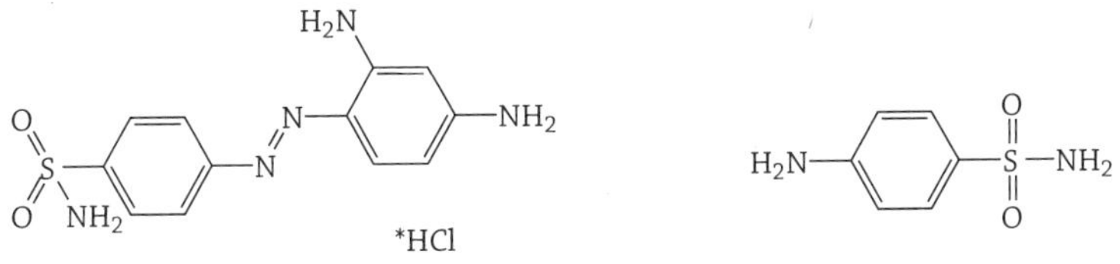

Prontosil red   Sulfanilamide

Figure 3.6:
Prontosil Red dye. The dye is metabolized *in vivo* to produce the antibacterial sulfa drug sulfanilamide.

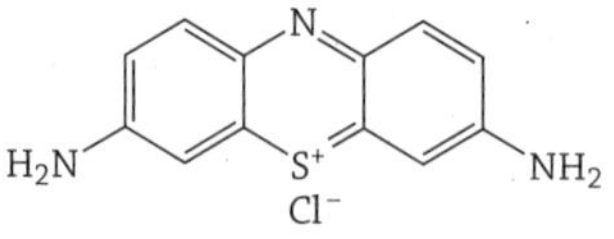

Lauth's violet
3,7-diaminophenothiazonium chloride

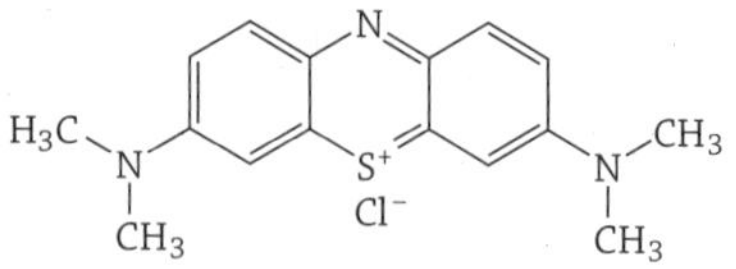

Methylene blue
3,7-tetramethyldiaminophenothiazonium
chloride

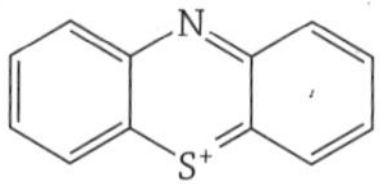

Phenothiazine

Figure 3.7:
The dyes Lauth's violet and methylene blue both contain the tricyclic phenothiazine structure.

indiscriminant manner but displayed striking selectivity. Ehrlich imagined, and quite correctly, that the dyes must actually combine differentially with tissues through specific chemical reactions. If that was the case it might be possible to find dyes that selectively interacted with microbes (or possibly cancer cells) and selectively kill them. This was the "magic bullet" hypothesis that became the basis for what is now known as chemotherapy.

One of the dyes that Ehrlich liked to experiment with was methylene blue. He found, for example, that when it was injected into animals it selectively stained nerve cells. Indeed, this association with nerve cells even sparked some early studies attempting to examine the effects of the dye on patients with psychiatric disorders, although this idea was not widely followed up at the time. In 1891 Ehrlich also observed that methylene blue was helpful in patients suffering from malaria, and suggested that drugs with this type of structure might act as "magic bullets" in such circumstances and could kill the infectious agent in the disease. During WWI, the Germans were cut off from their normal supplies of quinine and, in spite of William Perkin's and Ludwig Knorr's efforts, nobody had successfully synthesized it. However, it was thought that it would be a good idea to follow up Ehrlich's previous observations and see if methylene blue could be improved upon as an antimalarial drug.[9]

W. Schulemann and colleagues at Bayer began synthesizing analogues of methylene blue and found that the diethylaminoethyl derivative was more potent than the parent dye, but also had serious side effects. Schulemann persevered by attaching similar aminoalkyl side chains to other tricyclic ring systems and eventually, in 1931, synthesized mepacrine (quinacrine)—an effective, and for many years widely utilized, antimalarial drug (Figure 3.8).[8]

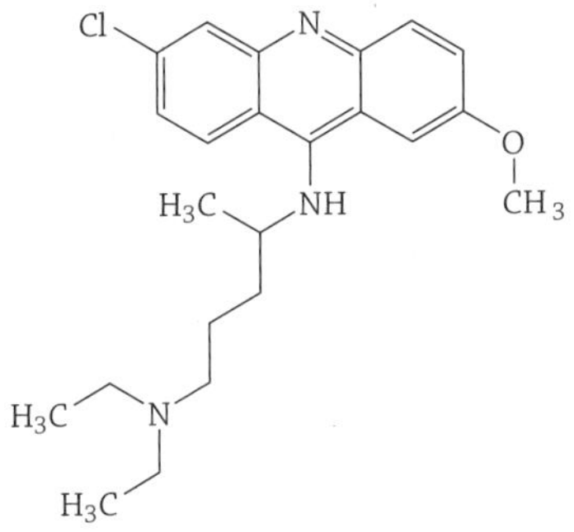

Figure 3.8:
The antimalarial drug quinacrine.

THE FALL OF THE GERMAN DRUG INDUSTRY

Quinacrine represents just one of the many triumphs of the German chemical and pharmaceutical industry in the late nineteenth and early twentieth centuries. However, a great tragedy was about to befall German science, one from which even today it has not completely recovered.[10] Following a visit to the United States, where he was impressed with the organization of various business cartels such as Standard Oil, Carl Duisberg, the head of Bayer and an extremely able scientist and businessman, set out to persuade his colleagues in the German chemical industry that adopting a similar cartel arrangement would be beneficial and end the cutthroat rivalry between the various drug and chemical companies. In 1925 several of the German companies including Bayer, BASF, Hoechst, and Agfa formed an official union as a new giant company named IG Farben, which stood for *Interessen-Gemeinschaft Farbenindustrie AG* (literally, Community of Interests of the Dye Industry) under the leadership of Duisberg and Carl Bosch of BASF. Bosch was the man who had helped to create the Haber-Bosch industrial synthesis for ammonia, for which he had won the Nobel Prize in chemistry. IG Farben was the fourth largest company in the world, employing over 100,000 people with a gigantic newly built headquarter complex in Frankfurt. It was clearly the world's dominant force in the chemical industry.

Unfortunately things took a tragic turn in Germany in the years after IG Farben was founded. Adolf Hitler understood how important the company would be to his overall ambitions, as the industrial base for the German war effort. As with other German companies, IG Farben became "Aryanized" and its many Jewish employees were dismissed. The old guard company leaders like Duisberg and Bosch, who had little time for Hitler and anti-Semitism, either died or retired leaving the company in the hands of a group of Nazi sycophants. Pharmaceutical research took a back seat to the industrial aims of the Nazi war machine. Worst of all was the Nazi plan to make synthetic rubber at a factory it built in Monowitz, adjacent to the Auschwitz concentration camp. IG Farben murdered hundreds of thousands of Jewish slave laborers in their basically unsuccessful attempts to supply Hitler with the rubber he needed. One irony of the situation was that it was left to an industrial chemist to produce one of the most poignant and revealing pictures of the crimes perpetrated by IG Farben and the Nazis. The Italian Jewish chemist Primo Levi survived a year at Auschwitz/Monowitz to tell the tale in his book *If This Is a Man*. After the war many of the IG Farben executives were put on trial for war crimes, for which at least some were convicted and jailed, and the company was put into liquidation. Nevertheless, its major components including Bayer and BASF were ultimately reconstituted and became part of the postwar German economic miracle, rising again to prominent positions in today's pharmaceutical industry.

CHLORPROMAZINE, THE FIRST ANTIPSYCHOTIC DRUG

However, outside of Germany, other important events during the Second World War and shortly thereafter provided the impetus for further drug development.[3,8,9,11] In particular the Japanese conquest of many parts of Southeast Asia cut off much of the available quinine source to the Allies, who then initiated their own program into research on antimalarial drugs. In the United States, Gilman and his colleagues produced a series of methylene blue analogues in which aminoalkyl chains were attached to the central nitrogen atom of the phenothiazine ring. Unfortunately, these proved to be ineffective as antimalarials and the negative results were published in 1944. Nevertheless the compounds were taken up, developed further, and tested by scientists at the Rhone-Poulenc drug company in France, who confirmed their lack of antimalarial activity.

However, Rhone-Poulenc had a very successful ongoing research program aimed at the development of drugs with antihistamine activity, which had already introduced powerful antihistamines such as phenbenzamine and chlorpheniramine. Interestingly, the Rhone-Poulenc scientists observed that several substances in the phenothiazine series they had produced, although ineffective as antimalarials, produced powerful antihistamine-like effects. This was particularly true of the phenothiazine derivative known as *promethazine*, which was then marketed for this purpose under the name

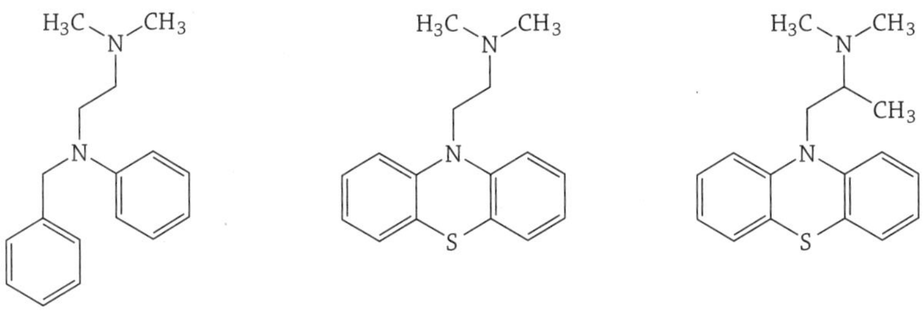

Figure 3.9:
Antihistamine drugs produced by the Rhone-Poulenc Company in the 1940s.

"Fenergan" (Figure 3.9). Of particular note, the Rhone-Poulenc researchers observed that promethazine increased the sleep time induced by barbiturates in rats, which was taken as an indication that it might also have some effects on the central nervous system.

The scene now switches to the town of Bizerte in Tunisia,[3,9] where in 1949 a French army surgeon named Henri-Marie Laborit was investigating drug combinations that could be used to counter surgical shock. On the advice of a colleague he tested promethazine and found that it was very effective when used in combination with an opiate, producing a "lytic cocktail" of drugs used for preparing patients for surgery. He noted that his patients seemed extremely calm and even somewhat "indifferent" to their procedures. The idea that you could prevent surgical shock using a drug that had a depressant effect on the central nervous system intrigued the Rhone-Poulenc scientists, who further analyzed all of their on-hand phenothiazine derivatives in an attempt to see whether any exhibited enhanced central nervous system effects. It quickly became clear that some of these substances, such as promazine and particularly its derivative chlorpromazine (CPZ), had a unique pharmacological profile when tested in animals (Figure 3.10).[3]

CPZ had a pronounced ability to decrease locomotor activity and increase barbiturate-induced sleep time. On the other hand, its effects on learning were quite different from the barbiturates. CPZ selectively inhibited the learned conditioned avoidance response to foot shock in rats, a test in which rats learn to climb up a rope in order to avoid an unpleasant electric shock. In contrast, depressant drugs like barbiturates just inhibited all of the animals responses including non learned behaviors. Thus CPZ seemed to have a much more specific effect on learned behaviors, further highlighting its effects on the brain. Another interesting effect which was noted was that CPZ was a very effective blocker of apomorphine-induced emesis in dogs, also a highly selective effect.

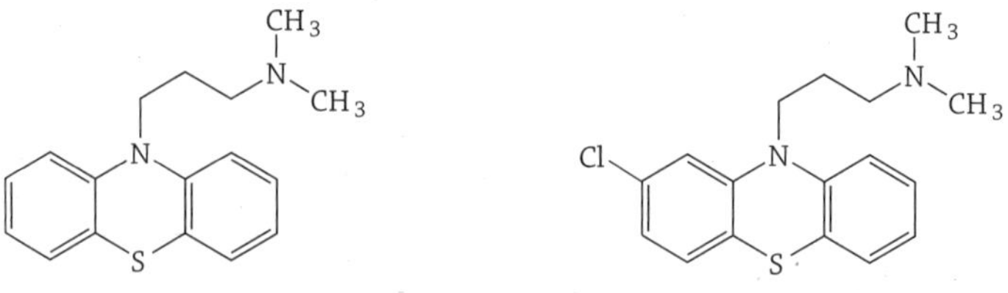

Figure 3.10:
Chlorpromazine, the first neuroleptic/antipsychotic drug.

The drug was distributed to various doctors including Laborit, who observed that it had a powerful calming effect on his patients together with hypnotic effects and an ability to reduce their metabolic rate and induce hypothermia. Overall, particularly when used together with known anesthetics and analgesics, he described these effects as "artificial hibernation," a state in which patients could better withstand the stress associated with surgery. Rhone-Poulenc marketed the new drug in 1952 under the name "Largactil" (meaning Large-broad, acti-activity) in an attempt to describe the drug's extensive range of pharmacological effects.[3,9]

And so it was that the psychopharmacological revolution was launched, because it was in the treatment of psychotic illness that CPZ would find its greatest utility. What exactly do we mean by this? The word *psychosis* is used to describe a constellation of symptoms where patients exhibit a gross disruption of their appreciation of reality.[11] Typically this may involve hallucinations, paranoid delusions, illusions, and generally disordered thought processes. The syndrome known as *schizophrenia* is a common form of psychotic illness affecting approximately 1% of the world's population. The various symptoms associated with schizophrenia coalesced into a defined syndrome in the mid nineteenth century when it was referred to as *dementia praecox*, literally meaning "early dementia." This was meant to indicate that it was a type of dementia that seemed to occur primarily in teenagers and young adults, as opposed to other dementias that occurred in the aged population. Subsequently, Bleuler coined the term *schizophrenia* in 1908. Since that time it has become clear that schizophrenia is probably a diverse illness with multiple causes, which can be manifest in different ways. Currently the symptoms associated with the different subtypes of the disease have been collected in the *Diagnostic and Statistical Manual of Mental Disorders* (4th edition text revision)[12] and it is generally assumed that these will be revised to some extent in the upcoming fifth edition of this publication, so our appreciation of the complexity of the disease is still evolving.

One way in which the symptoms of schizophrenia have been categorized is into what are known as "positive" and "negative" symptoms. The former symptoms apply to behaviors that are not displayed by normal people. These would include hallucinations and delusions. On the other hand, negative symptoms generally refer to normal behaviors that are deranged in schizophrenic patients, including lack of emotional affect, lack of motivation, and lack of normal social interactions. Problems of cognition are also regularly observed with schizophrenic patients, these being considered as a third type of symptomology. In the early 1950s, although there were many schizophrenic patients there was no really effective way of treating them. In the decades leading up to the 1950s, treatments such as sleep therapies, insulin shock therapies, and prefrontal lobotomies were introduced but were clearly more barbaric than helpful in most instances.[11] A more humane therapeutic approach to the treatment of the large number of patients in mental hospitals was something that was badly needed.

In Laborit's studies, CPZ was always administered as a cocktail together with other drugs for the general purposes of anesthesia and preparation for surgery. Nevertheless the profound calming effects of the drug were impressive, and so it was a logical next step to test it on mental patients who were frequently abnormally agitated. It was left to two French psychiatrists, Jean Delay and Pierre Deniker, to start examining the effects of CPZ on psychiatric patients when the drug was administered by itself.[3,9,11] They observed that CPZ had a significant calming effect on severely agitated and psychotic patients, particularly when used at somewhat higher doses than had been used by Laborit in his drug cocktails. They described the condition of patients as "characterized by a slowing down of motor activity, affective indifference and emotional neutrality," which they thought resembled a sort of "chemical lobotomy" and which they named a "neuroleptic syndrome" (from the Greek for "taking hold of the nerve"), descriptive of the drug's side effect of generally slowing down motor activity.

In 1952 Delay and Deniker proceeded to test CPZ on a large number of agitated schizophrenic patients and reported excellent results. For example, in one case:

"...Giovanni A, was a 57 year old manual worker with a long history of mental pathology, admitted for giving improvised political speeches, getting into fights with strangers, and walking along the street with a plant pot on his head proclaiming his love of liberty. After a 9 day treatment with CPZ he was able to maintain a normal conversation and within 3 weeks he was in such a calm state that he was able to be discharged."[3]

ANTIPSYCHOTICS SHIFT THE PARADIGM

Over the next couple of years the news of CPZs neuroleptic or "antipsychotic" effects spread throughout Europe, Canada, and the United States, and its success with patients began to be widely appreciated. A significant advance in this field was the first report in 1954 of a controlled, blinded clinical trial of the effects of CPZ compared to a placebo control, which was conducted by the psychiatrist Joel Elkes and his wife, then at the University of Birmingham in the United Kingdom.[3] This trial reported positive results of the effects of CPZ in approximately 40% of patients. The results of this study were extremely influential, not only because of the positive findings but also because of the methodology introduced into the field of psychiatry. In the opinion of some writers it ushered in the start of psychopharmacology as an independent discipline.

In Canada, CPZ was distributed by Rhone-Poulenc's subsidiary to several psychiatrists, such as Heinz Lehmann who experimented with it and reported positive outcomes.[11] The introduction of CPZ into the United States was basically driven by the efforts of Smith Kline & French Laboratories, which marketed the drug in 1954 under the name of Thorazine. Initially it was only sold as an antiemetic. However, the news of its antipsychotic effects led the families of schizophrenic patients to lobby for its use in psychiatry. Some resistance to this idea in the United States was the result of the fact that the predominant approach to psychiatric medicine in the country at that time was Freudian, and it was not considered reasonable by many psychiatrists that a "psychiatric aspirin" could really help the underlying psychopathology that caused psychotic illness. Generally speaking, however, psychoanalysts treated neurotic patients as outpatients in their offices—not psychotic patients, who were the provenance of mental hospitals, and so the use of antipsychotic drugs was not a big influence on office-based psychiatry at least to begin with. Hence the use of the drug did spread throughout the country, particularly driven by psychiatrists of the younger generation who were less influenced by the European psychoanalytic tradition.

Over the next few years, evidence for the antipsychotic effects of CPZ rapidly accumulated. Some studies even attempted to evaluate the effects of neuroleptics in schizophrenic patients when directly compared to psychotherapeutic approaches, and the results appeared to demonstrate the superiority of the psychopharmacological approach. It wasn't surprising that the pharmaceutical industry rapidly woke up to the possibilities of treating this large group of new patients. Numerous analogues of CPZ were produced, many of which were even more potent, if not more effective, than CPZ. The structural features necessary for neuroleptic activity of phe-nothiazine derivatives were precisely established, and drugs such as thio-ridazine (Mellaril) and trifluoperazine (Stelazine) also became widely used. Further studies demonstrated that the tricyclic phenothiazine nucleus was not actually essential for producing efficacious drugs, and that other tricy-clic ring systems such as the thioxanthene structure could substitute just as well, leading to further series of antipsychotics such as those typified by chlorprothixene and flupenthixol, which were introduced by the Danish company Lundbeck.

As time passed it became clear that all of these drugs really exhibited a new pharmacological profile. They were not just central nervous system depressants, but possessed highly selective effects on some of the primary positive symptoms of psychotic illness, as well as other useful actions including their powerful antiemetic effects. However, as with all classes of drugs, side effects eventually started to show up and, in the case of anti-psychotic drugs, some of these were evident from the very beginning.[11,13]

It became clear soon after these drugs had been introduced that they tended to produce a syndrome that resembled the symptoms of Parkinson's disease (PD), such as rigidity and difficulty making voluntary movements. Indeed, such effects are implied in the name "neuroleptic" originally used to describe these drugs. The PD-like effects became known as "extrapy-ramidal" side effects, acknowledging the part of the nervous system (the extrapyramidal system) which is compromised in PD. Other types of side effects were also noted, particularly in patients who had taken high doses of neuroleptics for extended periods or had recently stopped taking them. In this case, rather than the paucity of movement observed with the drug induced PD syndrome, something quite the opposite was observed—an excess of movement. Patients exhibited repetitive body movements, par-ticularly with their lips and tongue and sometimes with their extremities. In many ways these movements appeared similar to the tics exhibited by patients with the movement disorder known as Tourette's syndrome. Patients would also describe inner feelings manifest as extreme tension compelling them to move (akathisia). Such syndromes are known as *dys-kinesias,* and the syndrome associated with drug use became known as "tardive dyskinesia." Overall, therefore, it was observed that neuroleptics could produce different types of movement disorders depending on factors such as the dose and the length of time the drug was taken. As we shall see, these observations would have important implications in subsequent attempts to understand the molecular basis of neuroleptic drug action.

The 1950s really were revolutionary times in the development of psy-chopharmacology. Not only were antipsychotic drugs introduced, but also antidepressant drugs (Chapter 4). Moreover, drugs for treating anxiety were developed and became known as "minor tranquilizers" (Chapter 6). They were "minor" in so far as in the United States, drugs such as CPZ became generally known as "major tranquilizers" and later generally as "antipsychotics."

ANTIPSYCHOTICS: NEW STRUCTURES AND NEW MECHANISMS

In addition to the development of the phenothiazines, thioxanthenes, and other related chemical compounds, further discoveries also contributed to the establishment of antipsychotic drug therapy. Two major discoveries should be recognized in particular. One of these occurred in Belgium. Here, in 1934, Dr. Jan Janssen had established a relatively small drug company to distribute the products of the Hungarian chemical company Gideon Richter.[14] However, during WWII, Gideon Richter, the original founder of the company, had been murdered by the Nazis because he was Jewish and so Janssen had lost his supplier. He therefore started to try to develop his own products. Eventually his son Paul A. Janssen took over the company that was then headquartered in the Belgian town of Beerse. Like William Perkin, Paul Ehrlich, or Carl Duisberg before him, Janssen proved to be one of the giants of industrial chemical and pharmaceutical research. He was a genius when it came to the development of drugs, leading Sir James Black, who won the Nobel Prize for the development of the β-blocker propanolol and the antihistamine cimetidine, to call him "the most prolific drug inventor of all time."

In the years leading up to WWII, Otto Eisleb, a scientist at IG Farben, had synthesized a couple of novel analgesic agents (Chapter 6). One of these was pethidine (Meperidine, Demerol), the first completely synthetic opiate, and the other was methadone, which IG Farben marketed under the name Dolophine (in honor of Adolf Hitler!). Following the war, chemists at Janssen made some modifications to the methadone molecule and the company had marketed its own derivative dextromoramide (Palfium). The company then turned its attention to the pethidine molecule.

Initially the scientists at Janssen substituted a propiophenone group for the methyl group on the nitrogen atom of pethidine to yield another potent analgesic (R-951; see Figure 3.11). However, things started to get more interesting when they added a butyrophenone group instead. Now the resulting compound, R-1187, was clearly observed to have analgesic activity but also produced a profound cataleptic effect in animals, which

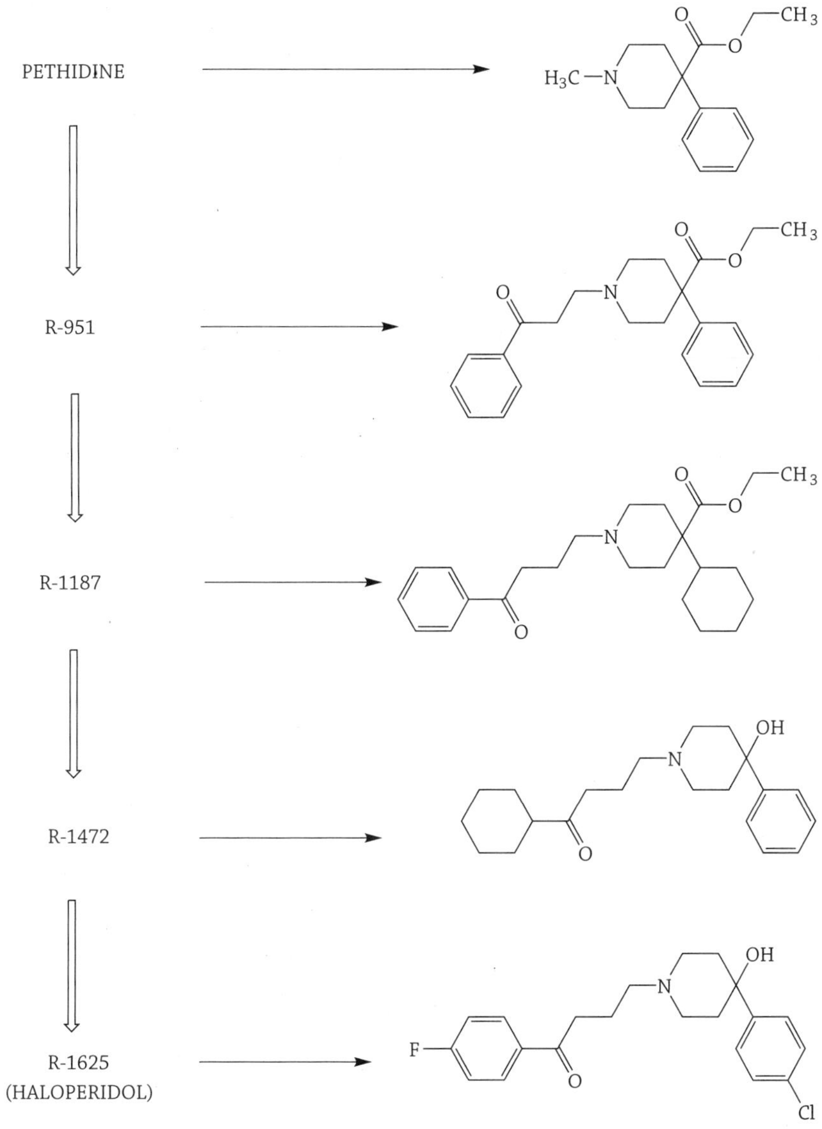

Figure 3.11:
How the Janssen Comany synthesized the first butyrophenone antipsychotic haloperidol starting with the opiate drug pethidine.[14]

reminded Paul Janssen of the effects that had been reported for CPZ. Janssen and his colleagues now made several hundred analogues of R-1187 in an attempt to dissociate the analgesic and possible neuroleptic effects they had observed. Finally they synthesized R-1625, which they named haloperidol because it contained two halogen atoms.

The properties of haloperidol were of great interest. First of all the drug produced a profound hypomotile cataleptic state in rodents, but at doses that were 50 times lower than CPZ. A second test was also very revealing. At the time a hypothesis existed connecting amphetamine abuse to the symptoms of schizophrenia. It had been observed that people taking high doses of amphetamines often exhibited symptoms of paranoia, hallucinations, delirium, and motor stereotypes that reminded some people of psychosis. Indeed, some of these were professional cyclists, a good number of these being from Belgium where the sport has a wide following, and Paul Janssen was certainly aware of this. Hence, a test had been established in which the "antipsychotic" effects of drugs were assessed based on their ability to antagonize the effects of amphetamine in rats, these being increased motor activity and repetitive stereotyped behaviors depending on the amphetamine dose. Janssen observed that haloperidol was extremely effective at reversing the effects of amphetamine in rats, and again that it was much more potent than CPZ. Hence, the scientists at Janssen predicted that haloperidol would exhibit potent antipsychotic activity in man.

Janssen distributed haloperidol to psychiatrists, first locally in Belgium and then throughout Europe. The antipsychotic activity of the drug was uniformly confirmed, together with its propensity to produce the same extrapyramidal side effects as previously associated with the phenothiazine antipsychotics. The introduction of haloperidol into the United States had to overcome some initial setbacks, but the drug was eventually marketed there as well—and with great success. Indeed, haloperidol became one of the most successful antipsychotic drugs ever discovered. Thus, the butyrophenones joined the phenothiazines and similar agents as primary therapeutic interventions in schizophrenia.

RESERPINE: THE NATURAL ANTIPSYCHOTIC

The third piece of the puzzle relates to the introduction of the alkaloid reserpine as an antipsychotic drug.[15] *Rauwolfia serpentina* is a tropical plant that grows in sub-Himalayan regions of India and has been used in folk medicine for centuries. For example, dried *Rauwolfia serpentina* root was used to calm the mentally ill in Indian folk medicine. In the early 1930s, researchers in India demonstrated that the *Rauwolfia serpentina* root decreased blood pressure and showed that it could be used to treat "insanity with violent maniacal symptoms." Clinical trials run in Western countries in the 1950s confirmed *Rauwolfia serpentina*'s hypotensive and sedative effects. In 1952 researchers at Ciba laboratories isolated the active prin-ciple, which they named *reserpine* (Figure 3.12) and which they marketed as a "tranquilizer-antihypertensive" agent. It was soon realized that reser-pine might well be a useful antipsychotic drug, and this was observed to be the case. Remarkably enough, its profile of effects proved to be very similar to those of CPZ, both in humans and animals. This included the ability to produce PD-like side effects. However, because reserpine had other actions, such as its cardiovascular effects and its tendency to produce severe depression in patients, its general use was quickly superseded by drugs such as CPZ.

THE DOPAMINE THEORY OF SCHIZOPHRENIA

By the early 1960s, then, there were at least three kinds of antipsychotic drugs that had been discovered, representing different types of chemical classes. These were drugs like CPZ and the other phenothiazines, drugs like haloperidol and the butyrophenones, and the unique alkaloid reserpine. It was natural for scientists to imagine that if they could elucidate actions that all three types of drugs had in common, then this might tell them something important about the pathophysiology of schizophrenia. One initial lead in this respect came from an understanding of the molecular basis of the action of reserpine.[15] During the 1950s it was gradually real-ized that what reserpine did was to produce a depletion of biogenic amine neurotransmitters from the nerve cells in which these molecules were nor-mally stored and released. By biogenic amines one is referring to 5-HT/ serotonin, which we discussed in Chapter 2, as well as the catecholamine class neurotransmitters dopamine, norepinephrine and epinephrine.

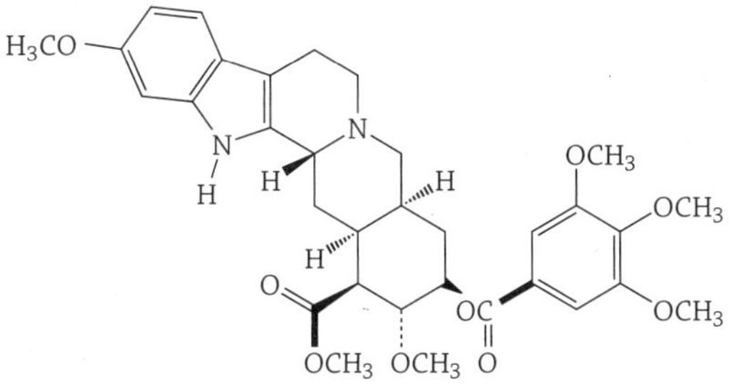

Reserpine

Figure 3.12:
The structure of reserpine, the active antipsychotic principle of the plant *Rauwolfia serpentina*.

Interestingly, it was also observed that if reserpinized animals were given the chemical L-dopa, which acts as a biochemical precursor to dopamine and then to norepinephrine, the ability of reserpine to produce hypoactivity and catatonia was reversed, implying that it was the depletion of these catecholamines rather than 5-HT that was responsible for this effect of reserpine. Subsequent studies also suggested that following L-dopa administration it was the formation of dopamine in particular, rather than norepinephrine, that was responsible for reversing the sedating effects of reserpine.

Indeed, around this time there was also a growing realization that dopamine in the brain didn't just act as a metabolic precursor to norepinephrine but had a life of its own. For example, the distribution of the two catecholamines in the brain proved to be quite different. In particular, nerves that innervated areas like the basal ganglia, which have an important role in the control of motor activity and movement, stored high concentrations of dopamine but not norepinephrine. It was therefore suggested that dopamine and norepinephrine might be separate neurotransmitters in the brain subserving different functions. Moreover, considering the high concentrations observed in the basal ganglia, one function that might be attributable to dopamine was in the regulation of motor activity. This idea led Hornykiewicz and his colleagues to study the concentrations of dopamine in the brains of postmortem PD patients. They demonstrated a considerable depletion of the catecholamine in the basal ganglia of these patients, opening the way to the idea that dopamine depletion was the primary cause of the symptoms of PD and that L-dopa might be used as a therapeutic intervention in the disease by resupplying the depleted neurotransmitter.

Based on such ideas it was also suggested that perhaps neuroleptic drugs acted in the same way as reserpine and depleted the brain of biogenic amines such as dopamine. This hypothesis could not be true, however, because it was shown that while the effects of reserpine could be reversed by L-dopa, the effects of CPZ (and subsequently of haloperidol) were not. Another mechanism was therefore also proposed. This was that CPZ and haloperidol blocked the receptors for dopamine. If that was the case, it would be easy to see why reserpine and antipsychotic drugs produced similar effects, because either depletion of dopamine (reserpine) or blockade of its receptors (CPZ and haloperidol) would both lead to an inhibition of dopamine-mediated neurotransmission.

Another important observation, as discussed above, was that drugs like CPZ and haloperidol could block the psychomotor effects of amphetamine.

At the time amphetamine was thought to act by directly stimulating cat-echolamine receptors, so this would be compatible with the block of dopa-mine receptors by these drugs. In fact amphetamine is not a direct activator of biogenic amine receptors, but acts by releasing these neurotransmitters from their nerve terminals (Chapter 8). Nevertheless, the conclusions as far as the actions of neuroleptics concerned were valid. All of these results pointed to the fact that blocking dopamine receptors in the basal ganglia was the way in which neuroleptic drugs produced their effects on the motor system, and phenomena such as hypomotility and catalepsy in animals and PD-like effects in humans.

But of course what everybody was really interested in was a hypothesis explaining how these drugs produced their antipsychotic effects, not their extrapyramidal side effects. For example in 1966 it was concluded by van Rossum that:

> "When the hypothesis of dopamine blockade by neuroleptic agents can be fur-ther substantiated it may have far going consequences for the pathophysiology of schizophrenia. Overstimulation of dopamine receptors could then be part of the aetiology. Obviously, such an overstimulation might be caused by overpro-duction of dopamine, production of substances with dopamine actions (methoxy derivatives), abnormal susceptibility of the receptors, etc."[15]

So, could the dopamine receptor blocking effects of drugs also explain their antipsychotic activity? Now, it should be recognized that there are several dopamine nerve systems in the brain. To begin with there are dopamine nerves that have their cell bodies in the substantia nigra of the midbrain and innervate the basal ganglia. It is these nerves that are compromised in PD, and it is the dopaminergic neurotransmission they provide which, when disrupted by neuroleptic drugs, produces their extra-pyramidal motor side effects. However, there are also dopamine nerves in other parts of the midbrain, such as the ventral tegmental area. These nerves don't innervate the basal ganglia but other structures, such as the nucleus accumbens, the amygdala, and the cortex. These nerves do not control movement but have other functions including roles in the con-trol of cognition, fear, and emotion. It was therefore hypothesized that it must be the dopamine receptors in these other areas whose overactiva-tion might then be responsible for the abnormal behaviors observed in schizophrenia. Indeed, the fact that one of the effects of amphetamine was "schizophrenic-like behaviors" was deemed to be consistent with such an idea.

ANTIPSYCHOTIC DRUGS BLOCK
DOPAMINE RECEPTORS

Conclusive data demonstrating that neuroleptic drugs could bind to dopamine receptors and block them had to wait until biochemical assays for such receptors became available. Scientists started to make use of the receptor binding assay technique which, as we discussed in the last chapter, had been introduced by Solomon Snyder and employed radioactive butyrophenones, like haloperidol or the potent drug spiroperidol, to label dopamine receptors in the brain. It was observed that both antipsychotic drugs and dopamine bound to these sites in the brain. In fact, the results indicated that there was more than one kind of dopamine receptor, and these were named *D1* and *D2*.[16]

It became clear that the interaction of neuroleptic drugs with D2 receptors was most likely to "explain" all of their observed antipsychotic effects. Indeed, the subsequent use of molecular cloning techniques has confirmed the existence of both D1 and D2 receptors. In fact, we now know there are probably 5 different kinds of dopamine receptors in the brain. However, it is the D2 receptor that seems to be the major target for traditional neuroleptic drugs. Thus the dopamine theory of schizophrenia was established and became the most influential way of thinking about the disease for many years. In truth, however, although the theory clearly explained why such drugs produced a variety of extrapyramidal effects, its extension to explain antipsychotic effects was something that was hard to really prove. And other events were to manifest themselves that were to further complicate the issue.

TYPICALS AND ATYPICALS

As it turned out, the coal tar legacy of the development of antipsychotic drugs had at least one more important twist.[17] The tricyclic chemical structures that had yielded antipsychotic drugs would also yield some of the first antidepressants, as we shall discuss in Chapter 4. The tricyclic ring system at the core of many such antidepressant drugs is called a *dibenzazepine* structure.

By analogy with the phenothiazines, thioxanthenes, and other drug classes, it was considered possible that novel drugs with interesting properties, possibly new antipsychotics, might be derived from tricyclic structures of this type. Around 1958, chemists at the Wander drug company in Switzerland started playing around with chemical structures of this type and synthesized a group of compounds based on the tricyclic dibenzodiaz-epine nucleus, which is obviously related to the structure of the antidepres-sant imipramine (Figure 3.13). They determined that some compounds in this class were "antidepressants but with neuroleptic properties." Further testing revealed that some of the compounds, such as clozapine, did seem to produce similar effects to CPZ in some tests but, interestingly, pro-duced few of the extrapyramidal signs associated with traditional neuro-leptic drugs. By 1962, clozapine had been given to over 100 schizophrenic patients. These trials confirmed the fact that it had clear antipsychotic actions in humans but, remarkably, seemed to produce few of the disabling neurological side effects associated with the use of traditional neuroleptic drugs. In 1967 the Wander company was acquired by Sandoz, who had to decide whether to develop clozapine further. Ironically, the lack of extra-pyramidal side effects was actually perceived by many investigators as a negative sign because by this time it was believed that such side effects and antipsychotic activity were inextricably linked. Indeed, Dr. Hippius, who was involved in much of the initial development of clozapine remarked:

"…we discovered to our surprise that clozapine, in contrast to all other com-pounds, had no extrapyramidal effects despite being a fully effective antipsy-chotic. This finding was almost unbelievable, because at that time it was a part of psychopharmacological dogma that extrapyramidal effects went in tandem with antipsychotic efficacy."[17]

So Sandoz felt their way forward cautiously. Clinical trials proceeded throughout the 1960s and continued to offer encouragement that clo-zapine had a unique therapeutic profile compared to previously used anti-psychotic drugs. Trials also began in the United States and, starting in

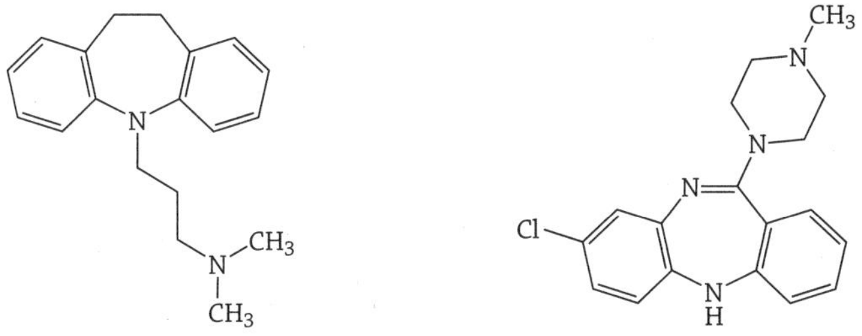

Imipramine

Clozapine

Figure 3.13:
The tricyclic antidepressant drug imipramine and clozapine, the first atypical antipsychotic drug.

1974, positive results were also obtained. However, the rise of clozapine as a novel antipsychotic then hit a bump in the road. It was reported in 1975 that during a clinical trial in Finland, eight patients who had been taking clozapine had developed a blood disorder called *agranulocytosis*. Under these circumstances the production of white blood cells by the bone marrow is decreased, reducing an individual's ability to fight infection and rendering even minor infections potentially lethal. Actually, agranulocytosis had been previously noted with other neuroleptics such as CPZ but nowhere near as frequently as reported in the Finnish study. Indeed, subsequent experience with clozapine has demonstrated that it does not generally appear to produce higher levels of this disease than other antipsychotic drugs. Nevertheless, the Finnish results were extremely worrying. Sandoz responded by stopping all clinical trial activity by 1976. However, the drug did remain available in the United States on a "compassionate need" ad hoc basis. This proved to be enough. The unique properties of clozapine and its effectiveness spread by word of mouth to a large number of doctors and patients. By 1982 it was also clear that any potential incidence of agranulocytosis could be effectively handled if it was observed early enough using the appropriate blood tests.

At this point Sandoz decided to reevaluate clozapine's potential. In 1984 they began a multisite trial in the United States named "Clozapine study #30," in which the effects of Clozapine were compared directly with those of CPZ. Several conclusions were made based on the results of the trial. First of all, clozapine showed a clear superiority to CPZ when assessed over a trial period of 6 weeks. Of particular interest was the observation that not only was clozapine more effective than CPZ in the treatment of the positive symptoms of schizophrenia, but it had also had a beneficial effect on the negative symptoms of the disease—something that was not generally observed with drugs like CPZ. Clozapine was also found to be helpful in improving the cognitive deficits noted with schizophrenic patients. Importantly, clozapine was often effective in patients who were resistant to the effects of traditional antipsychotic drugs. Combined with the lack of extrapyramidal side effects observed with clozapine, it was clear that the spectrum of effects it produced was "atypical," and so clozapine became the first example of a "second generation" or "atypical" antipsychotic drug.[18]

Armed with positive clinical data like this, and a scheme to monitor the possible liability of the development of agranulocytosis in patients, clozapine was marketed by Sandoz under the trade name Clozaril.[9,11,17] A race was now on between all of the large pharmaceutical companies to replicate the actions of clozapine by developing their own atypical antipsychotic drugs. As the 1990s got underway, Seroquel (quetiapine, ICI Pharmaceuticals/

Zeneca), Zyprexa (olanzapine, Eli Lilly), Geodon (ziprasidone, Pfizer) Risperdal (risperidone, Janssen) and most recently Abilify (aripiprazole) were all developed by rival companies. Some of these substances have chemical structures that clearly resemble clozapine (e.g., olanzapine), whereas some are completely different.

ATYPICAL ANTIPSYCHOTICS, ATYPICAL PROBLEMS

Atypical antipsychotics are now very widely used and have replaced traditional neuroleptics in many, but not all, situations. Numerous trials and meta-analyses have been carried out to try to determine whether in fact these drugs are truly better than a drug like CPZ, or indeed whether they are better than one another, and in what respects. Several things have emerged. Although it is clear that these newer drugs are effective antipsychotics, and there is a general feeling that they are better at addressing the negative symptoms of schizophrenia and helpful in patients resistant to traditional neuroleptics, with the exception of clozapine, demonstrating that they are more effective than CPZ has been difficult. On the other hand, there is no doubt that the newer range of drugs is a vast improvement when it comes to the occurrence of neurological side effects such as drug-induced PD and tardive dyskinesia.

Of course, no drug is free of side effects, and sure enough as time went on it became clear that atypicals produced their own set of problems. Many patients taking atypical antipsychotic drugs put on enormous amounts of weight and became quite obese. A "metabolic syndrome" which included obesity, glucose intolerance, dyslipidemia, and hypertension has been shown to be highly prevalent among patients with severe mental illnesses, leading to a greatly increased incidence of diabetes and heart disease and a reduced life expectancy in this population. These phenomena are greatly enhanced by some of the atypical antipsychotics, particularly by clozapine and olanzapine, and others to a lesser extent.[19] These adverse metabolic effects have been very widely observed with atypical antipsychotics and are viewed as serious problems, even leading to lawsuits being brought against pharmaceutical companies.

How do the atypical antipsychotic drugs help us to understand the neurobiological basis for psychosis? Do they help to support the dopamine hyperactivity theory of schizophrenia that held sway prior to their arrival? The basic answer to this is that they really don't. First of all, it appears that the D2 dopamine receptor is not the primary site of action for most of these drugs. A drug like haloperidol shows a considerable preference for the D2 receptor, having only relatively minor effects on other receptors. However, this did not prove to be the case for drugs like clozapine, which were found to exhibit a much broader spectrum of receptor interactions. In particular, many of these drugs showed significant interactions with the 5-HT2A receptor which, as we have discussed in Chapter 2, represents the major site of action for hallucinogenic drugs like LSD.[20] Perhaps this lack of strong interactions with D2 receptors was the reason atypicals didn't produce such pronounced extrapyramidal side effects? However, according to the dopaminergic theory of schizophrenia, the occurrence of such side effects was basically a *sine qua non* for effective antipsychotic activity and the two phenomena were inextricably linked. Prior to the arrival of atypicals there was a simple formula for making antipsychotic drugs—"make new substances that were powerful D2 receptor antagonists." That was the formula, pure and simple. It was true that there were side effects, and the idea was that we would have to deal with these independently. It was the price one had to pay for effective antipsychotic activity.

But what was the formula for making an atypical antipsychotic drug? There have been many suggestions as to what the basis of their activity might be. One of these, made by the influential psychiatrist Herbert Meltzer, is that there should be a particular balance between D2 and 5-HT2A antagonist activity, and much evidence suggests that this approach may have some validity. However, at the end of the day the waters have been muddied. There is no overall consensus as to why atypicals work the way they do. Because of this fact there can be no clear formula for making more of them, other than a sort of trial and error approach and creative screening for antipsychotic activity in animal models. Moreover, because we don't really understand how they work, they haven't really taught us very much about the basis of the disease that they treat. In fact, since the introduction of atypical antipsychotic drugs more than 30 years ago, there hasn't really been an appreciable advance in the production of new antipsychotic agents. Classic neuroleptics and atypicals remain the basis of pharmacological therapy for schizophrenia, even with all of their side effects. How are we to progress to produce better drugs and a better understanding of the cellular basis of schizophrenia? Which brings us to an important issue which is at the very heart of the problem. What is a good animal model for schizophrenia?[21]

HOW DO WE MEASURE PSYCHOSIS IN ANIMALS?

Obviously, in order to produce a new antipsychotic drug we need to have an animal model of psychosis. Now it is often possible to produce good animal models of diseases for drug development, or at least models that are adequate. For example, as we have discussed, we know that in PD one very important observation is that the dopamine-containing neurons that run from the substantia nigra to the basal ganglia (the nigrostriatal pathway) degenerate. When we destroy this pathway in a rodent using a toxin, this results in a movement disorder that mimics PD in many respects. Actually PD is a much more complicated clinical syndrome than just a movement disorder. But this is certainly a major part of the disease, and so the rodent model is of some help for developing new drugs. Similar things can be said with respect to a number of other diseases including stroke, amyotrophic lateral sclerosis (ALS), and multiple sclerosis (MS). But how about Alzheimer's disease (AD)?

Here we start running into some problems because AD is a disease that concerns higher cognitive functions in humans and, as we discussed in the previous chapter, it is clearly difficult to model these in rodents. On the other hand, in AD at least we have some leads in terms of precisely understanding the underlying neuropathology that gives rise to the disease. We can say that there are biochemical abnormalities in things like the enzymatic processing of a molecule called the *amyloid precursor protein* (APP). So, if we reproduce these in rodents we may at least hope that this may have some value as a model of the disease. Indeed, for better or worse, this is the current state of the art. However, schizophrenia is perhaps the hardest disease of all to model in animals. When the dopamine hypothesis of schizophrenia held sway, the prevailing animal models were really models of antipsychotic drug side effects, and the idea was that these were inextricably linked to the therapeutic actions of the drugs. So, if a drug produced side effects it would also produce beneficial effects. But once the atypicals arrived it was no longer possible to make this equation. Hence, it has become even more critical to establish reliable animal models of the disease. However, this requires some understanding of the neural substrate of the disease, something that is still only in its infancy. What exactly is wrong with the brain in schizophrenia? What neurons, pathways, or other neural substrates are not working properly, and why?

Let us therefore examine what kinds of newer animal models are available and how they may help in the further development of novel therapies for schizophrenia.[21] The first types of models to consider are what we might call "drug-induced behavior models," and we have already discussed two of the major ones. Considering that the positive symptoms of schizophrenia involve hallucinations and delusions, we would certainly be interested in what kinds of drugs produce such effects. Clearly amphetamine can produce a sense of paranoia, and LSD can certainly produce hallucinations. Hence giving these drugs to animals and examining their behaviors has been very widely employed as models of psychosis. Clearly amphetamine produces hyperlocomotor activity and stereotyped behaviors, whereas LSD, as discussed in Chapter 2, produces a "head twitch" response. Perhaps these behaviors reflect some of the positive symptomology of schizophrenia, such as psychomotor agitation and hallucinations. We have seen how these tests have been employed to produce traditional neuroleptic drugs, or even an atypical such as risperidone.[22] Nevertheless, it is clear that what is being measured here are not actually hallucinations but surrogate behaviors. It is likely that continued use of these tests will only generate more drugs with the same mechanisms of action that have already been obtained.

However, there is at least one other possibility that should be mentioned. Drugs such as phencyclidine (PCP, Angel Dust) are well known to produce hallucinations and dissociative behaviors in humans that also resemble schizophrenic symptoms. Indeed, PCP also produces a wide range of behaviors in rodents and has been used in various ways to produce an animal model of schizophrenia.[23] For example, PCP-induced hypermotility in rodents is widely used as a model of psychoagitation and the "positive" symptoms of schizophrenia. Now there are various things that are interesting about this. The first thing is the mechanism of action of PCP. So far, all of the neurobiological mechanisms we have discussed pertaining to schizophrenia and the action of antipsychotic drugs have concerned the actions of biogenic amines such as dopamine and 5-HT. But PCP doesn't work in this fashion. PCP is actually an antagonist of the actions of the excitatory neurotransmitter glutamate. The glutamate receptor in question is called the *NMDA receptor* because it is activated by the amino acid N-methyl-D-aspartic acid in addition to glutamate. It is these receptors that are inhibited by drugs like PCP. These observations start to allow us to move away from the link between biogenic amines and schizophrenia to a consideration of another neurotransmitter system. That this is the case should not surprise us, because the brain is a dynamic structure of interacting nerve pathways. If we disrupt the function of a major neurotransmitter such as glutamate, we may well be changing the function of nerves that utilize dopamine or 5-HT as well. However, we can at least say that it might be possible to use a drug that acts on the glutamate neurotransmitter system to produce changes in the brain that may induce or ameliorate psychotic behavior.

Another thing worth considering when thinking about animal models of schizophrenia is whether there are any true symptoms of the disease that can be reproduced in animals. In fact, this has proved to be possible. Let us consider some of the prevailing notions about what is going on with the human brain of a schizophrenic patient. At a behavioral level, attention and cognition have often been observed to be abnormal in schizophrenics, giving rise to the idea that a basic feature of the disease involves impairments in what is known as "sensorimotor gating." Normally we are continuously bombarded with all kinds of sensory stimuli and information, and we have to know on a moment-to-moment basis which things we need to filter out and which things we need to concentrate on. Schizophrenic patients are not very good at doing this. It seems that in schizophrenia intrusive, irrelevant, and ultimately overwhelming stimuli are not properly filtered out.

This can be demonstrated using a simple behavioral experiment. If a human subject or an animal is subjected to a sudden strong stimulus, such as a loud sound or a light flash, they exhibit what is known as a "startle response." We have all had this experience. Interestingly, it has been observed that if this strong stimulus is preceded by a weak stimulus called a "prepulse," then the amplitude of the startle response is reduced. It is as if the prepulse has alerted the organism for what is to come. This phenomenon is known as *prepulse inhibition* (PPI). PPI is not observed in schizophrenic patients to the same degree as in normal subjects. This loss of normal PPI is thought to result from the fact that schizophrenics cannot sort out and appropriately filter the normal flood of sensory stimuli to which they are subjected. Hence, it is thought that an animal model that reflects the deficiencies in PPI observed in schizophrenic patients would be extremely useful in elucidating the neurobiological basis of abnormal sensorimotor gating in schizophrenia.[24]

In fact, it has been demonstrated that lack of PPI can be produced in animals by a number of procedures. This includes giving them PCP, disturbing the development of their brains, or disturbing their interactions with their mothers during weaning. Thus defective PPI, which is observed in schizophrenics and which is known as an "endophenotype," can be directly compared in animals and humans; and this can then be used to examine the effects of potential antipsychotic drugs. Unfortunately, although patients with schizophrenia do exhibit deficits in PPI, patients with some other psychiatric and neurological disorders also exhibit similar deficits, so mimicking the phenomenon in an animal model cannot be said to exclusively model schizophrenia. Nevertheless, it is certainly considered an important advance.

GENES AND SCHIZOPHRENIA

Indeed, we may be able to produce an even more appropriate PPI model of schizophrenia. One question we can ask is what kinds of factors are really responsible for the manifestation of schizophrenia in a human? Presumably the disease is not due to people taking PCP, LSD, or amphetamine. Are all the factors that cause the disease genetic, are they environmental, or does the disease result from some complex interaction between these various factors? This is what is generally known as the nature versus nurture debate. It now seems clear that the manifestation of schizophrenia is usually due to an interaction between genes and environmental factors. For example, it is clear that there are aspects of the disease that can be inherited. The kind of data that supports this contention is to examine the lives of identical twins who were separated at birth, where one twin later becomes schizophrenic. It turns out that the other twin has a much greater chance than a person in the normal population of also developing the disease. Indeed, increased likelihood of having the disease is associated with different degrees of relationship to a patient. The more closely related the greater the likelihood. On the other hand, the fact that not all twins or relatives develop the disease illustrates the fact that other things such as environmental factors can modify whether it manifests or not. It is thought that some of these factors might be perinatal in nature, such as due to infection, diet, hypoxia at birth, or abnormalities in the maternal care of neonates.

Ideas such as these fit in with a currently influential hypothesis about the etiology of schizophrenia, which is that it has a strong neurodevelopmental basis. Both genetic influences and perinatal influences might certainly affect the subsequent development of the nervous system. Such considerations can also be factored into the development of an animal model for the disease. For example, when rat pups are reared in isolation from their mother from the time of weaning, they grow up to display behavioral abnormalities such as deficits in PPI. It is assumed that this is a model of how environmental factors may result in a schizophrenia-like behaviors. Such a model can then be used to test antipsychotic drugs, and indeed many types of antipsychotic drugs will prevent the deficits in PPI that normally occur in this situation. Because such a model is not produced through the effects of a specific type of drug (e.g., amphetamine, LSD, or PCP), we might expect it to give a fairly unbiased readout of antipsychotic activity when testing new drug candidates.

The idea that schizophrenia is a developmental disorder is also suggested from the observation that symptoms usually appear following adolescence up until around the age of 30. Furthermore, although there is no clear-cut gross neuropathological deficit that is associated with schizophrenia that can be compared to the lack of dopamine neurons in PD, the use of imaging techniques on the brains of live human schizophrenic patients have increasingly defined abnormalities in brain structure that could well have a neurodevelopmental basis,[25] such as a reduction in the thickness of the cortex and an increase in the volume of the ventricles of the brain. In addition, other studies have reported changes to individual populations of neurons, including alterations in the shape of the dendrites of cortical pyramidal neurons or the numbers of cortical inhibitory GABAergic interneurons. It has been suggested that these types of neuronal changes could be responsible for the cognitive impairment observed in the disease.

We would also hope that if we knew precisely what genes contributed to the disease, we might include these in animal models as well. Indeed, there has been some progress in identifying what genes may be involved. Several candidate genes have been identified by geneticists studying families of affected patients. For example let us consider the gene, disrupted in schizophrenia 1 (DISC1).[26] The way this gene was identified took advantage of an unusual situation. A large Scottish family was found that appeared to have a much larger than normal number of individuals who suffered from schizophrenia, along with a variety of other psychiatric disorders. Genetic analysis of this family allowed the gene DISC1 to be identified. Investigations so far have indicated that DISC1 is a "scaffold" protein. This means that its main job is to bring together other protein molecules that are involved in specific types of cell signaling. It seems that the proteins that bind to DISC1 may be involved with processes such as the development and migration of new neurons, which of course fits in nicely with the neurodevelopmental view of schizophrenia. Making mice that express the appropriate mutations in DISC1 are another way of modeling schizophrenia-like symptoms in rodents. So, as one can see, there are now several methods for producing animal models of schizophrenia that are based on an increasingly sophisticated appreciation of its pathogenesis. Hopefully, such animal models will allow for the screening and development of new types of drugs that will help to treat this terrible disease. Purple prose, indeed!.

NOTES

1. Thomas S Kuhn. *The Structure of Scientific Revolutions*. University of Chicago Press. 1962.
2. Turner T. Chlorpromazine: Unlocking psychosis. *British Medical Journal*. 2007, 334:S7.
3. López-Muñoz F, Alamo C, Cuenca E, Shen WW, Clervoy P, Rubio G. History of the discovery and clinical introduction of chlorpromazine. *Ann Clin Psychiatry*. 2005, 17(3):113–135.
4. For a detailed discussion of the life of William Perkin see: Simon Garfield. *Mauve: How one man invented a color that changed the world*. Norton Press. 2000.

5. Quinine history: See http://science.jrank.org/pages/5617/Quinine-History.html

   Irwin W. Sherman. *Magic Bullets to Conquer Malaria: From Quinine to Qinghaosu.* ASM Press. 2010.

6. Beer JJ. Coal tar dye manufacture and the origin of the modern research laboratory. *Isis.* 1958, 49:123–131.

7. Diarmuid Jeffreys. *Aspirin: The remarkable story of a wonder drug.* Bloomsbury Press. 2004.

8. Frank H. Clarke. *How modern medicines are discovered.* Futura Press. 1973.

9. Shen WW. A history of antipsychotic drug development. *Compr Psychiatry.* 1999, 40(6):407–414.

10. Diarmuid Jeffreys. *Hell's Cartel: IG Farben and the making of Hitler's war machine.* Metropolitan Books. 2008.

11. David Healy. *The Creation of Psychopharmacology.* Harvard University Press. 2002.

12. *Diagnostic and Statistical Manual of Mental Disorders* (edition number 4 text revision) is the current version of this manual. The manual describes the symptomology of diverse psychiatric disorders so as to try to maintain some consensus among psychiatrists. The use of this manual has now become extremely influential in terms of both the definition and diagnosis of mental disorders as well as how these things are handled by health insurance companies and other agencies. The next revision of the manual, DSM-5, has recently been published.

13. Kane JM, Correll CU. Pharmacologic treatment of schizophrenia. *Dialogues Clin Neurosci.* 2010, 12(3):345–357.

14. López-Muñoz F, Alamo C. The consolidation of neuroleptic therapy: Janssen, the discovery of haloperidol and its introduction into clinical practice. *Brain Res Bull.* 2009, 79(2):130–141.

15. Baumeister AA, Francis JL. Historical development of the dopamine hypothesis of schizophrenia. *J Hist Neurosci.* 2002, 11(3):265–277.

16. Marsden CA. Dopamine: the rewarding years. *Br J Pharmacol.* 2006, 147 Suppl 1:S136–144.

    Kebabian JW, Calne DB. Multiple receptors for dopamine. *Nature.* 1979, 277(5692):93–96.

17. Crilly J. The history of clozapine and its emergence in the US market: a review and analysis. *Hist Psychiatry.* 2007, 18(1):39–60.

18. Preskorn SH. The evolution of antipsychotic drug therapy: reserpine, chlorpromazine, and haloperidol. *J Psychiatr Pract.* 2007, 13(4):253–257.

    Meltzer HY. What's atypical about atypical antipsychotic drugs? *Curr Opin Pharmacol.* 2004, 4(1):53–57.

    Kane JM, Correll CU. Pharmacologic treatment of schizophrenia. *Dialogues Clin Neurosci.* 2010, 12(3):345–357.

19. Trollor JN, Chen X, Sachdev PS. Neuroleptic malignant syndrome associated with atypical antipsychotic drugs. *CNS Drugs.* 2009, 23(6):477–492.

    Pramyothin P, Khaodhiar L. Metabolic syndrome with the atypical antipsychotics. *Curr Opin Endocrinol Diabetes Obes.* 2010, 17(5):460–466.

20. Meltzer HY. The role of serotonin in antipsychotic drug action. *Neuropsychopharmacology.* 1999, 21(2 Suppl):106S–115S.

21. Nestler EJ, Hyman SE. Animal models of neuropsychiatric disorders. *Nat Neurosci.* 2010, 13(10):1161–1169.

Carpenter WT, Koenig JI. The evolution of drug development in schizophrenia: past issues and future opportunities. *Neuropsychopharmacology.* 2008, 33(9):2061–2079.

22. Colpaert FC. Discovering risperidone: the LSD model of psychopathology. *Nat Rev Drug Discov.* 2003, 2(4):315–320.

23. Mouri A, Noda Y, Enomoto T, Nabeshima T. Phencyclidine animal models of schizophrenia: approaches from abnormality of glutamatergic neurotransmission and neurodevelopment. *Neurochem Int.* 2007, 51(2-4):173–184.
Kargieman L, Santana N, Mengod G, Celada P, Artigas F. Antipsychotic drugs reverse the disruption in prefrontal cortex function produced by NMDA receptor blockade with phencyclidine. *Proc Natl Acad Sci U S A.* 2007, 104(37):14843–14848.

24. Swerdlow NR, Geyer MA, Braff DL. Neural circuit regulation of prepulse inhibition of startle in the rat: current knowledge and future challenges. *Psychopharmacology (Berl).* 2001, 156(2-3):194–215.
Geyer MA, Krebs-Thomson K, Braff DL, Swerdlow NR. Pharmacological studies of prepulse inhibition models of sensorimotor gating deficits in schizophrenia: a decade in review. *Psychopharmacology (Berl).* 2001, 156(2-3):117–154.
Swerdlow NR, Weber M, Qu Y, Light GA, Braff DL. Realistic expectations of prepulse inhibition in translational models for schizophrenia research. *Psychopharmacology (Berl).* 2008, 199(3):331–388.

25. Jaaro-Peled H, Ayhan Y, Pletnikov MV, Sawa A. Review of pathological hallmarks of schizophrenia: comparison of genetic models with patients and nongenetic models. *Schizophr Bull.* 2010, 36(2):301–313.

26. Lee FH, Fadel MP, Preston-Maher K, Cordes SP, Clapcote SJ, Price DJ, Roder JC, Wong AH. Disc1 point mutations in mice affect development of the cerebral cortex. *J Neurosci.* 2011, 31(9):3197–3206.
Johnstone M, Thomson PA, Hall J, McIntosh AM, Lawrie SM, Porteous DJ. DISC1 in schizophrenia: genetic mouse models and human genomic imaging. *Schizophr Bull.* 2011, 37(1):14–20.

CHAPTER 4

The House of the Sylvan Harmonies

"A screaming comes across the sky. It has happened before, but there is nothing to compare it to now."

Thomas Pynchon, *Gravity's Rainbow*

The Chinese house is called *Shen Ho Shih,* which means the "The House of the Sylvan Harmonies." This name is inscribed in Chinese characters on a tablet above the front door. Given the situation of the house, the name seems appropriate. From the back verandah one is confronted by thick woodlands with a small river running through the glades. The vista is reminiscent of a picture one might see on a Chinese screen or painting. The ceiling beams in the living and dining rooms are adorned with Chinese designs; the walls are painted celadon green, and yellow shantung drapes the windows. Fine Chinese furniture and artifacts are found throughout the house, including six scroll paintings depicting emperors of the Song dynasty. There is also a collection of pottery ranging from the Shang to the Qing dynasties, with examples from the Song dynasty being particularly well represented. This marks the owner as a man of excellent taste, as it is surely with the Song that the great tradition of Chinese ceramics reached its zenith.[1] There is only one strange thing about the house, and it is this: when one walks out through the front door and looks at the view, what one sees are not the plains of Shandong or Shanxi—but the prairies of Indiana.

The house belongs to Mr. Eli Lilly, who runs a pharmaceutical company in nearby Indianapolis that was founded by his grandfather, also named Eli Lilly. In addition to running his business, he has recently become interested in Chinese culture and in collecting Chinese artifacts. This led him to buy a former summer cottage on the banks of the White River near Indianapolis and to refashion it as his Chinese house. Sometimes he holds parties in the Chinese house, where the daughters of his Chinese colleagues wear the traditional *qipao* and act as waitresses. The effect is most authentic and visitors are always pleasantly surprised.[2,3]

Mr. Lilly has long been interested in history and archaeology and also serves as the chairman of the Indiana Historical Association. He has made several contributions to archaeological research in Indiana. However, his biggest project has been to purchase, restore, and develop the original house of William Connor, an important character in Hoosier history.

Connor settled in the Indiana Territory in 1801 and became a major Indian trader on the frontier. It was at his log cabin that representatives of the traders, local politicians, and the Delaware Indians would often meet. By 1823 Connor had become quite prosperous and built himself a two-story house made of brick, possibly the first brick house built in the whole of Indiana. In 1934 Mr. Lilly purchased the old Connor home together with four hundred acres of associated farmland. Over the years he renovated both the house and the land, and it became a well-known historical site. Connor Prairie is still active today and acts both as a pioneer village tourist attraction and as an important educational center for those interested in local history. It was next to the Connor Prairie, where in 1949 Eli Lilly purchased an additional 115 acres of woodland along the banks of the White river, that he found the abandoned cottage that became his Chinese house.

His interest in Chinese history and art began when he read F. S. C. Northrop's book *The Meeting of East and West,* which called for better mutual appreciation and understanding between Eastern and Western cultures so as to avoid future conflicts. As this was just after the end of the Second World War, Mr. Lilly's mind was very much concerned with the promotion of harmony in the world, and in Chinese culture he felt he had found a particular reverence for harmony and spirituality that was lacking in the West. As it happened, the head of the pharmacology department at Eli Lilly and Company was a Dr. Chen—an immigrant from China—and conversations between Dr. Chen and Mr. Lilly further enhanced his interest in all things Chinese. And so it was that Eli Lilly started to buy Chinese artifacts. It was recommended that he contact the dealer C. T. Loo, who had a gallery in New York and was well known for selling Chinese art to wealthy US families such as the Vanderbilts and Rockefellers. In 1947 Mr. Lilly visited C. T. Loo's New York gallery, saw a couple of Song vases that he liked, purchased them, and started to put together what would become one of the most outstanding collections of Chinese art in the United States.

Eventually all of this was bequeathed to the Indianapolis Museum of Art, where it resides today. It is well worth a visit.

THE ORIGINS OF ELI LILLY & CO.

The source of Eli Lilly's wealth was the pharmaceutical company of which he was the president. During colonial times Britain had been the major source of medicines imported into the United States.[4] However, after the American Revolution an independent US pharmaceutical industry started to develop. The country's western frontier was becoming settled, and the nascent pharmaceutical industry began to serve these rapidly developing national markets. The "cradle of pharmacy" in the United States was the city of Philadelphia, where the Philadelphia College of Pharmacy, the first such institution in the country, was founded in 1821. Soon afterward the first pharmaceutical companies started to form in the area.

Originally many of these developed from local apothecaries. John Smith founded what was eventually to become Smith, Kline and French in Philadelphia in 1830, and William Lambert founded what was to become Warner-Lambert in 1856. Generally speaking the pharmaceutical industry in the United States did not develop directly as an offshoot of the dye-making chemical industry as it had in Germany or the United Kingdom (Chapter 3). More often than not, US companies began with the sale of patent medicines and nostrums. These were remedies, often of questionable effectiveness, with exotic names whose ingredients were usually secret. However, in some parts of the country where there were large populations of German immigrants, companies were founded that did import a measure of German chemical know-how. This happened in New York, for example, where a German immigrant named Charles Pfizer founded a chemical company in 1848. Some established German companies also started to distribute their products through subsidiaries founded in the New York/New Jersey area for this purpose. Bayer, for example, started to do this in 1863. The New York area in general gradually began to challenge Philadelphia's lead in pharmacy and pharmaceuticals, with other companies such as Squibb being founded in 1859 together with a College of Pharmacy in New York City. As the US frontier expanded westward, so did the nascent pharmaceutical industry. The first Midwestern company to be founded was Parke-Davis in Detroit in 1866, with Upjohn founded in Kalamazoo, Michigan, in 1886 and G.D. Searle in Omaha, Nebraska in 1888.

The first Eli Lilly was born on July 8th, 1838, in Baltimore, to Gustavus and Esther Lilly, a family of Swedish origins, their original name having

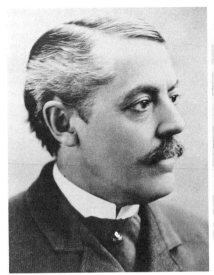
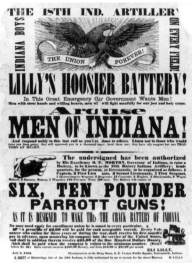

Figure 4.1:
Colonel Eli Lilly in 1885 and a poster recruiting men for Lilly's Hoosier Battery to fight in the Civil War.
(Images reproduced with permission of the Eli Lilly Co.).

been Lillja.[3] The family moved a couple of times, eventually settling in Greenfield, Indiana. It was here that, following his education at what was to become DePauw university, young Eli Lilly opened a pharmacy in 1861. However, fate intervened in the shape of the War between the States. Eli Lilly signed up and actively recruited a brigade from his local friends and acquaintances (Figure 4.1). Lilly and his troops fought in the Battle of Hoover's Gap (1863), and also in the Second Battle of Chattanooga and the Battle of Chickamauga. After many adventures he was captured and spent time as a Confederate prisoner of war. One of his most interesting adventures involved "The Republic of Jones." This was a group of Confederate deserters and desperadoes that declared an independent republic in Mississippi, a virtual state within the Confederate state.[5] Lilly and his men had been captured by the Confederates but fought with them to defeat the Jonesian army.

Following the war, Eli Lilly attempted to start several businesses. The first involved a cotton plantation in Mississippi. However, Eli's young wife died of malaria and he became depressed and could not continue with the enterprise. Returning to the Midwest, he then went back into the pharmacy business both in Indiana and Illinois. This went better, and he was able to put aside a little capital. He decided that what he really wanted to do was to manufacture drugs rather than to sell them. So it was that

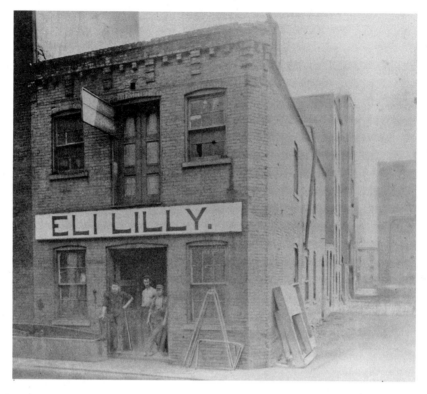

Figure 4.2:
The original building of the Eli Lilly Company (1876) at 15 W. Pearl St. in Indianapolis.
(Image reproduced with permission of the Eli Lilly Co.).

on May 10th, 1876, the same year as Custer's last stand, the 38 year old ex–army colonel opened a small pharmaceutical business on Pearl Street in downtown Indianapolis (Figure 4.2). It consisted of a two-story red brick building, eighteen by forty feet. The business was capitalized at $1400 and by the end of the first month had three employees. Eli Lilly's original products included things such as Bear's Foot, Black Haw, Cramp Bark, Hardhack, Life Root, Scullup, Sea Wrack, Squaw Vine, Wahoo and Wormseed.[3]

Nevertheless, Lilly's aims were somewhat different from those of his competitors. Being somewhat disillusioned with the quality of medicines he had encountered, especially during his wife's battle with malaria, he was determined to raise the standards of his products and, as far as was possible, to specialize in "ethical drugs" where the ingredients were clearly stated. By 1881 Eli Lilly had moved his gradually expanding business to a former chair factory on McCarty Street, where the company's headquarters are still situated. Lilly's new headquarters were to see the development of many important discoveries. As we shall see, one of these was the discovery of one of the most important antidepressant drugs ever made.

Entering Eli Lilly and Company through its McCarty Street entrance these days, and encountering the marble floors, gilt fittings, and high ceilings, one is perhaps reminded more of something built by the Sultan of Brunei rather than of the company's humble origins. However, over the years, the results of many sound business decisions concerning management and research has clearly brought its rewards. Eli Lilly & Co.'s first big hit at the end of the nineteenth century was Succus Alterans, sold as a remedy for venereal disease. Eli Lilly's brother first read about it in a newspaper. The potion was made by a Dr. Sims from Montgomery, Alabama, from such ingredients as bamboo brier, queen's delight, burdock root, pokeroot, and prickly ash. Eli Lilly journeyed to Montgomery to secure the rights to producing and marketing the medicine. It sold very well indeed, earning the young company a million dollars.

ELI LILLY MARCHES ON

By the time he died in 1897, Colonel Eli Lilly was a wealthy man whose company was steadily expanding and whose reputation was on the rise. Several innovations had contributed to this success including the hiring of a scientist to engage in pharmaceutical "research," a highly novel idea at the time. Eli Lilly & Co. also pioneered several advances in pharmacy, including newer methods for mass producing gelatin coated capsules for medicines. When the Colonel died, Eli Lilly and Company had over a hundred employees and a catalogue of some 2000 products. Among these was the company's version of tincture of cannabis. At that time there were few restrictions on what could be sold by pharmaceutical companies, and many of the effects produced by drugs were not really appreciated or understood. Tincture of cannabis was a very good seller and today the empty bottles, if you can find them, are considered to be "highly collectible" (Figure 4.3).

Following the Colonel's death, Eli Lilly and Company was taken over by his son Josiah Kirby Lilly Sr., generally known as "J. K. Senior". In the fall of 1880 J. K. Senior's father had enrolled him in a two-year course in the Philadelphia College of Pharmacy which, as we have seen, was the premier pharmacy college in the country at that time. J. K. Senior never forgot his pharmacy training and his introduction to pharmaceutical research, but spent most of his efforts in trying to guide the development of the business side of the company. Indeed, he was extremely successful in doing this over the years. World War I cut off the supplies of drugs that were imported into

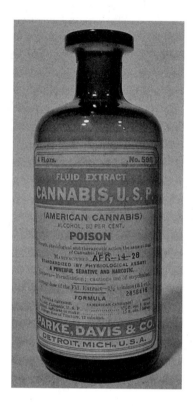

Figure 4.3:
Original Parke-Davis drug company tincture of cannabis bottle.
(Image reproduced with permission of Andrew Garret).

the United States from the large German pharmaceutical companies. This, together with the American government's abrogation of German patents, left the door open for US pharmaceutical companies to pick up the slack both in terms of research and production. In 1917 *Scientific American* was able to publish an article on Eli Lilly and Company describing the wonders of "the largest capsule factory in the world capable of producing 2.5 million capsules per day." However, as the twentieth century proceeded, some of the company's original products began to look a little dated. It was time to come up with a "blockbuster" product that would raise the company's reputation (not to say their profits) to the highest level. As it turned out, the discovery of such a product was just around the corner.

As we have discussed, Colonel Eli Lilly and J. K. Senior were both interested in promoting original research at the company, as well as other aspects of the business. In this respect they were somewhat ahead of their time and it was an approach that soon paid great dividends. In 1919 J. K. Senior announced that the company would initiate a Department of Experimental

Medicine. Recruiting the right man to run such a department was a critical step. Here, J. K. Senior made an extremely good choice.

THE ARRIVAL OF INSULIN

George Henry Alexander Clowes was born in Ipswich in the United Kingdom and underwent a rigorous training in pharmacy and pharmacology in the UK and Germany, after which he settled in the United States. His growing reputation as a researcher brought him to the attention of J. K. Senior, who offered him the position of head of the new Department of Experimental Medicine. Clowes wrote that Eli Lilly and Company "...have created a purely research position for me, in which, for the first time in my life, I am free to devote my attention to those fundamental problems on the border line field of physics, chemistry, biology and medicine... They have provided me with ample laboratory facilities and assistants and have arranged to let me carry on the biological side of my work at Woods Hole during the summer months." This certainly sounded like a good deal, and Clowes accepted the job. The fact was that although Clowes was rather an arrogant character, he was certainly a visionary and brilliant scientist who was always very conscious of all the current progress in basic research and how this might be developed in an industrial context.

On Christmas Day 1921, Clowes traveled to Yale University for a meeting of the American Physiological Society. Here he heard a paper read by Macleod, Banting, and Best from the University of Toronto entitled, "The beneficial influences of certain pancreatic extracts on pancreatic diabetes." The authors named their new extract *insulin*. Most of the audience was skeptical—but not Clowes, who cornered the authors immediately after their presentation and suggested a collaboration. They declined. However, by the next year the Toronto group found that they were having considerable difficulty making sufficient quantities of insulin to carry out all of their experiments. They remembered Clowes' interest and got in touch with him. In May 1922, Eli Lilly & Co. and the Canadians entered into an agreement for the commercial development of insulin.

By the next year scientists at the company had made several technical breakthroughs allowing them to produce large amounts of pure and stable insulin and were able to announce that they would be able to supply the hormone "to the entire world." The development of insulin was certainly one of those paradigm-shifting breakthroughs in medicine for numerous reasons. First of all, it provided an effective treatment for a terrible disease. Prior to the development of insulin there had been no treatment for diabetes. All of a sudden a large number of diabetic patients could be effectively treated and their lives saved. Second, the development of insulin provided the impetus for increasing understanding of the pathogenesis of diabetes. Indeed, Macleod and Banting received the Nobel Prize for their work. In addition, the development of insulin demonstrated how a basic science lab at a university and a pharmaceutical company could work together effectively. Indeed, Eli Lilly and Company benefited in numerous ways, and their profits increased enormously from the worldwide sales of insulin. However, there were also less tangible benefits, primarily the well-publicized role that the company had played in Nobel Prize–winning research and in providing a drug that truly benefited the human race. It's impossible to put a price on that kind of publicity.

ELI JUNIOR TAKES THE REIGNS

J. K. Senior was a family man. He and his wife Lilly Ridgely were married in 1882. They had two sons. The first, born in 1885, was named Eli Lilly, after his grandfather, and the second, named Josiah K. Lilly, Jr. (J. K. Junior) was born in 1893. It was expected that they would eventually enter the family's pharmaceutical business. Like his father before him, young Eli Lilly graduated from the Philadelphia College of Pharmacy in 1907 and joined the company that had been founded by his grandfather and was now managed by his father. He married Evelyn Fortune, his high school sweetheart and the daughter of a wealthy Indianapolis family. However, although young Eli's future career and happiness seemed assured, not everything went entirely according to plan. To begin with he had two sons, both of whom were named Eli, who both died in infancy. Then, in 1918, the Lillys had a daughter whom they named Evelyn ("Evie"). Unfortunately, as time wore on Eli's marriage to Evelyn Fortune began to disintegrate and eventually resulted in divorce in 1926. Eli was married again the next year to his secretary, Ruth Allison, a marriage that lasted until the end of his life. Unfortunately, his only child Evie was not to do well. Eli doted on his daughter and worried about the effect his divorce would have on her. He tried to use his wealth to improve her life. Although basically a modest and conservative person, he would break the bank for his daughter and do uncharacteristically wild and extravagant things. For example, he hired Benny Goodman and his band play at her debutante coming out ball—a madly sumptuous affair. Nevertheless, Evie gradually descended into depression and alcoholism and it was difficult for her to live an independent life. Ultimately Eli had to disinherit his daughter, as he could not in all good conscience leave his considerable fortune to her. Instead he created the Lilly Foundation, a charitable trust that even today is one of the largest in the world.

During the negotiations between Eli Lilly and Company and the Canadians over the development of insulin, J. K. Senior had been accompanied by young Eli, who rapidly acquired a sophisticated knowledge of the business for which he had been intended and who became more and more involved in research administration during the 1920s. In 1932 Eli Lilly took over from his father as the president of the company. The previous decade had seen Eli Lilly and Company move further and further away from its original products toward the development of new therapies with a clear chemical identity and more specific pharmacological effects. Apart from insulin, the company introduced Amytal (the first barbiturate produced in America), Merthiolate (an antiseptic), ephedrine (a stimulant and vasoconstrictor that could be used to treat asthma), and a liver extract that effectively treated certain forms of anemia. Like his predecessors, Eli Lilly proved to be a canny and innovative businessman. Eli Lilly & Co. was certainly in the vanguard when it came to labor relations; something which the company is proud of to this very day is that during the Great Depression not a single member of its staff was laid off—a truly remarkable statistic.

By the time Eli died, Eli Lilly and Company were one of the most successful pharmaceutical companies in the world. They had introduced influential drugs into the fields of antibiotics, cardiovascular medicine, and cancer, among other things. The company had spread from its Midwestern roots to encompass all parts of the globe. Research laboratories were set up in other countries such as the United Kingdom, and these too began to develop products. Furthermore, the company maintained its position as being a good place to work and had a continuing reputation for treating its staff well. The legacy of Eli Lilly's establishment of the Lilly Foundation meant that the company also remained a leader in philanthropy. When Eli Lilly died there was no obvious heir to inherit the business. However, like many multinational companies, capable CEOs were found to guide the company forward. Strangely, in spite of all of its success, Eli Lilly and Company had still not made its most important mark on the history of therapeutics. In 1977, the year Eli Lilly passed away, the company presented an NDA for a new product to the Food and Drug Administration. The name of the drug was fluoxetine, ultimately to be marketed under the name Prozac: the first drug to register more than a billion dollars a year in sales and to seal the name of Eli Lilly & Co. indelibly into the public's consciousness.

THE PSYCHOPATHOLOGY OF CLINICAL DEPRESSION

As we have seen, starting in the 1950s new drugs were introduced that were able to treat important psychiatric disorders such as schizophrenia (Chapter 3) and anxiety (Chapter 6) for the first time. Similar advances were also made at this time in the pharmacological treatment of major clinical depression and the related syndrome of manic–depressive or bipolar disorder.[6] Prior to the introduction of the antidepressant drugs in the 1950s, the syndrome of major clinical depression was not really defined as such. Of course, people with severely depressed mood had been identified and written about going back to ancient times. These patients were generally described as suffering from "melancholia." Indeed, many famous individuals are known to have suffered from bouts of such mood disorders. Winston Churchill, for example, referred to these periods as his "Black Dog."[7] However, the intermittent occurrence of mood disturbances did not generally prevent people from carrying out their normal everyday functions.

On the other hand, very severely affected patients, numbering perhaps 100 out of every million, were hospitalized, although effective treatments for such patients were generally lacking. The introduction of antidepressant medications in the 1950s, first to treat hospitalized individuals and then the population at large, helped to create "depression" as a new clinical entity affecting some 10% or more of the world's population. An ever more sophisticated and increasingly fragmented series of diagnoses are now used to characterize a wide spectrum of mood disorders. Although typically associated with depressed mood and low self-esteem, other types of symptoms including irritability, difficulty concentrating, insomnia, and anhedonia are commonly considered to be part of these syndromes. Various disease subtypes including milder forms of depression (dysthymia), seasonal affective disorder, postpartum depression, and a host of other entities are now also generally recognized.

There is a considerable comorbidity that has been recognized between depression and other types of psychiatric disorders such as anxiety, as well as other types of health problems such as diabetes. The time course of major depressive illness is quite variable, ranging from one or more isolated incidents to a continuous lifelong affliction. Overall, mood disorders of this type clearly constitute one of the world's greatest health problems, not only in terms of numbers of patients afflicted by them but also in the negative overall impact they have on an individual's career and relationships.

THE NAZI LARGESSE

As with many other advances in psychopharmacology, the origins of anti-depressant drugs are murky and unlikely. We might begin their story with Selfridges. Selfridges is one of London's best known luxury department stores, founded in the nineteenth century by William Gordon Selfridge, an American from Ripon, Wisconsin, who had settled in London following training with Marshall Field in Chicago. Like all big department stores, Selfridges became famous for its Christmas window displays. During the Second World War, Selfridges mounted particularly attractive displays as part of the general effort aimed at raising the spirits of blitzed Londoners. However, a V2 rocket hit the Red Lion Pub, which was situated just down the road from Selfridges, at 11pm, December 6, 1944, destroying Selfridges shop front and their entire Yuletide window display.[8] A restaurant in the store that was widely used by servicemen and customers alike was completely destroyed, killing 8 American servicemen and injuring another 32. Numerous British citizens were also killed or injured. I was born in Portman Square just across the road from Selfridges. They were still digging there in the early 1950s trying to finish repairing everything. There was still a big hole. "That's where the V2 hit," Mum used to say when we walked past (Figure 4.4).

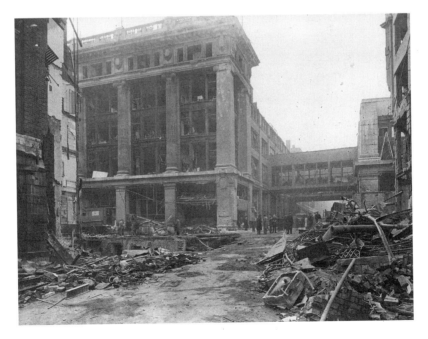

Figure 4.4:
The ruins of Selfridges following the World War II V2 rocket attack (1944).
(Image reproduced with permission of City of Westminster Archives).

The V2 was Hitler's last throw of the dice, his super-weapon with which he would bring doomsday to the citizens of Britain. Their predecessors, the VI flying bombs, or "doodle bugs," had previously caused a certain amount of trouble. However, you could always hear them coming and evasive action was often possible. Not so with the V2s, the world's first genuine ballistic missiles. Traveling faster than sound, there was no warning. They just arrived unheralded, bringing with them death and destruction. Fortunately the Germans didn't start launching the V2s until the war was nearly over. Nevertheless, over 2000 people in London were killed by them in a few months. The V1 and V2 rockets were developed and assembled at the German army's secret research center based at Peenemunde on the Baltic coast, run by the sinister Nazi rocket genius, Werner von Braun (Figure 4.5). In addition to the V1 and V2, we now know that a V3 intercontinental rocket was being developed to strike the United States, and perhaps Rocket OOOOO as well—a rocket so powerful that it could destroy the entire world. It is in Peenemunde that you will find the infamous "Test

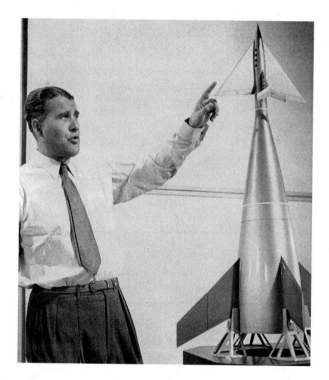

Figure 4.5:
Werner von Braun. Were the Nazis indirectly responsible for the development of anti-depressants?
(Associated Press).

Stand VII"—the site of the first V2 launchings—"the Egg the flying rocket hatched from, navel of the 50-meter radio sky."[9]

When Tyrone Slothrop,[9] or whoever it was, first entered Peenemunde as part of the Allied occupation in 1945, he found a lot of bombed out detritus, the ruins of Messerschmitts, rocket parts, and—what else? Large stores of C-stoff, a component of the V2 rocket propellant. In particular this contained highly reactive hydrazine, an oily, caustic, explosive liquid as one of its major ingredients.[10] And so it was that right after the Second World War an unprecedented amount of hydrazine became available at very cheap rates to the US chemical and pharmaceutical industries. This is certainly true. But is there more to this than meets the eye? We know that the major pharmaceutical companies always had contacts with the CIA. Recall that in 1953, Eli Lilly and Company had received a large grant for supplying LSD to the CIA for their use in their ARTICHOKE and MK-ULTRA projects (Chapter 2). We know that the CIA captured Werner Von Braun. We know that Werner Von Braun knew exactly where the hydrazine was hidden. We also know that von Braun had secret information on how to construct a new type of rocket capable of destroying the entire world. If the hydrazine could be sold to the pharmaceutical industry, then the proceeds could be channeled by the CIA through secret bank accounts in Lichtenstein and be used to bribe Von Braun and his colleagues into selling their secret information to the CIA, possibly saving the free world from Communism! (I have this information from several web sites with impeccable reputations for accuracy; for example, http://www.conspiracytheory.org).

THE FIRST ANTIDEPRESSANTS

Well, it was certainly nice to have all of this cheap hydrazine, but the question was what to try to make out of it? Hydrazine is a highly unstable substance that can be used as an intermediate in many chemical reactions. Derivatives of hydrazine, that is to say compounds known as hydrazines, were first discovered by the famous chemist Emil Fischer in the 1870s. As we have seen, Fischer was one of the students of the great Adolf von Baeyer (Chapter 3) and he first synthesized phenylhydrazine in 1874 while he was working in von Baeyer's laboratory in Strasbourg.[11] In 1912 two doctoral students, Hans Meyer and Josef Malley, synthesized isonicotinyl-hydrazine, although the compound was virtually forgotten for four decades until it was resynthesized in the 1950s as a result of the V2 hydrazine largesse. At that time, making drugs to treat tuberculosis was an important priority for the US pharmaceutical industry. The antibiotic streptomycin was certainly the major effective treatment for tuberculosis. However, the growing development of drug resistance was becoming a problem that limited its effectiveness. In order to test whether any new drug might be effective in treating tuberculosis, mice were first infected with *Mycobacterium tuberculosis* and then the new test compound was given to the mice to see if the progress of the disease could be prevented. Thousands of new chemical compounds were tested in this way by the US pharmaceutical industry. Chemical structures related to compounds known as thiosemicarbazones had been demonstrated to have some effectiveness in curing infected mice, and so many new compounds of this type were synthesized and tested.

In 1951, chemists working at the Squibb institute synthesized isonicotinylaldehyde-thiosemicarbazone as one of a series of thiosemicarbazones. Isonicotinylhydrazine was used as an intermediate in the synthesis. Amazingly, it was observed that isonicotinylhydrazine actually had far superior antitubercular properties to those of the final thiosemicarbazone product. Equally amazingly, the same observation was made at precisely the same time by a second research group at Hoffmann-LaRoche. This latter research started from the knowledge that nicotinamide, a group B Vitamin, had beneficial effects on tuberculosis. The chemists decided to combine this with a thiosemicarbazone. Again they made isonicotinylhydrazine as an intermediate, and again observed that it had more potent effects than its ultimate reaction product. The related product, isonicotinylisopropylhydrazine, was also synthesized and was also found to produce good antitubercular effects in mice. The medical potential of such substances, now renamed *isoniazid* and *iproniazid,* in the treatment of tuberculosis was quickly realized. They were rapidly tested on patients and their beneficial effects were soon confirmed. Indeed, the impact in the United States of the use of these new drugs was extremely significant. Tuberculosis-associated deaths fell from 188 deaths per 100,000 in 1904 to 4 per 100,000 in 1952, a year after the introduction of isoniazid and iproniazid (Figure 4.6).

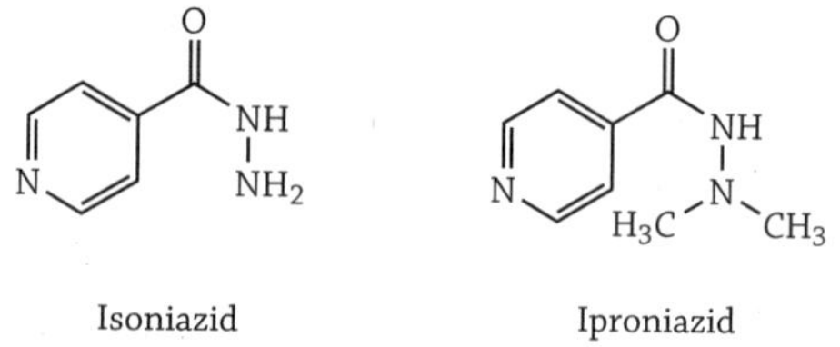

Isoniazid   Iproniazid

Figure 4.6:
Structures of isoniazid and the first real monoamine oxidase inhibitor antidepressant drug iproniazid.

However, the benefits of the new drugs were to extend far beyond their utility in tuberculosis. An inkling of what was to come was soon apparent. In a famous clinical trial carried out at the Sea View tuberculosis hospital in New York, patients were not only observed to improve after taking the new drugs but, after taking iproniazid in particular, seemed to exhibit a strange "side effect," this being the fact that they seemed to feel really, really good. No doubt this was partly due to the fact that they were delighted that their tuberculosis was in remission. However, their euphoria seemed to be quite excessive. It was reported that "A few months ago, the only sound here was the sound of victims of tuberculosis, coughing up their lives." Now the patients were "dancing in the halls tho' there were holes in their lungs."[10]

Iproniazid was marketed by Hoffmann-La Roche for the treatment of tuberculosis under the trade name Marsilid. Its psychological side effects were viewed as a potentially useful adjunct to the use of the drugs, in that they might improve the overall function of tuberculosis patients. However, it was not initially realized that iproniazid might actually help to improve the symptoms of patients who were just plain depressed and did not have tuberculosis. This leap of clinical insight was eventually made by Nathan Kline and his colleagues for good scientific reasons.

As we have discussed (Chapter 3), it had been recently observed that the drug reserpine could be useful in calming schizophrenic patients displaying excessive psychotic agitation. Reserpine also produced a general inhibition of motor activity in rats. Overall therefore, reserpine could be thought of as having a "depressive" effect. Now, what was required for the treatment of depression was something that did the opposite of this; that is, to selectively reverse depression. Nathan Kline thought that such a drug might be theoretically thought of as a "psychic energizer." So, Kline proposed that a useful experimental approach would be one that tested what kinds drugs might reverse the depressant effects of reserpine in rats and mice.

In 1956 Kline went to deliver a lecture at the Warner-Lambert drug company, where he met with Dr. Charles Scott. Scott told Kline that he had found that he could reverse the effects of reserpine with iproniazid. Kline realized that this was precisely the effect that might be expected from a "psychic energizer." Initially, Hoffmann-La Roche were not keen on letting Kline test out iproniazid on depressed patients. However, Kline was a most persuasive individual and eventually obtained supplies of the drug for this purpose. At the American Psychiatric Association meeting in Syracuse, New York, in 1957, Kline and his colleagues Harry Loomer and George Saunders reported the beneficial effects of iproniazid in a group of depressed patients, results that were rapidly confirmed by other research groups. The effects of iproniazid were widely reported in the *New York*

Times and other media. The floodgates had now opened and, within a year, some 400,000 depressed patients had been treated "off label" with iproniazid with generally positive results. As with the introduction of antipsychotic drugs at almost exactly the same time, this was a highly significant milestone in the history of psychiatry because no effective therapy had previously been widely available for the treatment of depression; and so there was a tremendous need for a new therapeutic agent of this type.

BIOGENIC AMINES AND MOOD

But why should iproniazid act as an antidepressant? To understand this we should return to the topic of the biogenic amines, dopamine, norepinephrine, and 5-HT, and their role as neurotransmitters in the brain. As we discussed in the previous chapter, the role of dopaminergic neurons in the mechanism of action of antipsychotic drugs has been widely discussed. When considering the antidepressants, it is norepinephrine and 5-HT which appear to be of prime importance. Just as the nerve cells in the brain that contain dopamine are restricted to relatively few groups of neurons or "nuclei," a similar picture has emerged as to the anatomical organization of the neurons that use norepinephrine and 5-HT as their neurotransmitters. In the former case, the vast majority of norepinephrine-utilizing neurons arise from a midbrain nucleus named the *locus ceruleus*. In fact, the number of these neurons is really incredibly small—around 13,000 in each nucleus, one on each side of the brain stem. However, the axons and terminals arising from these neurons are very widely distributed and course both upward and downward to innervate most areas of the brain and spinal cord. Thus, the influence of these few neurons on the functions of the nervous system is disproportionally large, regulating things such as the sleep/wake cycle, mood, and pain. The neurons that utilize 5-HT are also restricted to nuclei in the brain stem. These nuclei are somewhat larger than the locus ceruleus, the human brain containing several hundred thousand 5-HT utilizing neurons. Nevertheless, the number of these neurons is still extremely small compared to the huge number of neurons in the entire brain—perhaps a hundred billion in the human brain. The biogenic amine neurotransmitters, such as norepinephrine and 5-HT, are stored in small vesicle-like structures in the terminals of these neurons. When stimulated by an action potential, Ca ions enter the terminal and trigger the release of one or more of these vesicles into the synaptic space. The released transmitter then activates receptors on target cells. Once its job is done, the biogenic amine is removed. Some of the neurotransmitter may diffuse away and be metabolized. However, a great deal of it is taken up again by the nerve terminal and repackaged into the terminal's neurotransmitter storage vesicles.

These events are coordinated by a series of key molecules. First there are protein molecules in the nerve terminal that are responsible for the reuptake of biogenic amines following their release and activation of postsynaptic receptors. These are known as *biogenic amine reuptake molecules,* or transporters. Biogenic amines that are retaken up in this way, or new supplies of biogenic amines made by the nerves biosynthetic pathways, are pumped into the terminal's synaptic storage vesicles by a molecule called the *vesicular monoamine transport protein* (VMAT). Biogenic amines that are not effectively stored in synaptic vesicles are destroyed in the nerve terminal primarily by the enzyme named *monoamine oxidase* (MAO) (chapter 2). This enzymatic activity was first described in 1928 in liver, by Mary Hare of Cambridge University, and named *tyramine oxidase.* The enzyme was then further characterized by Richter and Blaschko and by Pugh and Quastel, who demonstrated that there were high concentrations of MAO in the brain, although the reason for this was unknown at the time. At a subcellular level it was shown that the enzyme resided on the outer membrane of the mitochondria, the organelles that supply much of the cell's energy in the form of the molecule ATP. By 1950 it was known that free biogenic amines in the nerve terminal were primarily oxidatively deaminated by MAO to produce their respective aldehydes. These were then rapidly converted to acids by enzymes known as *aldehyde dehydrogenases.* Thus, 5-HT and norepinephrine were converted by MAO to their aldehydes, and then to 5-hydroxyindole acetic acid and 3,4-dihydroxymandelic acid respectively. Similarly, in dopamine-utilizing neurons, the action of MAO and aldehyde dehydrogenase on dopamine yields 3,4 dihydroxyphenylacetic acid. Such biogenic amine metabolites are inert and do not activate the receptors activated by their parent molecules. A second enzyme called *catechol-O-methyl transferase* (COMT) may modify these products further by methylating a hydroxyl group to ultimately yield a wide variety of metabolic products.

Incredibly, just as the mood elevating effects of iproniazid were emerging in the early 1950s, the key to understanding these effects on the nervous system were also revealed when in 1952, Ernst Zeller of the Northwestern University Medical School in Chicago demonstrated that the drug was an excellent inhibitor of MAO.[11] Given this fact, it was not surprising when it was subsequently demonstrated that when iproniazid was given to animals it produced a rapid increase in their brain levels of 5-HT and norepinephrine. Now, it will be recalled from the previous chapter that reserpine produces the opposite effect; that is, a rapid decline in the brain's levels of biogenic amines (Chapter 3,[12]). The reason for this is that reserpine inhibits the activity of the VMAT protein responsible for accumulating biogenic amines in their nerve terminal neurotransmitter storage vesicles. Hence, if this protein is blocked by reserpine, biogenic amines remain unprotected in the cytoplasm of the nerve terminal, where they are metabolized by MAO as described above. However, if MAO is inhibited by iproniazid, then biogenic amines are protected from degradation and so accumulate in the nerve terminal. Hence, if all biogenic amine uptake into nerve terminal storage vesicles is prevented by reserpine, iproniazid would block all subsequent metabolism of these amines and so should prevent the effects of reserpine. This is, of course, exactly what Nathan Kline heard when he visited Scott at Warner Lambert.

THE RISE OF THE TRICYCLICS

So, by 1957 a new approach to treating depression had arrived together with a potential explanation of how such effects were produced. As we have seen, the antipsychotics were developed at precisely the same time, and reserpine played a significant role in both developments. Along with these new therapies, the key biological role of biogenic amines in the control of mood and in the development of psychiatric disorders was becoming more apparent every day. This was truly a revolution in medicine. Another fact that illustrates the importance and interrelated nature of all of these findings is that Nathan Kline won the Lasker Award (the American "Nobel Prize") twice—the only person ever to have done so. These awards were made for his pioneering work on antipsychotic and antidepressant drugs.

Iproniazid was certainly a paradigm shifting drug, but it wasn't necessarily the best version of this class of compounds and was quite quickly superseded by a variety of other monoamine oxidase inhibitors (MAOIs) including isocarboxazid (Hoffman-LaRoche), tranylcypromine (Smith, Kline & French) and phenelzine (Warner-Lambert), as well as other hydrazine derivatives (nialamide, mebanazine, and pheniprazine) or indole derivatives (etryptamine). Such drugs gradually became generally known as "antidepressants" rather than "psychic energizers." Although they were certainly effective in this regard, they did have some interesting and unfortunate side effects. As far as iproniazid was concerned, hepatotoxicity turned out to be an important problem. However, there was another problem that would eventually lead to MAOIs getting a bad reputation. This was the dreaded so-called "cheese effect."[13] It was observed that some people who were taking drugs like iproniazid would suddenly be subject to attacks of extreme hypertension, which could even be severe enough to trigger myocardial infarction or stroke.

The reason for this is as follows. We know that although biogenic amines function as neurotransmitters in the brain, they also have this function in the peripheral nervous system. Indeed, the role of norepinephrine as a neurotransmitter in the sympathetic nervous system is very well established and is of critical importance for many life subserving functions, including normal cardiac function and blood flow. Norepinephrine released from sympathetic nerves is a powerful vasopressor—that is, it causes constriction of blood vessels (vasoconstriction) and hypertension.

Now we know that norepinephrine is stored in neurotransmitter vesicles in the terminals of neurons such as sympathetic nerves, awaiting release. Certain substances such as amine tyramine (Figure 4.7) can also be taken up by nerve terminals and be stored in the same vesicles. Normally this doesn't happen to any great extent because there isn't much tyramine around in the body. Tyramine is produced by some bacteria in the gut, and it is also found in certain foods such as some cheeses. However, tyramine is destroyed by MAO in the gut and liver, and so it never enters the systemic blood circulation. However, consider what happens if you are taking an MAOI such as iproniazid. Now let's say you eat a nice piece of gorgonzola, which contains a lot of tyramine. The tyramine is not destroyed by MAO, which is inhibited by the iproniazid, and so it enters your blood circulation. It then enters the terminals of sympathetic nerves, where it is transported by VMAT into transmitter storage vesicles. Indeed, it actually displaces norepinephrine from these vesicles. So the vesicles fill up with tyramine, which acts as a "false transmitter." The nerve terminal is now flooded with norepinephrine. Normally this would be destroyed by MAO—but this is inhibited. So, all this displaced norepinephrine leaves the nerve terminal and causes massive vasoconstriction and hypertension. When these effects were first noted in some patients everybody panicked, and soon iproniazid was removed from the market. In truth, this was a severe overreaction, as

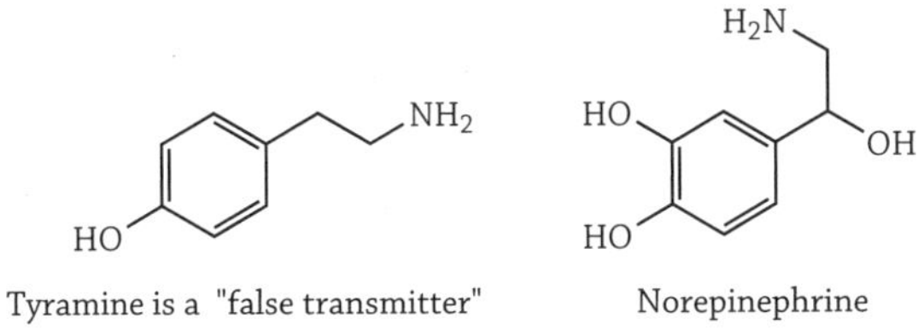

Tyramine is a "false transmitter"   Norepinephrine

Figure 4.7:
Structure of the neurotransmitter norepinephrine compared to that of the "false transmitter" tyramine. Tyramine was responsible for the "cheese effect" associated with the use of monoamine oxidase inhibitor antidepressant drugs.

the observed effects can easily be prevented with a few dietary restrictions. Over the years several different types of MAOIs have been produced to try and get round this type of problem.[13] However, generally speaking the use of MAOIs has been superseded by other classes of drugs, some of which were developed around the same time.

It will be recalled from our discussion of antipsychotics that in 1883, Berthensen at BASF had synthesized phenothiazine, which would ultimately give rise to chlorpromazine and the first antipsychotic medications (Chapter 3). Soon after the synthesis of phenothiazine, chemists at the Geigy company in Basel, Switzerland, synthesized the related structure iminodibenzyl (Figure 4.8). This substance originally found some use in dye making but was soon shelved and was left to gather dust in the Geigy basement. As we have also seen, after World War II the Rhone-Poulenc company in France had established a successful program for the development of antihistamines, and other companies were interested in following their lead. Robert Domenjoz, who was head of pharmacology, suggested that the Geigy scientists synthesize some phenothiazine-like compounds to test as antihistamines. Digging around in the basement they rediscovered

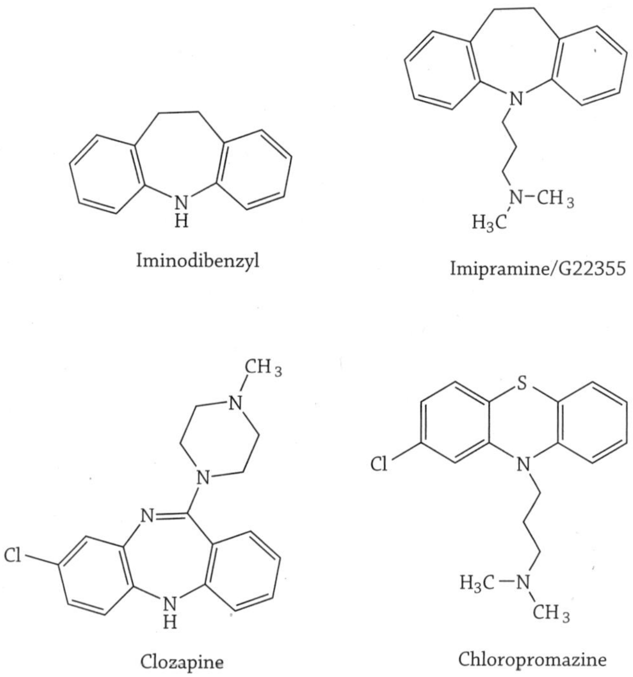

Iminodibenzyl

Imipramine/G22355

Clozapine

Chloropromazine

Figure 4.8:
Iminodibenzyl and the tricyclic antidepressant imipramine compared to the structures of the antipsychotic drugs chlorpromazine and clozapine.

iminodibenzyl and proceeded to make a chemical series based on this structure. Drug screening demonstrated that many of the compounds in this series did indeed have antihistaminergic potential, as well as a number of other properties. Some of the compounds were also sent to clinicians to be further examined on human subjects.

One analogue, named G22150, was dispatched to Dr. Roland Kuhn, who ran a psychiatric clinic on the shores of Lake Constance.[14] Kuhn obtained inconclusive results when testing the drug as a hypnotic. Subsequently, however, in 1952 the news began to emanate from France as to the highly novel antipsychotic effects of phenothiazines developed by Rhone-Poulenc. Every drug company obviously wanted a piece of the action. Kuhn asked Geigy if he could retest G22150, but was still unimpressed and requested further compounds, stipulating that if possible they should have some type of structural similarity to chlorpromazine. Geigy sent him G22355, one of the iminodibenzyl compounds that they had previously made in their antihistamine program, but with a dimethylaminopropyl side chain, as also found in CPZ (Figure 4.8). This compound was known as *imipramine*.

Kuhn was supposed to test the compound on schizophrenic patients. He did so and found that it was not helpful—if anything, it made them worse. However, he also took the opportunity of testing it on three patients suffering from major clinical depression and found that imipramine seemed to have beneficial effects. He then tested it on another 37 depressed patients, and again was impressed with the positive effects produced by the drug. He reported to the World Congress of Psychiatry in Zurich in 1957 that "The patients appear, in general, more animated; their voices, previously weak and depressed, now sound louder; they are more communicative, the lamentations and sobbing have disappeared. The depression, which had manifested itself through sadness, irritation and a sensation of dissatisfaction, now gave way to friendly, joyous and accessible feelings."[11] One may consider the timing of this report quite amazing, because it was exactly when Kline and others were reporting on the "psychic energizing" effects of iproniazid. How does one explain this kind of coincidence? It is certainly difficult, except to remark that since the arrival of the antipsychotics the "idea" of drugs for treating specific psychiatric disorders was in the air— the revolution was in progress. Instead of thinking of such disorders in a traditional psychodynamic manner, psychiatrists were now starting to think of them as specific disease states for which specific pharmacotherapies might be envisaged.

Based on the promising initial data, Geigy started to market imipramine in 1957 under the trade name Tofranil. As was the case with the MAOIs, imipramine was greeted with great enthusiasm and quickly became widely used in both the United States and Europe. In 1961, Merck in the United States started to market a similar drug named amitriptyline under the trade name Elavil, and over the next decade a large number of similar "tricyclic" antidepressants (TCAs) were developed by drug companies all over the world. Because of the perceived problems with the use of MAOIs, drugs like amitriptyline quickly became the drugs of choice for the treatment of depression. It is interesting to note the chemical structures of these drugs and compare them with the antipsychotics, including atypical antipsychotics such as clozapine (Figure 4.8). Even to the chemically untutored eye it will be clear that they are really quite similar, and yet the effects they produce are certainly different. Indeed, we might wonder what the site of action of the TCAs might be?

Clearly if both TCAs and MAOIs have antidepressant effects, we would imagine that at some point their mechanisms of action must be coincident. That this is indeed the case emerged from studies carried out in the late '50s and the decade of the '60s, leading to a new picture of the etiology of major depression. First it became clear that unlike MAOIs, TCAs did not inhibit MAO. Nevertheless, they did prove to interact with neurotransmission mediated by biogenic amines.

THE MECHANISM OF TRICYCLIC ACTION

It had been suggested as early as 1932 that many tissues could actively accumulate norepinephrine.[11] When radioactive biogenic amine derivatives became widely available in the 1960s, it became possible to follow the biological disposition and metabolism of these molecules more accurately. The Nobel Prize winning scientist Julius Axelrod demonstrated that if tritiated norepinephrine (that is, norepinephrine synthesized to contain radioactive tritium atoms) and tritiated epinephrine were injected into animals, they were removed from the circulation and accumulated in peripheral tissues. Indeed, the tritiated norepinephrine was observed to accumulate in areas with the densest sympathetic innervation, leading to the hypothesis that it was being taken up by sympathetic nerve terminals. Similarly, in the brain norepinephrine accumulated in areas with the greatest innervation by noradrenergic nerves. Destruction of noradrenergic nerves also resulted in a lack of norepinephrine accumulation. Such results suggested that it was the noradrenergic nerves that were responsible for the uptake and accumulation of norepinephrine, and we have discussed this when considering the "cheese effect."

Most tellingly, experiments carried out by Solomon Snyder, Leslie Iversen, and others using "synaptosomes," which are biochemical preparations consisting of pinched-off nerve terminals, directly demonstrated the accumulation of norepinephrine by these structures. Eventually it became clear that separate nerve terminal uptake systems were expressed in the terminals of the appropriate sets of neurons. Thus a selective norepinephrine uptake system was expressed in norepinephrine-utilizing neurons, a dopamine uptake system in the terminals of dopaminergic neurons, and a 5-HT uptake system in 5-HT neurons. What was the physiological role of these uptake systems? The idea developed that they were responsible for the termination of synaptic transmission following the release of these neurotransmitters. Thus, as we have discussed, once norepinephrine has been released and has stimulated noradrenergic receptors postsynaptically, it is retaken up by an active uptake system expressed in nerve terminals. So, what would be the consequence of a drug that blocked such a reuptake system? If biogenic amines are not removed once they have been released, then their synaptic actions would be prolonged and potentiated.

As it turns out, this is precisely the mechanism by which TCAs function. In particular, they inhibit the active reuptake of norepinephrine, 5-HT, or both of these molecules.[11] The knowledge that the two major classes of antidepressants, MAOIs and TCAs, both functioned by potentiating the synaptic actions of biogenic amines—either by blocking their metabolism or reuptake—naturally helped to support the idea that alterations in the normal functions of such amines might represent the basis for states of depression or other mood disorders [12]. Indeed, as the 1960s proceeded, biological psychiatric theories suggesting that depression resulted from such "chemical imbalances" became highly influential.

Eventually the proteins responsible for the uptake of biogenic amines into nerve terminals were fully identified.[15] These proteins are located in cell membranes, just like the ligand gated ion channels and GPCRs that we have already discussed. However, rather than being generally localized in the membranes of the postsynaptic cell, the uptake proteins are localized in the presynaptic nerve terminal membrane. Their structures have all of the telltale signs of membrane-associated proteins. In this case, 12 hydrophobic membrane spanning regions help the protein to thread its way in and out of the cell membrane. The three proteins responsible for the uptake of norepinephrine, dopamine, and 5-hydroxytryptamine are known respectively as the norepinephrine transporter (NET), and corresponding DAT (dopamine transporter) and 5-HTT (5-hydroxytryptamine transporter), and are clearly members of the same overall gene family. They share numerous amino acid sequences in common, in addition to their overall structure and function. Nevertheless they do demonstrate differences in substrate specificity, having relative selectivity for their designated neurotransmitter.

Moreover, they also exhibit selectivity in terms of the drugs that inhibit them. Even with the early TCAs, this was apparent from the fact that imipramine, amitriptyline, and clomipramine were more potent inhibitors of the uptake of 5-HT than that of norepinephrine. On the other hand, the related secondary-amine tricyclics desipramine, nortriptyline, and desmethylclomipramine were better at inhibiting norepinephrine uptake than uptake of 5-HT.[16]

Following their introduction, the TCAs rapidly became widely used for the treatment of depression. Of course, just as other classes of drugs they proved to produce their own set of side effects, generally things such as dry mouth and constipation owing to their frequently associated anticholinergic (antimuscarinic) actions, as well as some negative effects on the electrical conduction of cardiac muscle. Hence, it was natural for pharmaceutical companies to want to get away from the tricyclic structure and to produce newer types of antidepressants with fewer side effects. As the 1970s dawned, evidence had started to appear that highlighted the role of 5-HT in depression in particular. This included observations on reduced levels of the 5-HT metabolite 5-HIAA in the brains and cerebrospinal fluid of depressed patients who had died by committing suicide. Hence the idea of producing novel types of drugs that worked by specifically enhancing 5-HT-mediated neurotransmission seemed reasonable.

PROZAC: THE BILLION DOLLAR BABY

As we have discussed above, at this time the Eli Lilly company was a successful and well established pharmaceutical company. The company still kept up its good contacts with basic researchers in university departments, just as it had with the University of Toronto following their discovery of insulin. Each year the company would give out various awards for basic research by university professors, and the winners would be invited to Indianapolis to deliver a lecture. In 1971 Solomon Snyder visited the company and lectured on his research using synaptosomes to examine the actions of TCAs. The scientists at Lilly were struck by the fact that such preparations would make ideal assays for screening new compounds to see if they could block the uptake of biogenic amines into nerve terminals—obviously one major hallmark of antidepressant activity.[17] It was agreed to initiate a research program based on such an idea.

But where to start? It had been noted in the literature that apart from its properties as an effective antihistamine, the drug diphenhydramine (commonly sold in the United States as Benadryl) could also inhibit biogenic

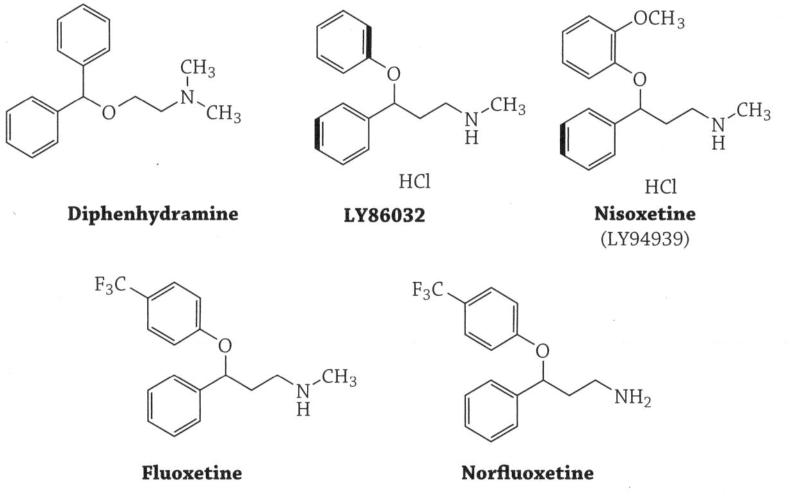

Figure 4.9:
The antihistamine drug diphenhydramine and several of the potential antidepressants prepared from it by the Eli Lilly Co including fluoxetine (Prozac).[17]

amine uptake into nerve terminals to some degree, and so it seemed that this might make an interesting starting point. A chemical synthetic program was started and initially produced several compounds, such as the phenylpropylamine derivative nisoxetine (Figure 4.9), which were found to be effective blockers of norepinephrine uptake but had much less effect on the uptake of 5-HT. In 1971 further studies revealed an interesting effect of adding certain substituents to the phenoxy ring. In particular, putting a trifluoromethyl group in the para position yielded a novel compound which showed high selectivity for blocking 5-HT uptake in comparison to norepinephrine. Similar properties were observed for its N-demethylated derivative. The compounds were named fluoxetine and norfluoxetine, respectively, and became the lead compounds for further examination and potential drug development.

Fluoxetine was then tested *in vivo* to see if its selectivity as a 5-HT uptake blocker was maintained in live animals, and this was found to be the case. The compound proved to be virtually completely selective for the 5-HT system. In 1973 Lilly had concluded that they should form a "team" within the company to oversee the further development of fluoxetine. The team included David Wong, Ray Fuller, and Brian Molloy, all key scientists who had been involved in the initial discovery of the compound. Fluoxetine was first tested for general safety by the toxicology department. In fact it did appear to produce a few odd effects, which slowed its further development for about a year. However, these effects were eventually explained and deemed to be harmless. So, in 1976 the company was ready to apply for an "IND" (investigational new drug) with the FDA which, as we have seen (Chapter 1), is the first step in the long road of clinical drug development in humans. These initial trials demonstrated that the drug was well tolerated and did indeed inhibit the uptake of 5-HT into human blood platelets, a type of blood cell that also expresses the 5-HT uptake transporter protein.

Going forward to Phase 2 trials to see whether the drug actually effectively treated depression in humans meant that clinical pharmacologists with particular experience in psychiatry were required to oversee this phase of the proceedings. Oddly, Lilly lacked such key personnel at the time and had to conduct a search to recruit the correct person, who then had to arrange sites for the trials. All of this activity took around 3 years. It will already be apparent from this example why it usually takes such a long time to bring a new drug successfully to the market. Eventually large-scale clinical trials were conducted, and fluoxetine proved to have significant beneficial activity in treating major depression. Interestingly, fluoxetine also proved to produce fewer side effects such as dry mouth, blurred vision, constipation, drowsiness, sedation, and direct effects on the electrical conductivity of the heart, which had plagued the use of traditional TCAs.[17] As described by David Wong in his memoir on the topic, "The clinical results of the fluoxetine trials were compiled in more than 100 volumes of 2-inch binders for the submission of an NDA to the US FDA in 1983. It had taken more than 7 years from the day of the first human dose to the day of submission of the NDA (New Drug Application')."[18] Actually fluoxetine was not the first selective serotonin (5-HT) reuptake inhibitor (SSRI) to be brought to the drug market. This was zimelidine, marketed by Astra in 1982. However, Astra was unlucky, as their drug proved to have a rare and unforeseen side effect of producing flu-like symptoms and had to be withdrawn. When fluoxetine was presented to the FDA they wanted to be reassured that the problems that had plagued zimelidine would not also be associated with fluoxetine. However, eventually the FDA concluded its deliberations and fluoxetine was approved for the treatment of depression on December 29, 1987. Lilly began the sell the drug under the trade name of Prozac.

THE SSRI PHENOMENON

It is safe to say that from Eli Lilly's point of view Prozac was a success. Who today has not heard of Prozac? Even if somebody doesn't actually know what it is or what it does, Prozac has become a metaphor in the public consciousness for all the drugs that are increasingly widely used by psychiatrists to treat an ever-expanding number of psychiatric syndromes. The notion that Prozac was an improvement on the previously used TCAs, and some canny marketing, was enough to propel its sales to stratospheric heights and by 1992 its annual sales reached $1 billion, the first drug ever to reach this landmark. Even greater success followed. By 2002 more than 40 million people had been prescribed Prozac and sales topped US$22 billion. Naturally the success of Prozac spurred other companies to produce their own "me-too" SSRIs, including sertraline (Zoloft), paroxetine (Paxil), and escitalopram (Lexapro) among others, all of which have been extremely effective from the sales point of view.

One development that has helped the general dissemination of SSRIs has been their extension to uses beyond major depression, illustrating the fact that the mechanisms of many of these syndromes may be closely related. For example, SSRIs are now widely used to treat eating disorders such as anorexia nervosa and bulimia nervosa, as well as post-traumatic stress disorder (PTSD), panic disorder, obsessive-compulsive disorder, and premenstrual dysphoria.[17] SSRIs have also taken over a large part of the anxiety market from benzodiazepines. Another unprecedented development has been the use of SSRIs to treat pets. If Fido gets a little anxious when you go away and chews up the furniture, it turns out that popping a Prozac is just what he needs. A story I once heard (for which I can find no supporting data, although it makes sense) is that Prozac is given to clams and oysters. Why, you may ask? It turns out that pearls are formed following the secretion of a mucus-like material from a gland in these animals. This secretion is under the influence of a 5-HT-utilizing synapse. Hence, in the presence of an SSRI, enhanced 5-HT mediated transmission occurs and more efficient pearl production ensues. So, happy as a clam, indeed! The idea of Prozac is now so firmly entrenched in our culture that it is the subject of numerous stories and jokes. For example, it has been reported that much of our water is now contaminated with significant amounts of SSRIs. One website asked readers to imagine what new dishes might be prepared from such Prozac-contaminated fish. How about Calm Chowder, Not so Bluefish, Fillet of Soleoft, or Bristol Myers Squid?[18]

Naturally, the success of SSRIs in the drug market and their associated widespread cultural influences have raised many important questions that have been widely discussed in popular books such as *Listening to Prozac*, *Prozac Nation*, *Let Them Eat Prozac*, *Talking back to Prozac*, and so on. At one extreme, for example, is the view that SSRIs don't really work at all and that they have been foisted on an unknowing and medically unsophisticated public by a cabal of drug companies and doctors who receive payoffs from promoting their use. Anybody who comes out and criticizes this status quo is immediately crushed by the huge financial resources available to the leaders of this international conspiracy. Another point that has been discussed is that, whether or not SSRIs really help people, there is data that they increase the likelihood that some individuals will think about and may actually commit suicide, and that such data has not been adequately considered or disseminated to patients and the public at large.

Another concern is that even if there are individuals who are helped by SSRIs, they are also given to huge numbers of people who don't really need them. This discussion is related to an ongoing debate about whether "cosmetic psychiatry" is really okay or not. Can SSRIs and other drugs be used to give people a leg up in a competitive society like ours? Is it reasonable to use performance-enhancing drugs in the widest sense of the word? This is not the place to discuss these arguments adequately. However, it would certainly be amazing if, with the vast profits at stake, pharmaceutical companies were not tempted to overstate their cases in some instances. As far as side effects like suicidality are concerned, this is certainly a serious issue. However, it is not unique to SSRIs. Numerous current lawsuits are attempting to support claims that many widely used anticonvulsant drugs also increase "suicidality." However, such effects are very small even if they do exist. We should always ask ourselves, what is the risk/benefit ratio? Should patients not take potentially helpful drugs because they cause side effects? This is always the question we must ask whenever a drug is prescribed, whatever the circumstances.

SSRIs BECOME SNRIs

Another question is, where we are going next in the pharmacological treatment of depression? One recent strategy is not all that innovative but may represent another small advance. The idea is that having removed norepinephrine from the equation when making the SSRIs, we should reintroduce it. After all, basic research and the action of the TCAs suggested that blocking norepinephrine uptake may also be a valid strategy. Indeed, as we have discussed, many of these drugs do block both 5-HT and norepinephrine uptake. While the SSRIs were being developed, certain other antidepressant drugs that don't primarily seem to work this way sneaked onto the market. Buproprion (Wellbutrin), for example, is not an SSRI but is one of the most widely prescribed antidepressants. The problem is that nobody really understands how it works, although prominent theories suggest that a major effect on norepinephrine uptake is part of the equation. Thus, many of the most recently introduced antidepressants are SNRIs; that is, "serotonin, norepinephrine reuptake inhibitors." If these sound a lot like TCAs, that is not surprising. Except of course they are not TCAs but completely different chemical structures. They don't necessarily have the same side effects as TCAs, and they may have a different balance of effects on the norepinephrine and serotonin uptake systems, which may indeed differentiate them from the original antidepressants. However, from the intellectual point of view they don't seem like a great advance. Nevertheless, drugs such as venlafaxine (Effexor) and duloxetine (Cymbalta) are now widely used and have even found some novel therapeutic indications. Thus, one should note the recent approval by the FDA for using duloxetine in the treatment of fibromyalgia.

Of course, just as with the other types of psychiatric disorders we have discussed, the development of fundamentally different approaches to the treatment of depression would be greatly helped by an understanding of the underlying neuropathology. Indeed, there are some odd things about the use of the available antidepressant drugs which nobody really understands. One of the major enigmas is the long period of time that it takes before the beneficial effects of the drugs manifest themselves. On the other hand, the effects of the drugs on biogenic amine uptake and metabolism in the brain occur immediately. Clearly, therefore, there is no direct one-to-one correlation between the degree of monoaminergic synaptic activity in the brain and mood.

As we discussed in the case of psychosis, modeling psychiatric disorders in animals with a view to furthering our understanding of these syndromes, as well as advancing drug development, is an extremely difficult task. Just as in the case of psychosis, there are animal models of depression. For example, there are tests like "learned helplessness." In such an experiment an animal is given a small negative stimulus like a mild shock from which it cannot escape. Eventually it gives up, and scientists imagine this is something akin to depression in humans. These animal models do have some validity, as they respond to currently available antidepressant drugs. Moreover, manipulations of animals using modifications of their genes in specific groups of neurons (specific gene targeting) has allowed scientists to learn more about the nerve pathways and molecules that are important mediators of depression. As we have also discussed, powerful animal models of disease often make use of genes that have been shown to be closely associated with the disease in question. In the case of schizophrenia, genes such as DISC1 are promising candidates, and animal models using these genes have been produced (Chapter 3). Unfortunately there are no such strong gene associations in the case of major clinical depression. This is naturally an extremely active area of investigation, and the genetics of the disease are slowly being unraveled. However, to date no major "depression genes" have emerged.

Animal models and human studies have started to define the neuroanatomical substrates for depression.[19] Areas of the brain such as portions of the cingulate cortex, amygdala, and hippocampus may exhibit changes in activity or cell volume. This makes a degree of sense, as such areas are known to be part of the brain's limbic system, which is an important mediator of mood and emotion. Translating such findings to humans, it has been shown that electrical stimulation of the cingulate cortex in some depressed human subjects produced a measure of relief from their symptoms. In the latest version of this type of experiment, mice were generated that had genes inserted into their prefrontal cortex that allowed the activity of these neurons to be stimulated by light. This is known as an "optogenetic" approach. Amazingly, when depression was induced in such mice using an animal model, the depression could be reversed by shining light on these nerve cells![20]

The involvement of limbic structures in depression fits well with the involvement of biogenic amines, because these brain areas are certainly innervated by neurons that utilize norepinephrine and 5-HT. However, as we have said, there is a pronounced temporal disconnect between the immediate effects of current antidepressant drugs on monoamine-mediated synaptic transmission and the weeks taken before their beneficial effects on the symptoms of depression become apparent. How can this be explained? The most likely explanation is that the development of antidepressant effects requires long-term changes in "synaptic plasticity" to occur. By synaptic plasticity we usually mean longer-term changes in the strength of synaptic communication. Among other things this may involve changes in the actual organization of synapses between neurons. Such alterations often require changes in the transcription of genes, translation of proteins, and synaptic morphology. These phenomena could be initiated by the increases in biogenic amines that are immediately produced. Downstream of these increases may be alterations in the expression of cytokines or growth factors in the brain that have been shown to be capable of producing changes in synaptic structure. The major candidate in this regard is a molecule called *brain derived neurotrophic factor* (BDNF).[20] Some studies have demonstrated that this protein molecule can produce effects in the nervous system which might be classified as "antidepressant." BDNF is highly expressed in the limbic system of the brain, and chronic stress—something that is generally associated with the development of depression—can reduce its expression. On the other hand, some antidepressant drugs tend to increase BDNF's levels of expression. BDNF exerts its effects by activating its receptor molecule TrkB, which is expressed by certain neurons in the brain. Activation of this receptor could then potentially drive the changes in gene expression that produce long-term changes in synaptic function. However, there is no simple relationship between expression levels of BDNF and the occurrence of depression. Indeed, other growth factors or cytokine-like molecules may act as modifiers of the effects of BDNF in specific areas of the brain, making its overall pattern of effects complex. Nevertheless, molecules like BDNF are good candidates for controlling the long-term synaptic changes initiated by monoamines in association with depression.

The role of such molecules may also help to explain another phenomenon observed in association with depression. It used to be thought that new neurons were not produced in the brain following the period of normal brain development. However, recent research has demonstrated that in a few areas of the brain there are residual populations of neural stem cells that are capable of producing new nerve cells in the adult brain—a process known as *neurogenesis*. In the dentate gyrus of the hippocampus, neurons are constantly dying and being replaced, fine-tuning the neuronal circuits associated with this key area of the brain. It has been consistently found that stress-related hormones such as corticosteroids reduce new neuron production in the adult dentate gyrus, and that this process can be reversed by some antidepressant drugs. Indeed, many of the major antidepressants such as Prozac actually require a degree of adult neurogenesis in order to be fully effective in animal models of depression. It is considered likely that these effects on adult neurogenesis are mediated by molecules like BDNF. Overall, the involvement of BDNF in depression is in line with current theories of both psychosis and depression, which are based on neurodevelopmental phenomena.

Although such research is certainly promising, it is not clear how long it will take before it can be "translated" into new therapies for treating human patients. My guess is that it will take a long time. In the meantime drug companies are struggling. The blockbuster drugs of the last 50 years are gradually going off-patent. What kinds of drugs will take their place? Making more blockers of biogenic amine uptake systems does not seem to be an alternative, as they are unlikely to be superior to those that have already been made. Since the 1970s the Eli Lilly Company has probably been the most successful in the world in developing new drugs for psychiatric disorders. Apart from Prozac, they have also marketed Zyprexa (olanzapine), an atypical antipsychotic, and Cymbalta (duloxetine), an SNRI that has also been marketed to treat fibromyalgia and several other syndromes. These three drugs have been fabulously successful but will all be off-patent in the not too distant future. Such a scenario is not unique to Eli

Lilly and Company, but is true for all the large pharmaceutical companies in the United States and Europe. It is hard to know where the new drugs will come from. Companies like Eli Lilly certainly do have many promising fields of research that have not yet been translated and could be productive in the future. There are certainly numerous neurotransmitter systems in the brain that have not yet been exploited pharmacologically and may yet prove to be important in the pathogenesis of depression. Interestingly, one of these is the glutamate system. Recent research appears to have shown that low concentrations of the glutamate receptor blocker ketamine may produce an antidepressant effect that is unusually rapid. However, the price of developing new drugs is becoming more and more expensive, leading to a possible scenario in which large pharmaceutical companies actually cease doing groundbreaking preclinical research in psychopharmacology and leave this task to others, their role reduced to developing and marketing promising new compounds discovered elsewhere. So are the days of the great pharmaceutical companies that generated the twentieth-century revolution in psychopharmacology coming to an end? *Quo vadis?*

NOTES

1. Stacey Pearson. *Song Ceramics: Objects of Admiration.* Percival David Foundation. 2003.
2. Sasha Su-Ling Welland. *A thousand miles of dreams: The journey of two Chinese sisters.* Rowman and Littlefield Publishing Group.
3. EJ Kahn Jr. *All in a century: The first 100 years of Eli Lilly and Company.* Eli Lilly Press. 1976.
   James H Madison. *Eli Lilly: A life 1885–1977.* Indiana Historical Society Press. 2006.
4. Maryann P. Feldman, Yda Schreuder. "Initial advantage: the origins of the geographic concentration of the pharmaceutical industry in the mid-Atlantic region." in *Industrial and corporate change.* 1996, 5:339–862.
5. The Republic of Jones. See http://yesteryear.clunette.com/jones.html.
6. David Healy. *Mania: A short history of bipolar disorder.* Johns Hopkins University Press. 2008.
   David Healy. *The creation of psychopharmacology.* Harvard University Press. 2002.
7. Carlo D'Este. *Warlord: A life of Winston Churchill at war, 1874-1945.* 2008.
8. Selfridges, Oxford Street. See http://www.westendatwar.org.uk/page_id__9_path__0p2p.aspx
9. Thomas Pynchon. *Gravity's Rainbow.* Penguin Books. 2006. The novel was first published in 1973. The ultimate "postmodernist" text, the novel has divided readers since it was first published between camps that think it is a masterpiece and those who think the entire thing is an enormous "put on." Tyrone Slothrop is the main protagonist in the novel.
10. Sandler M. Monoamine oxidase inhibitors in depression: history and mythology. *J Psychopharmacology.* 1009, 4:136–139.

11. López-Muñoz F, Alamo C. Monoaminergic neurotransmission: the history of the discovery of antidepressants from 1950s until today. *Curr Pharm Des.* 2009, 15(14):1563–1586.
López-Muñoz F, Alamo C, Juckel G, Assion HJ. Half a century of antidepressant drugs: on the clinical introduction of monoamine oxidase inhibitors, tricyclics, and tetracyclics. Part I: monoamine oxidase inhibitors. *J Clin Psychopharmacol.* 2007, 27(6):555–559.

12. Baumeister AA, Francis JL. Historical development of the dopamine hypothesis of schizophrenia. *J Hist Neurosci.* 2002, 11(3):265–277.

13. Wimbiscus M, Kostenko O, Malone D. MAO inhibitors: risks, benefits, and lore. *Cleve Clin J Med.* 2010, 77(12):859–882.

14. Healy D. Roland Kuhn (1912-2005). *History of Psychiatry.* 2006, 17:253–255.

15. Amara SG, Arriza JL. Neurotransmitter transporters: three distinct gene families. *Curr Opin Neurobiol.* 1993, 3(3):337–344.

16. Horn AS. The interactions of tricyclic antidepressants with the biogenic amine uptake systems in the central nervous system. *Postgrad Med J.* 1976, 52 (3 suppl):25–32.

17. Wong DT, Perry KW, Bymaster FP. Case history: the discovery of fluoxetine hydrochloride (Prozac). *Nat Rev Drug Discov.* 2005, 4(9):764–774.

18. http://theweek.com/article/index/205816/the-week-contest-fish-dish---august-13-2010

19. Krishnan V, Nestler EJ. The molecular neurobiology of depression. *Nature.* 2008, 455(7215):894–902.
Krishnan V, Nestler EJ. Animal models of depression: molecular perspectives. *Curr Top Behav Neurosci.* 2011, 7:121–147.

20. Covington HE 3rd, Lobo MK, Maze I, Vialou V, Hyman JM, Zaman S, LaPlant Q, Mouzon E, Ghose S, Tamminga CA, Neve RL, Deisseroth K, Nestler EJ. Antidepressant effect of optogenetic stimulation of the medial prefrontal cortex. *J Neurosci.* 2010, 30(48):16082–16090.

CHAPTER 5

ᴄᴠᴏ

The Cabinet of Doctor Snyder

"Who was the man who invented Laudanum? I thank him from the bottom of my heart, whoever he was. If all the miserable wretches in pain of body and mind, whose comforter he has been, could meet together to sing his praises, what a chorus it would be!"
Miss Gwilt, in *Armadale* by Wilkie Collins[1]

The eminent Victorian physician Sir William Osler once described the opiate drug morphine as "God's own medicine." Indeed, it is difficult to think of more influential drugs than opium and its derivatives. Opium has not only been important in therapeutics but in the entire world of recreational drug use. When we think of opium we tend to think of something mysterious, perhaps the opium dens in San Francisco's Chinatown or dank streets and alleyways in Victorian London. Indeed, it was on one foggy day deep into November that certain important facts concerning the nature of opium were revealed to me. It had been my habit, when visiting London, to spend some time rummaging around the used bookstores in Cecil Court.[2] My particular interests were in first editions illustrated by nineteenth-century artists. Many of these were children's books with drawings by Kate Greenaway, Walter Crane, and others. But not only children's books. Books of verse as well. On the afternoon in question, while stumbling through the mist, I found myself in Mr. Crompton's establishment where I purchased a book of verses by Edmund Spencer illustrated by Jessie M. King, an associate of Mackintosh and the Glasgow school. Mr. Crompton told me he had originally purchased it as part of a lot at Sotheby's from the estate of the late Mr. Aurelius Howard, a member of the famous Dorsetshire family. While going through it when I returned home, the following letter fell out from between its pages:

Euston Square, London, July 8th, 1869

Dear Mr. Collins

I must tell you how much I enjoyed meeting you again at your Bezique[3] evening in Portman Square last Thursday. It seems we are both quite obsessed with the game and it is a great pleasure for me to spend an evening with others similarly afflicted so that I do not have to pretend that I like it less than I do! The good Lord knows that there is no harm done when no money changes hands.

And that brings me to my subject, which is our obsessions and what we can do about them. This is something I did not want to bring up in company and would rather discuss privately as I now can. It seems that you make no secret about your use of laudanum ([4]). Indeed, what set me off was the comment made by Dr. Fergusson during the dinner. When you told him how much of the drug you routinely use at one time, he responded that this was enough to cause the death of every person seated around the table! Mr. Collins—like many others I have been an avid reader of your books over a number of years and have noted that opium frequently makes an appearance as a device which has an important role in the plot. Indeed, in your "Moonstone" it has pride of place and it could reasonably be said that the entire mystery revolves around its use. In "The Woman in White," an outstanding achievement I must say, opium plays a similarly important role and it makes cameo appearances in several of your other books. Clearly, therefore, you are certainly very well acquainted with opium and its effects. I think probably too well acquainted. It is with this in mind that I wanted to share with you some of my own experiences with the drug. Although you told us that you have taken it for many years for treatment of rheumatism and gout, I am sure that things have gone well beyond that stage at this point. Yes, I know it's for your nerves. You must have it! Indeed, as you know with these matters, you must have more and more of it all the time. It is clear that it has not had a detrimental effect on your prodigious imagination and your productivity. But will that always be the case? What happens during those times when you don't have quite enough of it at hand? The restlessness, sleeplessness, irritation and other phenomena—I have seen it in others who suffered from the same habit. And that is what I wanted to relate to you. Perhaps you have heard about some of it? My brother Gabriel and his wife Lizzie. Do you know what happened? I have written about it, although perhaps not everyone would understand this. You have to know where to look. But, I would like to explain to you the true nature of these events, what I have written, and my motivation for doing so. Perhaps it will give you some insight into your own situation, I do not know.

As you know Gabriel now has a secure reputation as a painter, at least with many people who have sophisticated taste. His work has been strongly supported by Mr. Ruskin, whose influence has helped bring the work of Gabriel and his friends into the public eye. But it was not always so. Like all artists in the beginning he had to struggle and had his share of criticism. Indeed, Gabriel and his coterie of friends deliberately provoked much of this. The group they formed and the manner in which they painted and even signed their work was designed to upset the *status quo*. Like many young artists they saw themselves as *agent provocateurs* and were certainly successful in this role. When he was first starting out as a painter one of his friends, Walter Deverell, introduced Gabriel to a model he had recently discovered. According to the argot of Gabriel's Preraphaelite brotherhood she was a "stunner." Deverell had espied Elizabeth Siddal working in a miliner's shop. After some persuasion she agreed to model for him and soon she was introduced to the rest of the Preraphaelite circle. Gabriel was immediately smitten with her, indeed the feeling was certainly mutual. When I first met "The Sid" I was also struck by her appearance, if not by her intellect. Not a beauty in the classic sense- but tall and slender with a straight back and a head of magnificent copper red hair. I tried to describe the effect in a poem.[5]

> She listened like a cushat dove
> That listens to its mate alone;
> She listened like a cushat dove
> That loves but only one.
> Not fair as men would reckon fair
> Nor noble as they count the line:
> Only as graceful as a bough,
> And tendrils of the vine:
> Only as noble as sweet Eve
> Your ancestress and mine
> And downcast were her dovelike eyes
> And downcast was her tender cheek
> Her pulses fluttered like a dove
> To hear him speak.

Lizzie was quickly taken up as the face of the Preraphaelites and, as I am sure you are aware, she appears in some great works. Millais' Ophelia is a case in point[6] (Figure 5.1).

I don't doubt her success as a model. Her striking looks certainly played an important role in the initial success of Gabriel and his friends. You may even have met her. I recall your brother Charles invited her to sit for him.[7] However, by that

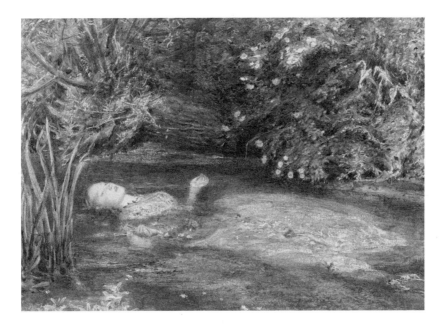

Figure 5.1:
Millais, Sir John Everett (1829–1896). Ophelia (w/c on paper).
Millais, Sir John Everett (1829–96) / Private Collection / Photo © Peter Nahum at The Leicester Galleries, London / The Bridgeman Art Library.

time she had become deeply involved with Gabriel in ways that had nothing to do with painting. His jealousy did not permit her to sit for others and she refused Charles saying she was too busy. Gabriel became totally obsessed with Lizzie and painted her to the virtual exclusion of everybody or everything else. Again I tried to explain the situation in verse—

> *One face looks out from all his canvases,*
> *One selfsame figure sits or walks or leans:*
> *We found her hidden just behind those screens,*
> *That mirror gave back all her loveliness.*
> *A queen in opal or in ruby dress,*
> *A nameless girl in freshest summer-greens,*
> *A saint, an angel—every canvas means*
> *The same one meaning, neither more or less.*
> *He feeds upon her face by day and night,*
> *And she with true kind eyes looks back on him,*
> *Fair as the moon and joyful as the light:*
> *Not wan with waiting, not with sorrow dim;*
> *Not as she is, but was when hope shone bright;*
> *Not as she is, but as she fills his dream.*[8]

I must confess I did not care for Lizzie, although on some level I understood the fascination she exerted upon my brother. What was she after all? A common girl, not from a class that made her Gabriel's equal in any respect. Indeed, most people in decent society would consider a girl who models as she did to be little better than a streetwalker. Nor was she his equal in talent or intellect. It is true that she had some aptitude for painting and poetry but it was not "immense" as Gabriel persisted in telling everybody. But then again her looks were striking and her manner could be ingratiating. In the end it was not just Lizzie who Gabriel loved, it was the poetry of his namesake Dante. He truly imagined himself to be that other Dante and Lizzie to be his Beatrice. His love for her was modeled on the ideal love of Dante for Beatrice with all its attendant frustrations. Lizzie was a fantasy. He didn't need Lizzie except perhaps as a model. She was a stone around his neck. I always looked after Gabriel and it was I that cared about him most. I repeat we didn't need Lizzie. Gabriel's relationship with Lizzie was a tragedy that we all watched unfurl act by act.

Lizzie was prone to great variations in her moods and she was often ill. There is no doubt that she was frequently depressed but whether her illnesses were real or figments of her imagination I cannot determine. One thing that was clear to me was that she used her illness to manipulate Gabriel. If ever he wanted to go away or do something she didn't like, she became "ill" and so he could not leave her. It is also true, however, that some of this was Gabriel's fault. In many ways she became completely dependent on him. Given the way she, an unmarried woman, was viewed by society she would have been completely destitute if he ever left her. Consequently she did her utmost to see that this never happened. She certainly would be more than insecure about the situation given the fact that he did not marry her. Whether I liked her or not it was clear that he had compromised her in every way and it was his duty to make her his wife. But he never did this, until it was too late....

Which brings me to Lizzie's use of laudanum, and its role in the course of events. She began taking the drug early on during her relationship with Gabriel, ostensibly for her diverse ailments and to help her with her depression. Soon, she could not do without it—a sentiment with which you, Mr. Collins, will I am sure have some sympathy. In the end it was not clear to me how many of her symptoms were being helped by the laudanum and how many were being caused by it. The complex interaction between taking the drug routinely, ceasing to take it and whatever ailments really afflicted her made all of this impossible to determine. At any rate her relationship with Gabriel declined along with her health; he being both greatly afflicted with feelings of guilt as well as whatever remained of his fantasy of Dante and Beatrice. Eventually Lizzie went down to Hastings to try to regain her health but her laudanum habit continued unabated. She became emaciated and paranoid. I am sure she believed above all that Gabriel would not be faithful to her while she was in Hastings and he was in London. Alerted to her sorry state he rushed down to Hastings and agreed to marry her. Indeed, to both Gabriel and Lizzie's great joy, she was soon pregnant, and the thought of their child seemed to alleviate her depression somewhat. However, it did not alleviate her laudanum habit.

Can you imagine trying to bear a child under such circumstances when one's body has been virtually destroyed by laudanum? I cannot and, of course, nobody was surprised when the tragedy entered its final act. The baby was stillborn. Lizzie was not to be consoled; she sank into the deepest melancholia and her laudanum use reached even greater heights in an effort to deaden the psychological and physical distress. Even the fact that she became pregnant once again could not divert her from the path which her life had finally taken.

One Monday evening in 1862 Gabriel and Lizzie decided to go out for dinner to one of their favorite haunts together with Swinburne[9] who was a very true friend to both of them. It seems as though the dinner went very well as a matter of fact. When it was over Lizzie and Gabriel returned home and it appears that she went to bed and fell asleep. Gabriel left her there and went out to attend to a teaching appointment. But Lizzie must have awakened while he was out and in her paranoid state she may have believed he was meeting a lover. When he returned he found her virtually comatose. Her bottle of laudanum, previously nearly full, was now half empty and a suicide note was pinned to her nightgown. In spite of the efforts of doctors and friends it proved impossible to rouse her and by the next morning she was dead. She was 32 years of age and pregnant. Gabriel was devastated as were many of their close friends. Swinburne wrote—"To one at least who knew her better than most of her husband's friends, the memory of all her marvelous charms of mind and person—her matchless grace, loveliness, courage, endurance, wit, humor, heroism, and sweetness—it is too dear and sacred to be profaned by any attempt at expression." For my part, however, if I am true to the Good Lord, I have to admit to a profound feeling of relief that my brother was free of this woman and for that I will be eternally guilty.

But of course he was never entirely free from her. Indeed, the story had a strange epilogue. At the inquest Gabriel did everything in his power to deflect any suspicion that Lizzie had died by her own hand, something that would prevent her from having a Christian burial. Thanks to his efforts she was buried in our family plot at Highgate. In accordance with his Dantesque fantasies, Gabriel placed a book of verses he had recently composed along with a bible entwined in her beautiful hair in her coffin. Yet even that was not the end of matters. Just this year Gabriel was persuaded by his publisher to attempt to retrieve the book of verses he had buried with Lizzie. In order to do so an application had to be made to the Home Secretary which was granted. This was all accomplished with the greatest secrecy and without my knowledge or that of Gabriel's mother or any other members of our family. Indeed, so as not to attract attention it was done in the dead of night. Gabriel did not have the presence of mind to attend. However, from what he subsequently learned and I have been told, a surprising sight awaited the few people who carried out the task by firelight. First Lizzie's corpse was still well preserved but naturally somewhat emaciated. However, when the lid was lifted from the coffin the contents gleamed so brightly in the light of the fire that the workmen had to shield their eyes. What could be responsible for such a phenomenon? It was, of course, Lizzie's hair that had continued to grow after her death and had eventually occupied the entire casket. Her copper locks, so famous in her life, were still triumphant in her death.

I have always been greatly disturbed by the role laudanum played in Lizzie's destruction ever since I became initially aware of the problem many years ago. I felt it necessary to write about it and perhaps give a warning to people who would neglect Our Lord's laws and abuse the use of drugs to this degree— something that appears very common these days. I had pondered this matter until one day I was visiting the Royal Academy, as I did on a regular basis. It was I believe in 1857. There I saw several pictures painted by Mr. Fitzgerald.[10] These pictures dealt with many things, but certainly laudanum was a central theme.

In one painting Mr. Fitzgerald depicted a scene which particularly caught my attention. The scene is highly reminiscent of Lizzie Siddle's death[11] (Figure 5.2).

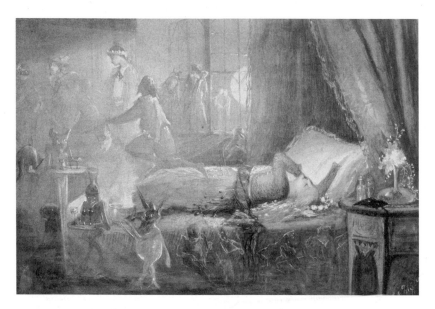

Figure 5.2:
Fitzgerald, John Anster (1832–1906). "The Stuff that Dreams are Made of" (w/c on paper). (see also 109712), Fitzgerald, John Anster (1832–1906) / Private Collection / Photo © The Maas Gallery, London / The Bridgeman Art Library.

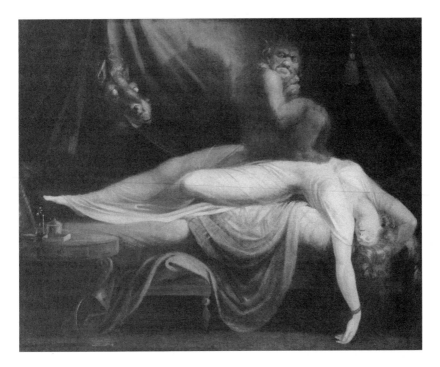

Figure 5.3:
Henry Fuseli (1741–1825). The Nightmare, 1781 (oil on canvas).
Detroit Institute of Arts, USA / Founders Society purchase with Mr. and Mrs. Bert L. Smokler / and Mr. and
Mrs. Lawrence A. Fleischman funds / The Bridgeman Art Library.

It reminded me of an earlier work painted by Mr. Fuseli many years ago[12]
(Figure 5.3). A young woman appears prostrate on her bed afflicted by night-
mares in both paintings. However, in Mr. Fitzgerald's picture laudanum has been
added as a factor that contributes to her dreams. As in Lizzie's case, the laudanum bottles can be observed on the young lady's side table. And here I also noted
something altogether remarkable—the agency by which the laudanum was given
to the victim. Goblins. These creatures are responsible for dispensing the drug to
her. Mr. Fitzgerald clearly feels that it is demons like these that must be responsible for urging us to sample laudanum and ensnaring us with it. Indeed, another
painting showed Mr. Fitzgerald himself also in a drug induced reverie with the
same goblins serving him his awful medicine[13] (Figure 5.4).

These images stirred my imagination and suggested a way in which I could
make the dangers of laudanum apparent by the use of poetic allegory. The result
was my poem called "Goblin Market."[14] I own that there are naturally many ideas
that are expressed in this poem, but the use of laudanum and my observation of
its effects upon Lizzie are certainly paramount among them. As I know you have
read the poem, there is no need for me to go over it in detail, but I shall take the
liberty of pointing out certain things.

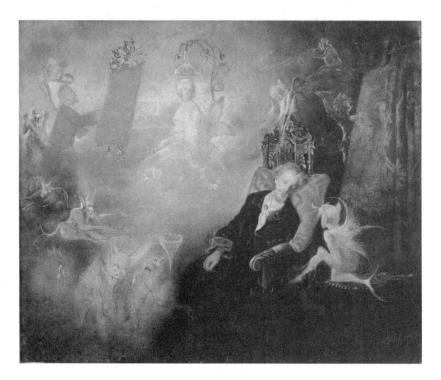

Figure 5.4:
Fitzgerald, John Anster (1832–1906). The Artist's Dream, 1857 (oil on millboard).
Private Collection / Photo © The Maas Gallery, London / The Bridgeman Art Library.

In the poem goblins attempt to seduce two young sisters into buying their "fruits." While the girls are out walking in the evening the goblins cry:

> *"Come buy our orchard fruits,*
> *Come buy, come buy:"*

The fruits they offer are not of an ordinary kind but magnificent and luscious to a fantastic degree. Laura is curious and impulsive, but Lizzie is cautious, remembering their friend Jeanie who had fallen prey to the goblins the previous year and had eaten their fruits but then:

> *"But ever in the moonlight*
> *She pined and pined away:*
> *Sought them by night and day.*
> *Found them no more, but dwindled and grew grey:"*

This is my warning to learn from others in which we have observed the terrible effects of laudanum.

Lizzie cautions Laura—

"*Their offers should not charm us,*
Their evil gifts would harm us."

Laura does not heed the warning. But she has no money. Now the goblins have her. They want to possess her body and soul, just as laudanum does. So Shylock like they demand corporal payment for their wares.

"*You have much gold upon your head,*
They answered all together:
Buy from us with a golden curl.
She clipp'd a precious golden lock...."

Laura gorges herself on the goblins' fruit. And then in a laudanum like trance—

"*And knew not was it night or day*
As she turn'd home alone."

But Laura is now trapped and can never find the goblins again or obtain satisfaction from their fruits.

"*Day after day, night after night,*
Laura kept watch in vain
In sullen silence of exceeding pain
She never caught again the goblin cry:"

Instead, she shows the signs of being caught in laudanum's net.

"*But when the noon wax'd bright*
Her hair grew thin and grey;
She dwindled, as the fair full moon doth turn
To swift decay and burn
Her fire away."

And:

"*She no more swept the house,*
Tended the fowls or cows,
Fetch'd honey, kneaded cakes of wheat,
Brought water from the brook:

But sat down listless in the chimney-nook
And would not eat".

But Lizzie can still hear the goblins call. She goes to them and proffers not her curls but real money to buy fruit to take to her sister. The goblins of course have other ideas—

"One may lead a horse to water,
Twenty cannot make him drink,
Though the goblins cuff'd and caught her,
Coax'd and fought her
Bullied and besought her,
Scratch'd her, pinch'd her black as ink,
Kick'd and knock'd her,
Maul'd and mock'd her.
Lizzie uttered not a word
Would not open lip from lip . . . ."

In the end the goblins do not get Lizzie or her money. Their spell is broken. She returns home covered with the juice and pulp of fruits used by the goblins in their assault. She is met by Laura:

"Lizzie, Lizzie, have you tasted
For my sake the fruit forbidden?
Must your light like mine be hidden,
Your young life like mine be wasted
Undone in mine undoing
And ruin'd in my ruin . . . "

Laura embraces Lizzie kissing her and sucking the fruit pulp from her body. But it is of no avail. She is the slave of laudanum. She needs it but will never again obtain real satisfaction from it. Laura suffers the pangs of her final humiliation by the goblins and their evil arts. She "dies" and is resurrected the next day finally cured.

Here then you will see the seductiveness of laudanum, how it seems to cure but later only to enslave. How I saw this happen to Lizzie Siddal. How its spell is so hard to break. How one needs the greatest help and support to do so. Mr. Collins would you not wish to be free of your slavery to laudanum? I believe you would. And there is one who would help you. The Lord Jesus is your greatest friend and source of help in your trials. It is to Him you must look.

It has seemed to me that a substance as dangerous as laudanum is far too easy to obtain. Indeed, this issue has been widely discussed. As you may be aware a law was just passed in the Parliament restricting its sale, so that one may only obtain it from a professional pharmacist. I worry however, that this might not give rise to a class of people who would sell it illegally in our backstreets. Then indeed a new class of goblins will have been born.

I wish you well

Sincerely,

Christina Rossetti[15]

OPIUM AND THE ANCIENTS

We have discussed the fact that the practice of psychotropic drug taking must be extremely ancient and how a good argument can be made for the use of natural hallucinogens in the development of religion (Chapters 1 and 2). However, some drugs, such as opium and its major active constituent morphine, have a special place in the history of drug use. Opium is not only one of the most ancient drugs, but it is also the most effective drug ever discovered for combating the most basic of all human complaints: pain. Whatever advances are made in medicine, nothing could really be more important than that. Not only does morphine occupy this fundamental place in therapeutics, but additionally the economies of several countries depend on the production of opiates. Opiates have a special place in the history of recreational drug taking and in the influence of drugs on artists and their works while simultaneously constituting a huge social and criminal problem throughout the world. Overall, I can say without any hesitation that morphine is the most significant chemical substance mankind has ever encountered.

The use and cultivation of poppies is very ancient.[16] Remains of poppies, such as their seeds, have been found in Neolithic tombs in Switzerland and other parts of central and southern Europe dating back to 4000 BC or even earlier. However, it is not clear how these poppies were being used. One should be aware that, although morphine probably occurs in at least small amounts in most kinds of poppies, it is only found in pharmacologically significant quantities in what is known as the "opium poppy," *Papaver somniferum*.[17] Moreover, even in *P. somniferum* opium is concentrated in certain parts of the plant, which don't really include the seeds. Different kinds of oils and other preparations that could be of practical importance can also be made from poppies; therefore, just finding the remains of the plant doesn't necessarily mean it was being used for its modern pharmacologically recognized properties.

Nevertheless, there is a story that suggests that this was indeed the case. It is clear that poppies were cultivated in ancient Sumer. What appear

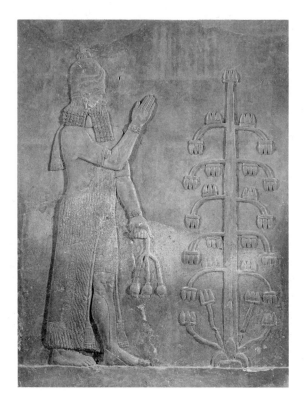

Figure 5.5:
Bas relief of a Genie carrying a poppy. Khorsabad 10th–6th BCE.
(Lessing Photo Archive)

to be opium poppies are pictured in certain Mesopotamian bas reliefs (Figure 5.5).

In the 1920s several tablets were recovered from the palace of the Assyrian king Ashurbanipal at Nineveh. These tablets were dated to around 1700 BC, but some appear to contain the Sumerian names of drugs copied from around 3000 BC. The poppy is included in these records. This might also indicate the antiquity of the poppy, although it is not clear that the plant that is referred to in these records is *P. somniferum* rather than a non-narcotic wild poppy such as *Papaver rhoeas*. In addition, a clay tablet ideogram dating from Nippur in the third millennium BC appears to describe the poppy. It is said that this ideogram can be translated into English as "joy plant." If this were truly the case then we would imagine that the Sumerians knew a thing or two about the psychological effects of opium. This interpretation has been widely disseminated. I would like to believe it but unfortunately, as we have seen from the work of John Marco Allegro (Chapter 1), translating Sumerian is not a straightforward business. Some scholars have translated the Sumerian ideogram for poppy as "bitter melon" or possibly "cucumber" which isn't quite as interesting. Others have claimed the Assyrian bas reliefs do not illustrate opium poppies but fly swatters[18] (Figure 5.5)! Further evidence that the ancient Egyptians used opium is similarly equivocal. So, all we can really say is that the ancients certainly knew about poppies and cultivated them, and that with any luck they were aware of their psychological effects as well. At any rate it makes a good story.

By the time we get to the Hellenistic and Roman periods, however, there is no doubt that opium poppies were being cultivated for more or less the same purposes as they are used today. Clear indications of this exist in the sophisticated writings of Greek and Roman medical practitioners.[16],[19] Nevertheless, there are still mysteries. In the Odyssey, written around 800 BC, Homer refers to nepenthe, the drug that "chases away sorrow." Just as with soma in the Rigveda (Chapter 1), a large literature has speculated about the true nature of this drug. Opium appears the clear winner in this debate, but here again we will never know for certain. Around 70 AD the Greek physician Dioscorides of Anazarbus composed his *Materia Medica,* one of the most important works in the entire history of medicine, in which he described the many uses of opium. Some of these are strikingly modern. For example, he described a process in which poppy capsules are first boiled in water. This extract was then boiled again with honey to produce syrup. This could then be cooled to form individual tablets that could be sucked for relief of pain, cough, or diarrhea. The analogy with modern cough drops that can be purchased in a drug store is certainly quite obvious. Indeed, from this point of view things have changed little over several millennia.

Dioscorides also describes something else that has basically not changed over the years, and that is the method of harvesting what is known as crude opium from the poppy. The highest concentration of opium is contained in a milky sap or "latex," which is found throughout the plant but mostly in the seedpod.[17],[19] Once the delicate petals of the plant have fallen off, a small pea-sized seedpod is revealed. This matures in size over the next couple of weeks, after which time it is ready to harvest. In Dioscorides' day the traditional method for doing this was to slash the seedpod with a special knife. If this is done in the afternoon, some of the latex will have oozed out and this exudate ("poppy tears") will congeal on the seedpod and can be scraped off the next morning (Figure 5.6).

This technique is known as "tapping" and a virtually identical method is still used today in places like Afghanistan. To stop any buildup of latex on the knife, which would result in its inefficiency, the blade is frequently

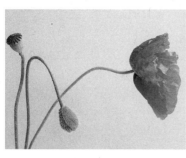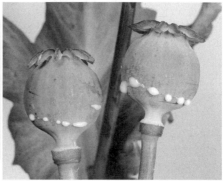

Figure 5.6:
Papaver somniferum, the opium poppy.
(Matka Wariatka © Photoscom)
Poppy "tears" of poppy latex during the opium harvest.
(Nigel Cattlin / Alamy)

washed. In many places, however, the peasant farmers who carry out this work will just lick the blade instead—one of the bonuses of the job. The latex is then sun dried for several days, after which it is shaped into balls or squares and stored. Prior to further use such as smoking, the crude opium is "cooked" by macerating it in boiling water and removing any detritus. The aqueous extract can then be further concentrated by evaporation to form a thick paste. Such opium is now ready to be smoked or processed further. These days, poppies grown for the modern pharmaceutical industry may bypass the traditional opium harvesting technique, and dried opium pods along with other parts of the plant (a preparation known as "poppy straw") can be directly used instead.

The most influential of all of the Greek physicians was certainly Galen of Pergamon (born AD 129), whose 20-volume *Opera Omnia* collected virtually all of the medical knowledge of his day.[19] The ideas he described became the basis for the way medicine was practiced from Roman times through the Middle Ages and beyond. Galen taught that disease was due to an imbalance of the four basic humors, an idea that he developed from Hippocrates' works. He also taught that bringing these humors into balance once more could cure diseases. Drugs like opium could be employed for this purpose. Among other things Galen acted as a physician to the emperor Marcus Aurelius. Galen writes that the emperor used to take medicines known as *Mithridatium* or *Theriac*. These were basically a mishmash of various herbs and other ingredients, of which opium was certainly one of the most important. Galen would regulate the opium content of the preparation according to the daily dictates of Marcus Aurelius' life—for example, whether he needed a good night's sleep or to feel very energetic. However, although the emperor regularly took opium-containing mixtures he was apparently not addicted to the drug, Galen saying that he could always cut back if he wanted to.

OPIUM AND ALCHEMY

Following the decline of Roman influence, opium trading was taken up by other nations including the Arabs, Venetians, and Portuguese. Galenic theories of medicine were still generally in the ascendancy during this time, although this began to change somewhat in the sixteenth century with the influence of alchemists such as the famous Phillipus Aureolus Theophrastus Bombastus von Hohenheim (aka Paracelsus). Paracelsus wrote extensively on topics ranging from magic to something akin to a genuine approach to therapeutics.[20] He encouraged the use of specific drugs to treat specific diseases, rather than an approach based on the balancing of humors. In this way his approach to medicine can be seen as more recognizably modern. He suggested things such as the use of different metals including zinc and mercury for treating diseases, and he was also very keen on the use of opium, which he now formulated in a new way. Paracelsus extracted opium with alcohol to form a tincture to which other ingredients could also be added. He called this preparation "laudanum" from the Latin *laudare,* to praise, and encouraged its use for a variety of purposes. Indeed, at that time opium was one of the only drugs available that might at least have been of some value under a variety of circumstances. As it was a liquid, laudanum was also easily administered and its popularity grew under the influence of Parcelsus and his many disciples. However, it should be noted the drug was used as a medicine rather than for any purely recreational purpose. Different individuals formulated their own versions of laudanum by adding diverse ingredients, but the basic ingredient was always opium extracted into alcohol. The English doctor Thomas Sydenham, regarded as one of the founders of modern medicine, devised a laudanum recipe consisting of 2 ounces of opium, 1 once of saffron, a dram of cinnamon and cloves, all dissolved in a pint of Canary (Spanish) wine. Sydenham and his colleagues throughout Europe recommended the use of laudanum for a wide variety of complaints, and its use in therapeutics began to increase rapidly.

One can get some kind of idea as to how the use of laudanum was viewed around this time from an account written in 1700 by Dr. John Jones in his book *Mysteries of Opium Reveal'd,* perhaps the first book to be entirely devoted to this topic.[21] Dr. Jones reveals himself to be "Chancellor of Landaff, a Member of the College of Physicians in London and a former Fellow of Jesus College, Oxford." It is clear from his book that he must have been very well acquainted with the effects of opium, as he describes both its good and bad effects with great accuracy. Jones also paid attention to the psychological effects of the drug, which was rather an original consideration at the time. Perhaps he was himself an addict? Indeed, one can assume that along with the increasingly wide use of laudanum at that time came an increasing addiction problem, although it was not necessarily considered as such in a modern sense. Dependency upon opiates was more or less regarded as just a side effect of the drug, and would not necessarily be perceived as problematic. Jones was clearly aware of both the acute and chronic effects of opiate use. When considering the acute effects of opium, Jones recommends them to us in the following terms.

"It causes a most agreeable, pleasant, and charming sensation about the Region of the Stomach, which if one lies, or sits still, diffuses it self in a kind of indefinite manner, seizing one not unlike the gentle, sweet Deliquium that we find upon our entrance into a most agreeable Slumber, which upon yielding to it, generally ends in Sleep: But if the Person keeps himself in Action, Discourse, or Business, it seems (especially when given in a Morning, after a moderate Rest at Night) like a most delicious and extraordinary Refreshment of the spirits upon very good News, or any other great cause of Joy, as the sight of a dearly beloved Person, etc. thought to have been lost at Sea, or the like, causing such a pleasant Ovation of the Spirits, Serenity, etc. as we find after a competent Measure of generous Wine ad Hilaritatern, (as Men use to say.)"

On the other hand, he says that if one has been taking the drug for some time and then stops—

"Great, and even intolerable Distresses, Anxieties, and Depressions of Spirits, which in few days commonly end in a most miserable Death, attended with strange Agonies, unless Men return to the Use of Opium; which soon raises them again, and certainly restores them; if it has time to operate, before they die; which it soon does in a liquid Form. Or, if they have not Opium, or will not take it, they must use Wine very plentifully, and often as a substitute to the Opium, tho' it doth not perform half as well as Opium."

It is really not possible to find a better description of the acute and chronic effects of opiates even today.

THE INVESTIGATION OF OPIUM

Thus, during the eighteenth century laudanum was being widely used in Europe as an analgesic, as well as a treatment for sleeplessness, diarrhea, vomiting, cough, and a number of mental and nervous complaints. The eighteenth century also ushered in the dawn of modern scientific attempts to explain opium's mechanism of action, part of the awakening of recognizably modern scientific approaches and methodologies that followed the writings of Francis Bacon in the previous century. Of course real progress was difficult to make because of the nonstandardized preparations of opium used in these studies, which presumably contained widely differing amounts of active ingredients. Nevertheless, even in the late seventeenth century some "experiments" had been performed with opium, although these were generally directed to discovering novel methods for administering the drug rather than understanding its mechanism of action per se.[19] In fact, no lesser lights than Christopher Wren and Robert Boyle actually utilized a primitive form of intravenous drug administration by using the quill of a pen to inject opium into the vein of a dog, which they reported became extremely "stupefied." A similar study was carried out in Germany at around the same time by Major and Elsholtz, who injected opium intravenously into dogs. The dogs seemed to fall asleep. In order to ensure that this was truly the case, Elsholtz came up with what he considered to be a critical test. He argued that as these were very well trained German hunting dogs, they would always obey their masters. He therefore bellowed hunting commands at the dogs. The dogs slept on. Hence, Elsholtz concluded that the dogs were indeed in a deep sleep and the drug must have been fully effective.

In the eighteenth century one interesting view of the action of opium developed in the context of what was known as the Brownian, or Bruonian, system or theory of medicine developed by the Scottish physician Dr. John Brown around 1780.[22] The fundamental principle in Brown's system, as detailed in his *Elements of Medicine,* was that of "excitability." By this he meant a basic quality of living matter resulting in "a capacity to perceive outside impressions and the ability to respond to them." Brown suggested that some diseases were the result of a lack of excitability, which he called "asthenia," as opposed to an adequate degree of excitability or "sthenia." Indeed, Brown believed that most diseases represented states of asthenia and that they could be corrected by agents that increased excitability. The Bruonian system was widely adopted in the practice of medicine and was extremely influential throughout Europe, even influencing the early German Romantics such as Novalis who wrote several essays on the topic. Brown suffered greatly from gout and had found opium to be a very effective treatment. As he thought that gout was due to a state of asthenia, he recommended that opium was "the strongest and most diffusible stimulant" capable of powerful excitation and the correction of asthenia. This "explained" the widespread effectiveness of the drug for the treatment of so many diseases.

True pharmacological research on the mechanism of action of opium in the modern sense began around 1742 with the work of Charles Alston, Professor of Botany and Materia Medica at the University of Edinburgh.[19] Alston performed studies in which he compared the effects of opium in normal frogs to those that had been experimentally manipulated in some manner (extirpation of the heart, decapitation, or pithing). He concluded that the initial site of action of opium was on the nerves rather than by diffusion through the bloodstream. Such a hypothesis was supported by other observations demonstrating that following oral administration of the drug to animals, virtually all of the material remained intact in the stomach even though a strong drug response was observed. Hence it was believed that nerves innervating the stomach must be where the drug exerted its effects. On the other hand, the ability of the drug to produce effects when administered directly into the bloodstream must be due to effects on nerves that innervated the blood vessels. However, later work challenged this view and suggested that opium first had to be absorbed and enter the blood that would carry it to its site of action. In the end a combined model arose that contained elements of both these previous theories and suggested that opium first entered the blood that carried it to its site of action on nerves. Such a conclusion allows us to see the first inklings of what we might consider a theory of drug action in the modern sense of the word.

However, it was in the nineteenth century that our understanding of the mechanism of opiate action really progressed, and when the manner in which the drug was used in Western society changed irrevocably. There were two important breakthroughs in the early years of the nineteenth century with respect to the future of opium use. The first was scientific and the second was cultural. The first breakthrough answered the question as to the identity of the active chemical principles contained in opium. This led to the development of new opiate drugs and provided precise scientific information as to how opiates produced their effects. The second breakthrough occurred in the context of the use of opium by artists and an appreciation of its psychological potential.

THE IDENTIFICATION OF MORPHINE

By the start of the nineteenth century the science of organic chemistry was in its infancy and just starting to emerge as a powerful method of scientific investigation (Chapter 3). One branch of this subject that was extremely active involved trying to address the question as to the identity of important chemical components that could be isolated from natural products. In this way it was thought that one might isolate the active principles from sources like the opium poppy or cinchona bark, the source of quinine, these being two of the most important drugs available at the time. Solvent extraction of natural products followed by crystallization was one of the new methods utilized in these investigations. In the late eighteenth century the great Swedish chemist Carl Wilhelm Scheele had isolated gallic, malic, oxalic, and citric acids from various plants by using such methods. These studies gave rise to the notion that active substances isolated from natural products were acidic in nature. Interestingly, although it was originally thought that the best way to test the activity of such compounds was by self-experimentation, the realization that some of them might be toxic led to the decision to perform animal testing instead. This led Rudolf Bucheim to set up what was virtually the first university pharmacology laboratory in Dorpat, Estonia. He was succeeded there by his student Oswald Schmiederberg, who eventually moved to the University of Strasbourg where he established the leading school of experimental pharmacology in the nineteenth century and went on to train many of the scientists who contributed to Germany's dominance in this subject, which lasted up to the start of the Second World War (Chapter 3).

In contrast to the notion that active plant constituents were acidic in nature, Charles Louis Derosne, working in Paris in 1803, crystallized a substance from opium which appeared to have alkaline properties, although he was unsure what to make of this and thought that his results might be due to some contamination by potash used in the preparation. On the other hand, a couple of years later, a young German pharmacist named Wilhelm Friedrich Serturner also extracted and crystallized a substance from opium, whose narcotic activity was demonstrated by administration to dogs.[16,19] Serturner described the substance as having "an almost alkali like character." However, his discovery failed to cause much of a stir because it was published in a "low impact" journal (alas, some things never change). Serturner named his new substance *morphium*, after Morpheus the god of sleep from Ovid's *Metamorphosis*. Over the next decade Serturner published a series of papers further describing the properties of morphium, particularly the ease with which it reacted with acids to form readily crystallizable salts. Further studies in which he and three students all took 100mg of morphium, resulting in the symptoms of opium poisoning over the next few days, were also reported. At this point one of Serturner's publications was read by Joseph Gay-Lussac,

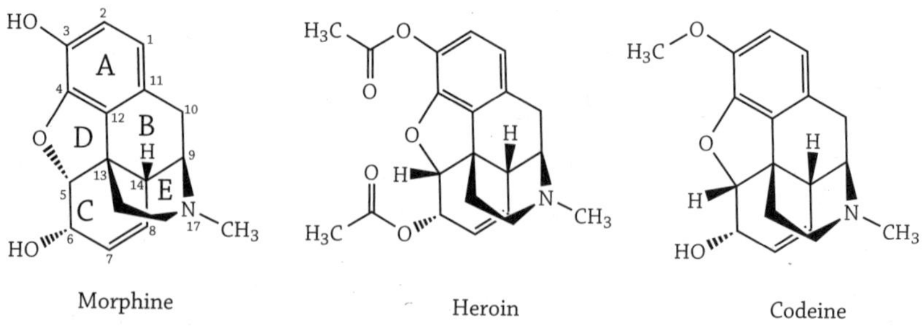

Figure 5.7:
Morphine, its diacetyl derivative heroin, and its methoxy derivative codeine.

the most prominent living French chemist, who had it translated into French and published in a high-profile French journal. Now the work was widely read and its importance appreciated. Gay-Lussac also had the foresight to predict that morphium might be the harbinger of an entirely new class of plant-derived molecules with basic characteristics. He suggested that the names of such compounds should all end in the suffix "ine." So, *morphium* became *morphine* (Figure 5.7). A few years later the term *alkaloid* was suggested to describe this new class of plant-derived basic molecules.

Serturner's work and approach stimulated a search for similar types of natural products from other sources that was met with considerable success, including the isolation of quinine by Pelletier in 1820 and cocaine by Neimann in 1860. It should come as no surprise that the drug that had been used for millennia as "opium" is anything but a pure substance and actually contains an enormous number of active molecules.[17] However, the major narcotic effects of opium are due to the presence of morphine and, to a somewhat lesser extent, to a closely related molecule named *codeine,* which was isolated from opium by Robiquet in 1832 (Figure 5.7). In the same year another related alkaloid named *thebaine* was also isolated. Thebaine has no narcotic activity but has played a key role in further chemical development of opiate drugs. In fact, the actual chemical structure of morphine was not elucidated until 1923 by Gulland and Robinson at the University of St. Andrews, and its total synthesis was first achieved by Gates and Tschudi at the University of Rochester in 1950. There are numerous other alkaloids found in opium, many of which have biological activities of one kind or another and may contribute to the overall experience of taking opium. However, morphine is clearly the most important of these, and morphine and codeine are the only constituents that have the characteristics of narcotic drugs.

DE QUINCEY AND THE RISE OF ROMANTICISM

A second important change that occurred at the end of the eighteenth and start of the nineteenth centuries concerned the recreational use of opiates. The use of opiates by artists in the nineteenth century and their "discovery" of its psychological effects should be considered in the context of simultaneous discoveries concerning the nature of the subconscious in general, not only in the development of psychiatric medicine but also in the arts.[27] The Romantic Movement, which developed around the start of the nineteenth century, was a reaction against the Classicism of the eighteenth century. Romanticism encouraged artists to give vent to their emotions and sensory responses to events. Artists turned their attention inwards and began to explore their inner psychological landscape as a source of material for their work. In this respect, dreams and other subconscious phenomena began to take on particular importance. The association of opium with sleep and dreaming meant that it became a tool, albeit sometimes an unwitting one, in shaping an individual's dream world, and much has been written and speculated upon concerning the influence of opium on the output of many nineteenth-century artists.[23,27]

Indeed, many of the artistic movements of the last two centuries, including Romanticism, Symbolism, and Surrealism, have been concerned with aspects of the subconscious. Artists of every type became fascinated by the nature and purpose of dreaming as well as other manifestations of subconscious activity, and opium and other psychotropic drugs were certainly influential in this development at every step of the way.[27] Pride of place must go to two great writers, the poet Samuel Taylor Coleridge and the essayist Thomas De Quincey. Coleridge was a highly experimental person in all aspects of life, and in his youth was a close friend of the pioneering doctor Thomas Beddoes, who discovered "laughing gas" (nitrous oxide), about which Coleridge wrote extensively. Coleridge was prescribed opium for medicinal purposes early in his life, and he became heavily addicted to the drug. The role of opium-infused dreaming in the genesis of *Kubla Khan* and the *Rime of the Ancient Mariner* have long been discussed.[23]

De Quincey pushed the envelope even further. Instead of being an influence on the subject matter used by the author, opium became the subject matter. In the 1820s De Quincey published a series of articles in the *London* magazine, which were then collected together the next year as *The Confessions of an English Opium Eater*. Some years later De Quincey took up this theme again in his unfinished *Suspiria de Profundis*. In these books De Quincey described his very personal experiences with opium, not as a medicine but in terms of its effects on his psyche.[23,24] He recounts that on one

Sunday afternoon in 1804, while he was an undergraduate at Oxford, he was visiting London. He had been troubled by painful neuralgia for some time and went into a chemist's shop in Oxford Street and purchased a small amount of laudanum. He says that not only did it help with his pain but allowed him to enter "an abyss of divine enjoyment." He relates how, under the influence of laudanum, he would wander around London exploring the streets and describes his descent into the demimonde, including how he consorted with and befriended prostitutes. He also describes attending events like the opera and how laudanum allowed him to deepen his experience and to appreciate such things more profoundly.

De Quincey was a regular although not heavy user of laudanum over the next decade and certainly not an addict. However, after he left Oxford (without a degree in spite of his brilliant performance) he went to live with his friend, the great romantic poet Wordsworth. Here he suffered diverse health and personal problems and began to use laudanum much more heavily, eventually becoming entirely addicted to it. His involvement with laudanum then ebbed and flowed over his lifetime, ranging from astronomically high levels of addiction and dependence to stringent efforts to abstain from the drug altogether, something he never succeeded in accomplishing.

During all of this time he married, had a family, and managed to carry on an active career as an essayist and critic addressing many issues with considerable wit (e.g., "On murder considered as one of the fine arts").[24] In the extreme depths of his addiction, De Quincey also experienced many of the negative effects of the drug, including horrifying dreams, a degree of paranoia, and sometimes the effects of partial drug withdrawal. *The Confessions of an English Opium Eater* is essential reading for anyone interested in the history of recreational drug taking. Additionally, the 1962 movie *Confessions of an Opium Eater,* directed by Albert Zugsmith (whose other efforts included such things as *Sex Kittens Go to College* and *The Private Lives of Adam and Eve*) may well be worth your time. The movie stars Vincent Price as Thomas De Quincey, who gets involved in an adventure in San Francisco that includes drug trafficking and an Asian sex slaves racket.[25] One might argue that the director has taken certain liberties with De Quincey's original conception—but I digress.

ARTISTIC ENDEAVORS

With De Quincey we have clearly encountered a paradigm shift in the practice of drug taking. His descriptions of the personal psychological effects of the drug pointed the way toward the next logical step. After this, others argued that although Coleridge and De Quincey may have originally taken laudanum for medicinal purposes, and then have experienced artistically interesting "side effects," why not discard the medicinal component altogether and just take the drugs for their side effects? This theme was particularly championed by the members of the Club des Hashischins (literally the "Club of the Hashish Eaters") in Paris, who experimented widely with the use of cannabis and laudanum as an aid to their artistic endeavors. Charles Baudelaire, a key member of the Paris group, actually translated De Quincey's work into French and it was used virtually as a bible by him and his colleagues.[26] Indeed, De Quincy can be seen as a key figure in the development of recreational drug taking in Europe and the United States. Much has been written on the use of laudanum by numerous other nineteenth-century artists including Wilkie Collins, whose novels frequently employ laudanum as a key plot device. Poe also frequently utilized opium in his stories, using it to produce a Gothic romantic atmosphere. Examples also exist of the influence of opium-taking in music. The example always quoted, and it is certainly a good one, is Berlioz's *Symphonie Fantastique*. Here Berlioz supplied a specific program that went along with his symphony, describing it as the reveries of a young rejected lover who had "Poisoned himself with opium."

The influence of opium in nineteenth-century painting is also easy to see, even when it is not explicitly stated. Sleep, often used as a metaphor for death, as well as dreams are frequently portrayed. The atmosphere is sensual and ponderous—everything is very still. The heavy lidded, somnolent models beloved of the Pre-Raphaelites, and the dreamy canvases of symbolist painters such as Puvis de Chavannes, all suggest the influence of opiates[27] (Figure 5.8).

There are several other important events to consider when describing the practice of opiate use in the nineteenth century. Although laudanum remained the preparation used for many years, the isolation of pure morphine by Serturner meant that use of the pure drug eventually began to take over as the preparation of choice. The invention of the hypodermic syringe by the Scottish physician Dr. Alexander Wood in 1853 provided a much more direct method of drug administration. The use of laudanum gradually declined with the arrival of pure morphine, as well as some of its semisynthetic derivatives. Opiate use has remained a powerful influence on artists up to the present day. The works of William Burroughs and Irvine Welsh spring immediately to mind. However, in the twentieth and twenty-first centuries most opiate-influenced literature is no longer devoted to the effects of opium and laudanum but to the effects of their modern manifestation, the drug heroin.

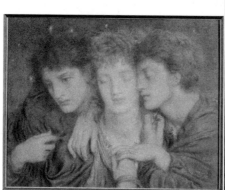
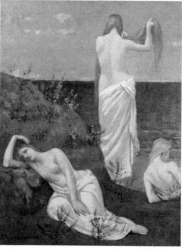

Figure 5.8:
Examples of dreamy opiate-influenced paintings from the latter part of the nineteenth century. Right: Puvis de Chavannes, Pierre (1824–1898).
Young Girls by the Sea, before 1894 (oil on canvas).
Musee d'Orsay, Paris, France / Giraudon / The Bridgeman Art Library.
Left: Solomon, Simeon (1840–1905). Sleepers and One that Waketh, 1871 (w/c on paper).
© Leamington Spa Art Gallery & Museum / The Bridgeman Art Library.

OPIATES AND THE INDUSTRIAL REVOLUTION

I do not wish to suggest that the widespread use of opium and laudanum in the nineteenth century was entirely the provenance of artists. Nothing could be further from the truth. Opiate use was extremely widespread at all levels of society, and opiates were much more freely available than they are today, even after laws were passed in 1868 attempting to restrict their sales to trained pharmacists. The problem was that the law didn't cover numerous patent medicines that contained opium as their major ingredient. This included things such as Dover's Powders, Paregoric, or Dr. Collis Browne's Chlorodyne—the latter actually a mixture of tinctures of opium and cannabis, originally designed as a medicine for those suffering from cholera.

In the United States, opiate-containing patent medicines were also widely used, particularly in the context of the bloody Civil War when wounded soldiers frequently availed themselves of these preparations (both for pain relief and for their antidiarrheal effects). The use of opiates in the United States at this time was so great, and drug addiction among the military so common, that it became known as "soldier's disease." Many of the patent medicines available were relatively cheap and were therefore affordable by all members of society both in Europe and America.

Of course, the development of nineteenth-century society and its habits cannot be dealt with adequately without due consideration of the effects of the Industrial Revolution.[16] This produced vast population movements from the countryside to industrial centers such as Manchester, where many migrant workers were employed in factories, frequently under extremely poor conditions. Young mothers had to go to work, leaving their children at home to be cared for by elderly relatives or other minders. On returning home these unfortunate women might only think about how to get a good night's sleep rather than the stresses of looking after their children. Medicines were therefore developed specifically intended to keep children quiet. These included things such as Godfrey's Cordial and Mrs. Winslow's Soothing Syrup (Figure 5.9). The effects of the latter were commemorated by the composer Edward Elgar, whose Adagio cantabile for Wind Quintet was so named—the smooth chromaticism of the piece clearly intended to invoke the tranquility produced by the narcotic concoction. Such patent medicines contained large amounts of opiates, and so the children taking them were apt to be very quiet indeed and spend a great deal of their time in an opiate-induced slumber. Hence by the dawn of the twentieth century it can be seen that the use of opiates in one form or another was endemic to all parts of Western society—the rich and the poor, poets and peasants.

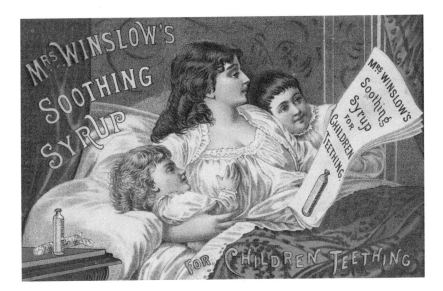

Figure 5.9:
Mrs. Winslow's soothing syrup. One highly regarded opiate containing nineteenth-century patent medicine widely used for "calming" babies.
(Associated Press)

As we shall discuss, the recreational use of opium per se is not common these days in Western countries—other opiates like heroin are used instead. Nevertheless, the concept of "opium" has become deeply ingrained in our collective consciousness and it is associated with several important Romantic aspects of our lifestyle. Imagine, for example, that you are running a large cosmetics company and you have a new multibillion dollar perfume to bring to market. You would have to be extremely careful as to what you called it and how you presented it. One of the most successful new perfumes in recent decades was Yves St. Laurent's Opium. The advertising campaign for the perfume was very clever indeed. Consider the model pictured in one of these advertisements (Figure 5.10). Now consider Dante Gabriel Rossetti's famous painting "Beata Beatrix." Rossetti painted this portrait of his wife Elizabeth Siddal, who had killed herself by taking an overdose of laudanum. Elizabeth is portrayed as Dante's Beatrice and the manner of her death is commemorated by the presence of the bird carrying an opium poppy in its beak. The model in the Opium campaign, with her obviously Pre-Raphaelite sensibilities, clearly harks back to romantic images of this type. One may also note that the container for the perfume is in the form of a netsuke, indicating an oriental association. Of course, we know that the British were responsible for much of the production and marketing of

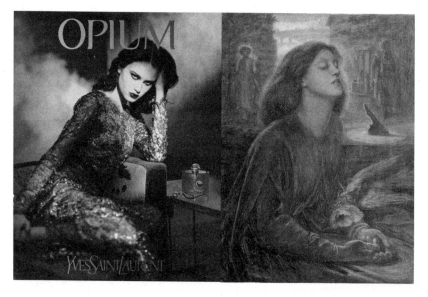

Figure 5.10:
Right: Dante Gabriel Rossetti (1828–1882). Beata Beatrix (oil painting).
Royal Pavilion, Libraries & Museums, Brighton & Hove / The Bridgeman Art Library.
Left: A Pre-Raphaelite influenced advertisement for Opium perfume.
(courtesy of the Advertising Archives)

opium in the Far East and fought several wars with the Chinese to ensure their preeminence in this regard. The association of opium with the romantic and mysterious East is something that everybody understands, and so the advertisement taps into our collective subconscious.

HEROIC ACTS

In parallel with all of the changes in the way opiates were regarded and used in the last two centuries came changes in the opiates themselves. As we have seen, the natural opiate products isolated from the poppy are morphine and codeine. Following their identification it was not long before chemical changes to these molecules were introduced in an effort to try and improve them. In this particular case "improve" meant, above all other things, discovering opiates that were as effective as morphine but which were not addictive.

One of the first attempts to do this also proved to be one of the most significant.[29] Although not the first semisynthetic derivatives of morphine to be produced (which was its quaternary ammonium salt), Charles Alder Wright prepared esters of morphine and codeine, including acetylcodeine and mono- and diacetylmorphine, and reported studies on their properties in 1874. These new derivatives were not reported to produce any particularly remarkable effects in animal tests, and the work basically went unnoticed.

Several other tests were performed over the next few years on diacetylmorphine, and reports as to its analgesic activity remained somewhat variable. E. Merck and Company in Germany next synthesized ethylmorphine, a structure very similar to that of codeine, and observed that it had cough-suppressant properties similar to those of codeine, which was already being widely used in the treatment of coughing.

Merck and Company marketed ethylmorphine in January of 1898 as a cough suppressant, making it the first semisynthetic derivative of morphine to reach the market. In 1895 a team led by Arthur Eichengruen at Bayer also began preparing derivatives of morphine, and rediscovered diacetylmorphine in 1897. Heinrich Dreser at Bayer tested diacetylmorphine and demonstrated that it slowed and deepened respiration in rabbits. He therefore imagined that, like codeine, it might be used to treat respiratory complaints. He tested the molecule as a cough suppressant and found it to be highly effective, especially in tuberculosis patients. The story goes that Dreser also tested what was probably rather a large dose on himself and his colleagues, who thought that it made them feel "strong" or "heroic," which is *heroisch* in German. From this Bayer derived a name for their new drug—"Heroin" (diamorphine; see Figure 5.7).

The biological activity of the morphine molecule is dependent on the fact that the –OH groups in positions 3 and 6 are not substituted. If one of these positions is modified, as in codeine (Figure 5.7), narcotic activity is reduced but not abolished. Modification of both groups, as in thebaine, yields an essentially inactive molecule.[29,30] As both of these groups are modified by acetylation in heroin, where does its potent activity come from? It turns out that there are enzymes in the brain that can easily remove the acetyl groups from heroin, yielding first 6-acetyl morphine and then morphine itself. However, the presence of the two acetyl groups makes it much easier for the molecule to pass into the brain in the first place, something that morphine doesn't actually do all that easily. So basically, heroin is an intercontinental ballistic missile system for rapidly delivering morphine into the central nervous system. Once in the blood, heroin easily enters the brain where it is readily converted to morphine, which is then responsible for its biological activity. In fact, one might describe heroin as a "prodrug" for morphine.

So it was that in 1898 Bayer put heroin on the market as a cough suppressant, saying that unlike morphine or codeine, it was nonaddictive—certainly one of the greatest blunders in the history of pharmacology. 1898 was truly a remarkable year for Bayer and for pharmacology. Acetylating substances to come up with new drugs was a paradigm that the company was very fond of at the time. At the same time Bayer put heroin on the market as a new cough suppressant, they also marketed their newly discovered antipyretic and analgesic drug—the acetyl derivative of salicylic acid also pioneered by Arthur Eichengruen, which they named "Aspirin"[31] (Figure 5.11).

The use of heroin for the treatment of cough and other respiratory disorders basically deflected people's attention away from its other opiate-like properties, at least for a time.[29] Heroin was introduced into the United States in 1898 by a New York doctor named Morris Manges, who reported that it was "100 times safer than codeine." The next year Dr. Heinrick Leo also reported on the specific respiratory effects of heroin, and that "as a general narcotic, morphine and codeine far exceed heroin in action..." Thus heroin was introduced into the United States as a "respiratory specific—much less toxic than codeine, and without morphine's systemic side effects or habituation." The manner in which heroin was used in the first decade of the twentieth century also helped to mask its addictive liability. If a patient had a respiratory problem because of an acute infection, this would soon clear up and so the drug was not taken for a long enough time for its addictive liability to become apparent. If the patient had a chronic problem like tuberculosis, on the other hand, they would also take heroin chronically but would never stop taking it and so would

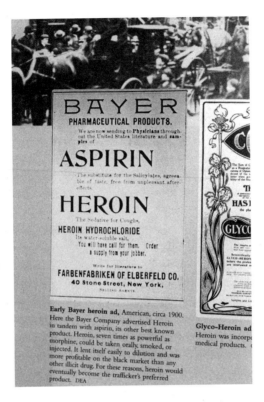

Figure 5.11:
Bayer advertisement shortly after they had launched their two new drugs, Aspirin and
Heroin, in 1898.
(Associated Press)

not go into withdrawal. Moreover, as they were taking the drug orally, tolerance and dependence would occur relatively slowly. Eventually, however,
reports of heroin addiction and withdrawal started to surface, leading to
a wide range of medical opinions about its safety. By the second decade of
the twentieth century it was well established that heroin was a danger-
ously addictive drug, and its medical use had basically ceased. Heroin had
become a "street" drug.

In New York City as elsewhere, heroin addicts needed money in order
to buy the drug. They noticed that there was a class of people in the city
who would make their living by collecting and then reselling valuable
pieces of discarded junk (e.g., an old piece of discarded furniture). In the
United Kingdom this business is known as the "rag and bone" trade, but in
New York these folks were known as "junkers." Realizing the commercial
potential of reselling junk, heroin addicts started to do the same thing and
became forever known as "Junkies."[16]

THE HOLY GRAIL

Because the use of new semisynthetic derivatives like heroin had clearly not solved the problem of producing nonaddictive opiates, several efforts were initiated in the early twentieth century to try and solve this problem. After all, it was argued, it had been possible to make procaine as an analogue of cocaine (Chapter 8), producing a useful local anesthetic that was free of the euphoric and addictive effects of cocaine, so why couldn't similar things be achieved with morphine? This seemed like a reasonable and highly persuasive argument.

There were several concerted attempts made to produce nonaddictive opiates. Elucidation of the chemical structure of morphine by Gulland and Robinson in 1925 opened the door to performing logical chemical analysis and structure activity studies on modifications to the basic structure of the molecule. A particularly influential series of studies took place in the United States starting in 1929 and funded by the Rockefeller Foundation. Over 200 morphine derivatives were synthesized and tested in a pharmacology lab by Dr. Nathan Eddy, who also developed quantitative techniques for measuring the diverse effects of opiates both in animals and humans.[32]

Clinical testing of any promising lead compounds was performed on addicted inmates at the federal penitentiary at Lexington in Kentucky, presumably without informed consent. Here again, reliable quantitative measures for the effects of opiates and their addictive potential in human subjects were developed. By the late 1950s it was concluded that the results of this program had not really been successful, and it had not been possible to dissociate the analgesic effects of opiates from their addictive potential. Nevertheless, as we shall now discuss, an enormous amount had been discovered about the pharmacology of opiates, and several interesting new classes of compounds had been produced. This information was one of the keys to the subsequent development of our understanding of the basic mechanisms of opiate action at a cellular and molecular level.

Let us consider the chemical structure of the morphine molecule[30] (Figure 5.7). It can be described as a "pentacyclic" alkaloid. In other words, it has a basic character and is made up of 5 ring systems. Morphine is related to the simpler 3-ring structure, phenanthrene bridged across the 4,5 positions by oxygen and the 9,13 positions by an ethanamine chain. Another feature of the molecule is that it contains asymmetric centers at positions 5,6,9,13 and 14. This is a fairly typical feature of complex organic molecules, and means that a molecule can exist in different forms that are mirror images of each other but are otherwise precisely the same shape. It is the same situation with your left and right hands. If you look at them you would conclude that they are the same shape. Now try to put one exactly on top of the other. You can't! They are mirror images of each other, just like the "stereoisomers" of morphine. It turns out that the poppy only makes one of the mirror images of morphine, which is designated (-)-morphine. The mirror image molecule, which is designated (+)-morphine, does not exist in nature but can be made synthetically in a laboratory. If this is done, and the properties of the two "stereoisomers" are compared, it turns out that the (+) isomer is completely inactive. As we shall see, the fact that all of the typical pharmacological effects of morphine are associated with the (-) isomer is an important clue in understanding how the drug works.

A second question we might ask is, how can we modify the morphine molecule and produce new compounds that work better or worse? We have already noted that altering the two hydroxyl groups at positions 3 and 6 that give us codeine-like and thebaine-like molecules leads to a decrease in activity. Heroin doesn't really count, because the acetyl groups on these two positions are removed *in vivo*, giving us morphine back again.

Modifications of the C ring of morphine (Figure 5.7) and codeine can produce new molecules that retain their opiate-like activity. Such chemical modifications have produced several important drugs, including hydromorphone, a semisynthetic opiate that is still widely used today, particularly to control pain following major surgery (Figures 5.12 and 5.13). It is sold under the name Dilaudid—the name coming from laudanum. Hydrocodone, oxycodone, and oxymorphone are also important opiates which are used clinically. One popular way of doing this is to mix a drug like hydrocodone with a non-opiate analgesic like acetaminophen (Tylenol). The resulting drug combination is widely utilized under the names Vicodin or Norco. Another important result was the synthesis of compounds in which the 6 and 14 carbon atoms of ring C are bridged by a bimethylene chain. Compounds such as etorphine (Figure 5.12) are among the most potent opiates ever made, being thousands of times more potent than morphine. Unfortunately, such incredible potency does not result in better drugs from the clinical point of view because they are not safer or less addictive than morphine. However, ultrapotent opiate drugs like etorphine have found a specific use—immobilizing large animals in game parks. Basically, if an excited elephant or rampant rhino is charging toward you, firing an etorphine dart at it usually stops it in its tracks.

Another important question to answer is whether the entire morphine structure is really necessary to produce the effects of the drug—do we really need all five of those rings, or would something simpler do (Figure 5.12)? It would certainly be easier from the synthetic point of view if one could find

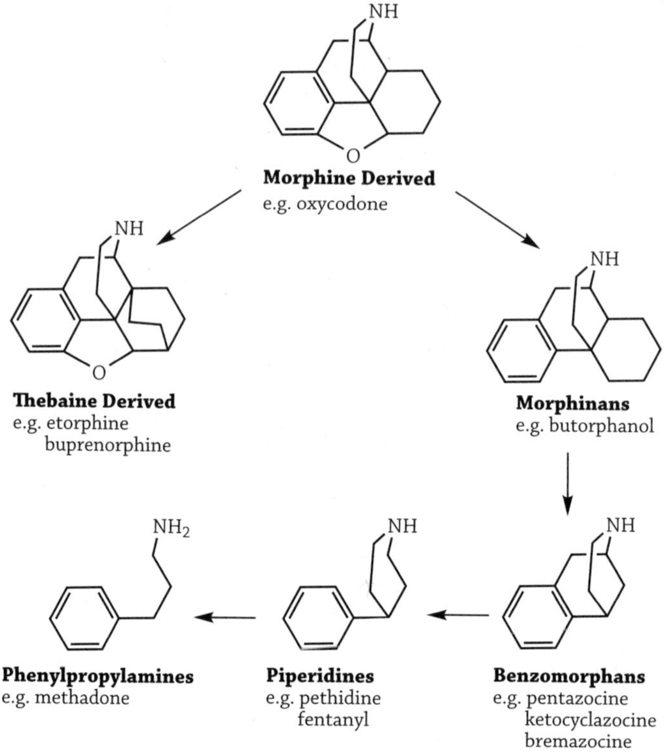

Figure 5.12:
Deconstruction of the morphine molecule by gradual simplification still produces powerful opiate drugs.[30]

an effective molecule with a simpler structure. So for a start, what happens if we dispense with the oxygen bridge?[30]

The resulting structures are called *morphinans* (Figure 5.12) and are obviously very similar in structure to morphine. It was observed that substances of this type, such as levorphanol, behaved as potent opiates just like morphine. The stereochemistry of levorphanol is similar to that of (-)-morphine. Its enantiomer (optical isomer) is called *dextromethorphan*, which is analogous to (+)-morphine and has little opiate activity. However, the small degree of activity it does have has made it useful as a cough suppressant and it is found in many nonprescription cough medicines. A further simplification of the morphine structure is represented by 6,7-benzomorphans, ring C in these molecules being replaced by methyl or other alkyl fragments at the C-5 or C-9 positions (Figure 5.12). Here again it is clear that molecules of this type can exhibit potent morphine-like effects. Agents such as metazocine, phenazocine, cyclazocine, and pentazocine are

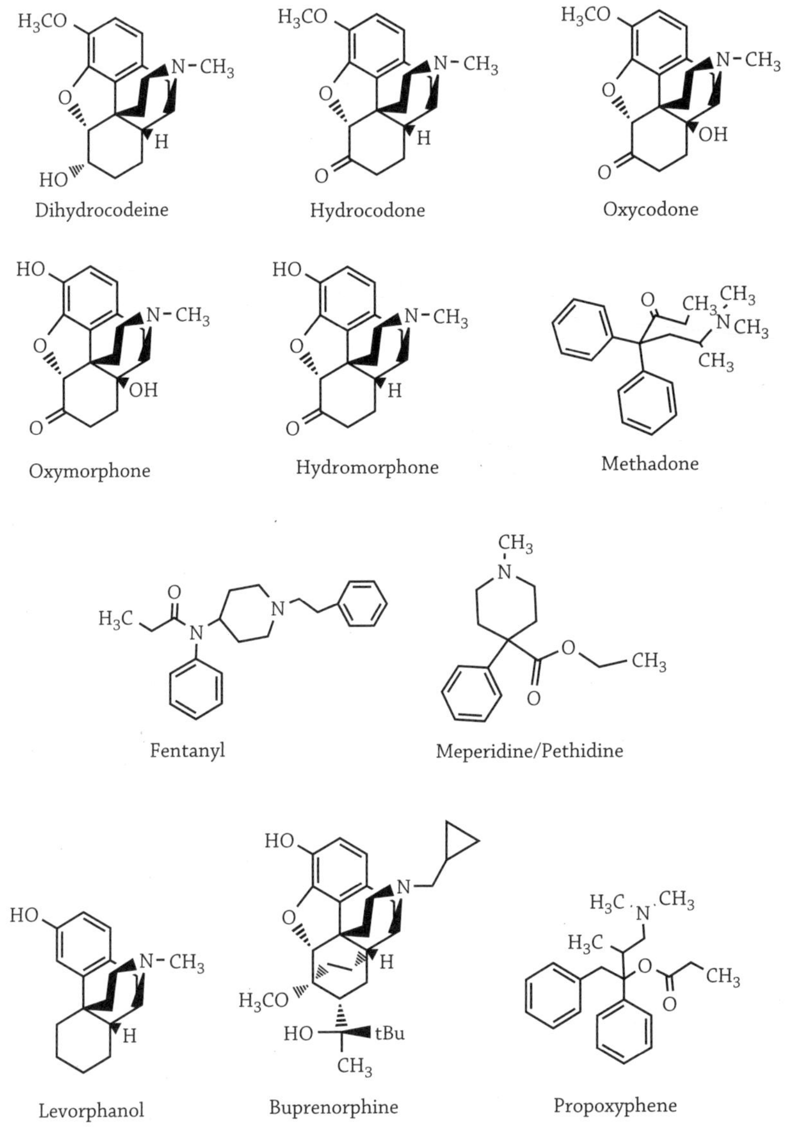

Figure 5.13:
Structures of several important clinically used opiate drugs.

potent analgesics but have other interesting properties as well. Some of these molecules, such cyclazocine and ethylketocyclazocine, produce dysphoric hallucinogenic effects in addition to analgesia, an observation which will be further explained below.

These studies demonstrated that one could dispense with at least two of the rings in the structure of morphine and still produce compounds that act as potent analgesics. In fact, even simpler structures that retain morphine-like activity are possible. As noted in our discussion of antipsychotic drugs (Chapter 3), in 1926 Otto Eisleb, working for IG Farben, synthesized pethidine (Figures 5.12 and 5.13) as one of a series of agents designed to act as antispasmodic substances, not analgesics. Indeed, the structure of pethidine is loosely based on that of the anticholinergic drug, atropine.[33] However, when the substance was tested in mice it was observed to produce a Straub tail reaction. This is a phenomenon is which mice hold their tails erect, something that is typically caused by morphine-like drugs. This alerted Eisleb to the fact that the new compound might have opiate-like activity, which indeed proved to be the case.

Based on the fact that the chemical structure of pethidine doesn't really have a close resemblance to that of morphine, except for the similarity that they both posses a 4-phenylpiperidine moiety, he naturally predicted that it would act as a nonaddictive analgesic. But, of course, as with all the other morphine-like substances that have been made, this proved to be a false dawn, and pethidine was found to have the same benefits and problems that had been associated with other opiate analgesics. Pethidine (known in the United States as meperidine and sold under the name Demerol) has been consistently used in the clinic and is still widely used today. IG Farben proceeded to synthesize numerous analogues of pethidine and, just prior to the Second World War, synthesized a potent opiate analgesic with a related simple structure. This compound was further developed after the war in the United States and was given the name methadone (Figure 5.13). Further analogues such as propoxyphene (Darvon) have also been made and used clinically (Figure 5.13). As we have discussed (Chapter 3), the Janssen Pharmaceutical company also produced related structures after the war and synthesized molecules such as fentanyl and alfentanil, opiate analgesics of very high potency that are widely used in anesthesiology (Figure 5.13).

As one can see by comparing the structure of morphine to that of pethidine or methadone, it is clear that many of the elements of the original chemical structure are not required in order for a drug to exhibit both the properties of a strong opiate-like analgesic as well as strong addictive potential. Considerable structural simplification has been achieved when considering some of these "synthetic" opiates. However, the problem of addiction and related phenomena are just as prevalent with these molecules as with the original drug. Nevertheless, these extensive studies produced numerous useful opiate drugs, and essential information about the relationships between opiate structure and function.

INHIBITING MORPHINE

A further important breakthrough was provided by experiments that examined what happened when the N-methyl group in morphine was modified in different ways.[34] In 1942, scientists at the Merck Institute at Rahway, New Jersey, substituted the nitrogen in morphine with an N-allyl group to yield nalorphine. They found that this drug acted as an antagonist of the effects of morphine (for example, it blocked morphine-induced suppression of respiration), although it did itself posses a degree of analgesic activity. Such properties indicated that it might be something along the lines of an opiate partial agonist. Curiously, it also produced strange dysphoric, hallucinogenic effects as observed with some of the 6,7-benzomorphans discussed above. However, a similar N-allyl derivative of oxymorphone named *naloxone* proved to be a potent pure antagonist of the action of morphine (Figure 5.14) and was free of hallucinogenic activity. If a methylcyclopropyl group was added to the nitrogen instead of an allyl group, the resulting compound known as *naltrexone* also proved to be a potent opiate antagonist (Figure 5.15). A methylcyclobutyl group was similarly effective. This same chemical trick yielded partial agonists or antagonists when applied to the basic structures of other opiate-like molecules. Thus, addition of a N-allyl to the morphinan levorphanol produced levallorphan, which clearly exhibited antagonist properties. The methylcyclopropyl-containing molecule buprenorphine is a potent partial agonist that is related to etorphine (Figure 5.12). In fact, in 1915 Julius Pohl had synthesized the N-allyl derivative of codeine and had reported that it could antagonize the effects of morphine on respiration. However, his observations were not taken up by the research community at large for another 30 years, illustrating the fact that even if an observation is very important it won't necessarily lead

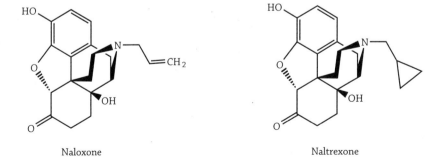

Naloxone   Naltrexone

Figure 5.14:
The opiate antagonists naloxone and naltrexone.

to anything if the scientific community at large doesn't understand its significance.

By the 1960s, over 50 years of intense activity on the medicinal chemistry of opiates had yielded much important structural information, although attempts to dissociate opiate activity from addictive liability had not succeeded. However, the following conclusions could be made and pointed the way forward to further understanding the cellular basis of opiate action.

First, the complex 5-ring structure of morphine was not required for opiate activity and much simpler synthetic molecules could do more or less the same job, although arguably none of them were superior to morphine in terms of its painkilling ability or addictive liability. Numerous studies had been carried out describing exactly how changes to the chemical structure of morphine affected the opiate-like properties of the resulting molecules. Second, there was the extreme stereospecificity of morphine and related molecules. Thus (-)-morphine and levorphanol had much higher biological activity than (+)-morphine or dextromethorphan. Also of great importance was the fact that molecules with partial agonist or pure antagonist properties, such as naloxone, could be produced.

THE OPIATE RECEPTOR CONCEPT

These observations put important constraints on the properties of the molecules that were thought to be expressed by nerve cells and to mediate the effects of the opiates—the opiate receptors. Indeed, over the years the characteristics of the presumed opiate receptors had been the subject of considerable speculation. Initially it had not been clear that opiates acted through "specific" interactions with protein receptor molecules rather than through less specific interactions with the lipid bilayers that contributed to the structure of the cell membrane. However, the structural chemical data that had accumulated suggested that specific opiate receptors, presumably proteins, did exist.

Another type of observation that propelled the field of opiate research forward in the second half of the twentieth century was the increasing use of bioassays (Chapter 1). Such assays would typically involve the use of an isolated smooth muscle preparation that expressed the receptor of interest and responded in a predictable way when receptor agonists were applied. Pharmacologists had used such preparations to great effect during the first half of the twentieth century to define the characteristics of neurotransmitter receptors and drugs that interacted with them. In 1917 Trendelenburg had observed that the peristaltic reflex of the isolated guinea pig ileum was inhibited by low concentrations of morphine. However, this was not the case in other species such as the rabbit. In the 1950s Paton and his colleagues at Oxford demonstrated that the depressant effect of morphine in a preparation of electrically stimulated guinea pig ileum was due to inhibition of the release of the neurotransmitter acetylcholine by nerves within the preparation.[35] Once released from these nerves, acetylcholine is responsible for the observed contraction of the muscle. Apparently the cholinergic nerves within the preparation expressed the mysterious opiate receptor which, when activated, decreased the release of acetylcholine and so also decreased the observed muscle contraction.

Traditionally, the way that opiates had been tested was to use live animals ranging from dogs and mice to Heinrich Dreser's friends at Bayer or prisoners in Lexington. However, a small piece of innervated smooth muscle from a guinea pig was a great improvement on this in terms of convenience. The preparation was easy to set up. Different concentrations of a drug, or even of different drugs, could be sequentially added to the tissue and their effects accurately assessed, producing important information on drug dose–response relationships, receptor affinities, and other basic pharmacological data. Partial agonist and antagonist effects of drugs could also be easily and accurately monitored. Generally speaking, the effects of drugs in the guinea pig ileum assay correlated very closely with their activity in whole animals. The exception to this rule would be a drug like heroin, which would appear to be completely inactive in the bioassay but strongly effective when tested on a live animal. However, this was an unusual situation. The guinea pig ileum became the method of choice for examining the effects of drugs on opiate receptors. Also, it turned out that the guinea pig ileum was not the only opiate-sensitive smooth muscle preparation. Hans Kosterlitz and his colleagues demonstrated that opiates also suppressed the electrically stimulated contractions of the mouse vas deferens.[36] In this case the presumed opiate receptor was expressed on nerves that released norepinephrine rather than acetylcholine. The fact that such smooth muscle preparations seemed to express bona fide opiate receptors, whose activity could easily be monitored, increased the comfort level of scientists who thought that such a specific receptor molecule must truly exist.

DR. SNYDER'S BREAKTHROUGH

In the early 1970s little was known about the biochemical identity of receptors in general.[37] Furthermore, because such molecules were assumed to exist in very low concentrations there was no real technology available for potentially purifying them. In the 1960s Earl Sutherland and his colleagues had started to define some of the biochemical consequences of receptor activation, including the production of the second messenger molecule cyclic AMP, but the biochemical nature of the receptor molecules themselves remained elusive.

Around 1970, however, Jean Pierre Changeux and his colleagues introduced a new approach to the problem. They showed that they could identify the nicotinic receptors for the neurotransmitter acetylcholine by examining the binding of a snake toxin that potently interacted with these receptors and blocked them. To do this they made the toxin highly radioactive by chemically attaching radioactive iodine to it, and chose a tissue from the electrical organ of an eel where the receptor was found in extraordinary abundance (Chapter 8). This approach was a resounding success and led to purification and characterization of the properties of nicotinic acetylcholine receptors. But how could this method be applied to other receptors whose concentrations in brain tissue were clearly very low, orders of magnitude lower than that of nicotinic receptors in the electric organs of eels?

Attempts to identify the opiate receptor using radioactive drug binding studies had been previously attempted and had not been successful. Enter Sol Snyder. There were several technical problems associated with the identification of the opiate receptor, but fortune and brilliant intuition favored Snyder's approach to the problem. He was fortunate to work at Johns Hopkins Medical School in the laboratory next to Pedro Cuatrecasas, an outstanding biochemist who was himself involved in the identification of receptors, particularly those for the hormone insulin, and the two labs had already started to collaborate with one another.

The first question was, what radioactive drug to use in attempts to produce an opiate receptor binding assay? Snyder and his graduate student Candace Pert picked the opiate antagonist naloxone. This turned out to be an inspired choice, because the way these assays were performed preserved the high affinity of antagonists for their target receptors, whereas the affinity of agonists was reduced. Snyder also realized from his work with Cuatrecasas that another issue of central importance would be the ability to identify genuine drug binding to its receptor, rather than nonspecific interactions with other molecules. He argued that because these "background" interactions would generally not be of high affinity, they might be removed by rapid and extensive washing while the high affinity receptor interactions would be preserved.

Snyder and Pert arranged for naloxone to be labeled with radioactive tritium to as high a level of radioactivity as possible at the time. They then prepared nerve cell membranes from the brain and incubated them with the radioactive drug to see if "specific" binding could be observed. Their approach was an immediate success. A large amount of radioactive naloxone binding to the nerve membranes displayed the precise characteristics expected for the presumed opiate receptor. The binding was of high affinity, which means it was very tight and could not be easily washed away. And it was saturable—that is to say, there were a limited number of these binding sites, not too many. Most persuasively, the drug binding sites exhibited exactly the required pharmacological specificity. For example, addition of morphine to the incubation competed with, and so reduced, the binding of the radioactive naloxone in a potent manner. Levorphanol showed high affinity interactions but dextromethorphan did not. Pert and Snyder reported their results in *Science* in 1973 and the rest, as they say, is history.[38]

At the same time that Pert and Snyder were performing their studies, two other laboratories were carrying out similar research and the results from all of the three laboratories fundamentally agreed with one another. However, in Snyder's case, his report was only the tip of a very large iceberg. He realized that if his approach had worked with opiate receptors it should work for other drug and neurotransmitter receptors as well. Over the next few years he successfully identified receptors for many drugs and neurotransmitters, including those for glycine, GABA (chapter 6), the muscarinic receptors for acetylcholine, dopamine (Chapter 3), 5-HT (Chapter 2), ATP (Chapter 8), and many others. These studies ushered in the modern study of receptors as molecular entities and had enormous influence on the entire field of pharmacology. From the point of view of the mechanisms of opiate action, the biochemical identification of the receptor rapidly produced many new insights. Adapting the drug-binding assay in the anatomical domain using the paradigm of autoradiography allowed an appreciation of the distribution of these receptors in different parts of the brain and other tissues. In addition, manipulation of the conditions of the binding assays revealed subtleties in the interactions of agonists and antagonists with opiate receptors, allowing these properties to be predicted for newly synthesized opiate molecules.

ENKEPHALINS AND ENDORPHINS

The identification of opiate receptors also raised some interesting problems. It should be noted that for most of the studies discussed above, the identification of the receptor sites for a drug also implied the identification of the receptor sites for a neurotransmitter. Snyder used radioactive derivatives of the drugs strychnine, QNB, LSD, and spiroperidone to aid in the identification of receptors for the neurotransmitters glycine, acetylcholine, 5-HT, and dopamine. But what about radioactive naloxone? The neurotransmitter that normally acted on opiate receptors was what, exactly? Why should these receptors exist? What was their *raison d'etre*?

Snyder's studies had also demonstrated that opiate receptors were expressed in evolutionarily ancient animals, including ancient vertebrates such as the hagfish. Why should evolution have preserved a specific binding site for a chemical derived from a poppy? These questions raised a tantalizing possibility. Perhaps opiate receptors were really receptors for a neurotransmitter that had never been discovered? Perhaps a neurotransmitter existed that was chemically like morphine, and that routinely concerned itself with controlling the many phenomena associated with the action of morphine, ranging from pain to pleasure? Many laboratories around the world now started to hunt for this elusive substance. Again the race was tight.

In 1975, reports appeared from the laboratories of John Hughes and Lars Terenius demonstrating that extracts of the brain appeared to contain true endogenous opiate-like activity.[39,40] In Hughes' experiments the semipurified extract inhibited the stimulated contractions of the guinea pig ileum and mouse vas deferens just like morphine. But of course, lots of different things could do that. The clincher was that the effects of the unidentified material were completely blocked by the specific opiate receptor antagonist naloxone, indicating that they must truly be due to the activation of opiate receptors and not some other mechanism.

However, there were some major surprises. Naturally, everybody had expected the endogenous opiate neurotransmitter would be a small molecule with a structure something like one of the known opiate drugs, such as morphine. However, Hughes demonstrated that without doubt the active material was a small peptide; that is, a string of amino acids. Nothing could have been more surprising than such a revelation, as virtually nothing could resemble an opiate drug less from the chemical point of view. Then, in 1975, Hughes, Kosterlitz, and their colleagues published a paper in *Nature* demonstrating that the opiate activity they had measured was actually a mixture of two different pentapeptides with structures Tyr-Gly-Gly-Phe-Met (TGGPM) and Tyr-Gly-Gly-Phe-Leu (TGGPL).[40] Stringent tests showed that these peptides genuinely acted as opiate agonists. The authors of the paper suggested the name *enkephalin* for these substances—from the Greek for "in the head." Presumably the enkephalins acted as the endogenous neurotransmitter molecules that normally activated the opiate receptors described by Pert and Snyder a couple of years earlier.

The idea that endogenous opiates acted as neurotransmitters was further supported by experiments demonstrating that stimulation of a certain part of the midbrain known as the *periaqueductal grey* produced analgesia in animals which could blocked by naloxone, precisely the signature one would expect if the analgesia were being produced through the release of an endogenous opiate-like neurotransmitter. Moreover, the goal of producing a nonaddictive opiate analgesic was revived once more. It was argued that we couldn't be "addicted to our own opiates" and so the enkephalins must be nonaddictive. Moreover, the enkephalins represented an entirely new chemical class of opiate agonists that might help medicinal chemists move away from the traditional opiate chemical structures, typified by morphine and pethidine, that had not been successfully utilized to produce nonaddictive drugs.

These arguments may seem rather naïve in retrospect, and indeed the situation rapidly became much more complicated. The floodgates had opened. Hard on the heels of the discovery of the enkephalins came a large number of other reports describing the discovery of other endogenous opiates, all of which appeared to be peptides.[41] For example, the highest concentration of endogenous opiate activity in the body surprisingly proved to be the pituitary gland, from which a large peptide was isolated and named β-endorphin, whose sequence began with the motif Tyr-Gly-Gly-Phe-Met; that is, methionine enkephalin; and was then followed by another 26 amino acids. Longer versions of leucine enkephalin were also reported, including a class of peptides known as *dynorphins* that began with the motif Tyr-Gly-Gly-Phe-Leu followed by eight more amino acids. Gradually a consensus was reached by which the name *endorphin* was used for any endogenous peptide with opiate-like activity, whereas other names, such as enkephalin or dynorphin, were reserved for particular families of peptides within this general group. A further 17 amino acid peptide that started with the amino acid sequence Phe-Gly-Gly-Phe –Thr (PGGPT) was also shown to exist and was named *nociceptin*. However, structural studies with the enkephalins had demonstrated that the N-terminal tyrosine residue was required for opiate activity, and so it proved that although nociceptin had several biological activities it was not opiate-like. Thus nociceptin appears to be a related but non-opiate-like peptide neurotransmitter.

The hopes were quickly dashed that the endorphins might lead to the development of nonaddictive opiate drugs. Generally speaking, most endorphins are biologically fairly unstable and are rapidly degraded by enzymes. However, they can be easily stabilized by artificially modifying their amino acid sequences. For example, the synthetic molecule Tyr-D-alanine-Gly-Phe-D-Leu, containing unusual D amino acids substituted into the second and fifth positions, proved to be a relatively stable analogue of Leu-Enkephalin and could therefore produce extended effects *in vivo*. As with morphine, a new generation of medicinal chemists now produced a huge number of novel molecules such as this, based on the enkephalin structure. However, these all proved to exhibit addictive potential indicating that they activated opiate receptors the same way as morphine. Presumably we are not addicted to our own endorphins because they are rapidly disposed of once they have been released and performed their functions *in vivo,* and so do not activate receptors for long periods of time.

MULTIPLE OPIATE RECEPTORS

Armed with the enormous number of opiates that had been produced in the first 70 years of the twentieth century and the equally enormous number of new opiate peptide derivatives, together with the use of traditional pharmacological bioassay techniques and Sol Snyder's receptor binding assays, it was time to revisit the entire notion of opiate receptor pharmacology. Indeed, some investigators had already suggested that there might be more than one opiate receptor. Recall, for example, that opiates such as the 6,7 benzomorphans ketocyclazocine and ethylketocyclazocine, as well as the partial agonist nalorphine, had been reported to produce strange dysphoric hallucinations. So, perhaps there was some truth to the multiple opiate receptor suggestion.

Whereas Sol Snyder was the leader of the new wave of molecular neuropharmacologists, Hans Kosterlitz was the *éminence grise* of the older generation of opiate pharmacologists. Born and educated in Germany, Kosterlitz had come to the United Kingdom in 1934 and had settled in Aberdeen, where he developed an interest in opiate pharmacology and in the use of smooth muscle bioassays in particular. A courteous Old World gentleman, Hans Kosterlitz could play his tiny pieces of twitching muscle like Fritz Kreisler could play the violin. He was always coaxing new information out of them. Indeed, his role as mentor to his younger colleagues such as John Hughes, and his role in their instruction in these techniques, had been one of the keys to their success in identifying the enkephalins.

Kosterlitz and his colleagues started to examine the responses of the guinea pig ileum and mouse vas deferens preparations in detail. They demonstrated that relative to morphine, peptides like the enkephalins were more potent in the vas deferens than in the guinea pig ileum, suggesting that the receptors in the two tissues might be different. Binding assays carried out by Sol Snyder's lab, using radioactive enkephalins as well as radioactive naloxone, confirmed this idea, leading to the notion that there existed a δ opiate receptor that had particularly high affinity for the enkephalins and a μ opiate receptor that constituted the basic receptor site for drugs like morphine. Further studies identified a third receptor type, named the "κ receptor," which showed high affinity for dynorphin and for hallucinogenic opiates such as ethylkeotcyclazocine. Ultimately, cloning of the three separate opiate receptors together with an additional receptor for nociceptin proved the accuracy of these predictions. All of these receptors proved to be GPCRs (Chapter 2), and their sequences suggested that they formed a family of evolutionarily related proteins.[37, 39, 41]

When all the dust had settled, what we were left with was an entirely new neurotransmitter system reflective of the known effects of opiates in the nervous system—surely one of the most fascinating discoveries of modern science. There are analogies here that can be drawn with other neurotransmitter systems such as the catecholamines. The three catecholamine neurotransmitter molecules, epinephrine, norepinephrine, and dopamine, are all closely related chemically. They act on a family of receptors: α-receptors, β-receptors and dopamine receptors. Each receptor shows a preference for a particular catecholamine agonist, although this is not absolute and some cross-reactivity occurs. Anatomically the distribution of the nerves that use each catecholamine, and the expression patterns of their receptors, are unique. The catecholamine-using nerves exercise a wide influence on the brain at all levels up and down the neuraxis.

A similar description can be applied to the opiate peptide neurotransmitters. It proved to be the case that the enkephalins were most selective for the δ receptors and the dynorphins for the κ receptors. As far as the ligand for the μ receptor was concerned, β-endorphin seemed to fit the bill, although like the catecholamines some cross-reactivity between peptides and receptors exists. Amazingly, however, just when we had got the endorphins more or less sorted out, a new type of opiate peptide was isolated known as an *endomorphin*. The two related endomorphin tetrapeptides had sequences Tyr-Pro-Trp-Phe-NH2 and Tyr-Pro-Phe-Phe-NH2. These peptides also proved to have potent opiate agonist activity, particularly at μ receptors, and so could represent their main endogenous peptide ligands.[42] It is clear from anatomical studies that the enkephalins, dynorphins, and β-endorphin are all expressed in unique sets of neurons that traverse the entire length and breadth of the nervous system. Drugs are now available that act as fairly specific agonists and antagonists at the various receptor types. These drugs, in addition to lines of mice in which the genes for the different opiate receptors have been "knocked out," should allow investigators to ultimately understand the precise biological roles of each separate endogenous opiate peptide neurotransmitter system.

WASSON'S OPIATE

One interesting observation also illustrates how the world of natural products is always likely to surprise us and can often supply new leads for the production of novel drugs. It will be recalled that Gordon Wasson was one of the first people in recent times to venture into Central America and rediscover the use of hallucinogenic substances by Amerindians (Chapters 1 and 2). The story of his meetings with Maria Sabina and his use of psilocybin-containing mushrooms is well known (see Chapter 2). However, while visiting Maria Sabina with Albert Hoffmann, Wasson also encountered something else. This was another kind of hallucinogenic plant that also produced profound effects, and which the curanderos of the Mazatec people also used in their religious ceremonies. The plant was a species of the sage family known by various names. The local Mazatec Indians, following the tradition of combining their ancient traditions with their ultimate conversion to Christianity, had named the plant Maria Pastora or "La Maria," and viewed it as an incarnation of the Virgin Mary. In more common parlance the plant is known as *Salvia divinorum* or "magic mint." *S. divinorum* was utilized by the Mazatec Indians by chewing, smoking, or by brewing a bitter tea. Its effects were known to begin rapidly and the entire experience to be intense but somewhat short-lived. The use of *S. divinorum* has spread in recent times and it has gained quite a large following in the United States and Europe. Apart from its interesting hallucinogenic properties, another attraction was that until recently it was perfectly legal and easy to obtain in head shops or over the Internet.

Experiments designed to isolate the psychoactive molecules from *S. divinorum* resulted in some surprising and exciting results. An entirely new class of molecules was isolated and named the *salvinorins* [43] (Figure 5.15). The major psychoactive molecule of the class appears to be salvorinin A, other molecules being present in smaller amounts and possibly representing metabolites of salvinorin A. Testing pure salvinorin A in animals and man has shown that it reproduces the psychoactive effects of the plant. Of particular chemical interest is the fact that salvinorin A is not an alkaloid and does not contain the basic nitrogen atom that is so often found in psychologically active molecules isolated from plants. Salvorinin A is a diterpene, and is more related to the psychoactive constituents of cannabis (Chapter 7) than it is to morphine. Attempts to define the molecular basis

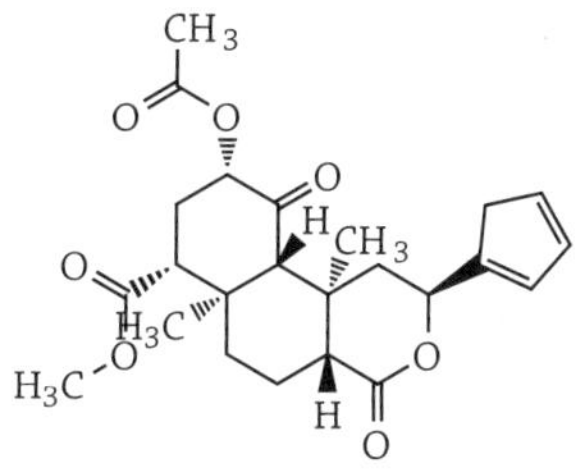

Salvinorin A

Figure 5.15:
Structure of Salvinorin A, a naturally occurring κ-opiate receptor agonist isolated from the Magic Mint, *Salvia divinorum*.

for the action of salvinorin A were also surprising. When screened against a wide range of GPCRs, it exhibited extremely selective interactions with κ opiate receptors. As it is known from studies with semisynthetic opiates that drugs that activate κ receptor have hallucinogenic effects, this result seems entirely reasonable. The unique chemical structure of salvinorin A is now being utilized in attempts to make further novel agents that interact with κ opiate receptor. This relatively recent finding illustrates that the continued search for unique natural products in providing leads for new therapeutic agents is likely to be a fruitful endeavor for many years to come.

OPIATES, NEUROTRANSMISSION, AND PAIN

In keeping with the many effects of morphine, μ opiate receptors are widely expressed in the nervous system. This includes areas of the brain such as the cortex that are involved in the conscious experience of pleasure and pain, areas involved in drug reward and addiction (the dopamine neurons of the midbrain), in cough and respiration (the respiratory nuclei and cough centers in the medulla and brainstem), in the regulation of incoming pain sensations from the viscera and periphery (spinal cord), and in the regulation of gastrointestinal motility (the nervous system of the gut).

One of the clues to understanding how morphine inhibits pain has already been discussed. If we think about the effect of a drug like morphine in the guinea pig ileum bioassay, this will provide us with an important clue. The drug is able to reduce the outflow of the neurotransmitter acetylcholine that is released from the cholinergic nerves innervating the smooth muscle strip used in the assay. Normally the acetylcholine causes this muscle to contract. However, if morphine reduces the amount of acetylcholine that is released then the contraction will be smaller. In fact, if we look at all of the different places in the nervous system where morphine produces its effects we will find more or less the same thing. Morphine-like opiate drugs inhibit the activity of the nerves they act upon, and so will reduce their release of neurotransmitters and will inhibit neurotransmission in this way.

How does this help us to understand morphine's ability to act as an analgesic?[44] It turns out that μ opiate receptors are expressed in exactly the right places in the nervous system for this to be possible. Let us consider the neuronal pathways that contribute to pain. Pain information is carried into the central nervous system from the skin or viscera (organs) by special nerves called *nociceptors*—meaning nerves specialized to carry "noxious" stimuli such as too hot, too cold, too much pressure, anything that is likely to produce tissue damage. In fact, avoiding tissue damage is the basic physiological function of the pain response. Put your hand in the fire and pain tells you to remove it right away, otherwise there will be dire consequences. Painful stimuli cause these nociceptive neurons to fire action potentials, and they transport information in this way into the spinal cord. Here they contact different types of "second order" neurons. Some of these are fibers that ascend to the higher structures of the brain, particularly the thalamus, and from there to the cortex where these signals are decoded as the conscious experience of pain. Other nerves trigger rapid spinal reflexes causing you to remove the part of your body that is in danger, for example your hand in the fire, without even thinking about it. These, then, are the pathways that bring pain information into your nervous system.

At the same time the brain has other neuronal pathways that serve to modulate incoming pain information. These are pathways that descend from the brain down into the spinal cord and inhibit the same second-order neurons that are also excited by incoming painful information, thereby forming a negative feedback loop regulatory system. These descending inhibitory pathways originate in areas of the brain such as the periaqueductal gray (PAG) and the rostroventral medulla (RVM). Now consider the places where μ opiate receptors are found in the nervous system. They are expressed by the incoming nociceptive neurons and by the second-order ascending neurons in the spinal cord. Activation of these receptors by morphine inhibits neurotransmitter release from the incoming nociceptors and also inhibits the firing of the second-order neurons. Both of these effects will inhibit pain transmission from the periphery into the brain. This will certainly result in an analgesic effect.

However, not only does morphine have such effects but it also activates the descending nerve fibers from the brain that have an inhibitory effect on pain. The μ receptors are expressed in the periaqueductal gray (PAG) and the rostroventral medulla (RVM), and their stimulation leads to activation of these descending pathways. At first glance this may seem odd. Doesn't morphine inhibit the firing of nerve cells? If that is the case, why are these descending pathways activated? The answer here is that the μ opiate receptors expressed in the PAG and the DVM are not actually expressed by the descending nerve fibers themselves. In both areas there are small inhibitory interneurons that use the inhibitory neurotransmitter GABA and that normally keep a brake on the firing of these descending pathways. The μ receptors are actually expressed by these inhibitory interneurons. Thus, when morphine activates these receptors it will inhibit these inhibitory interneurons and will remove their influence on the descending pathways, thereby activating them. So, as one can see, the expression of μ receptors allows morphine to simultaneously inhibit incoming ascending pain information and also to activate the brain's own descending pain inhibitory pathways. This double effect is one of the reasons why activators of μ receptors like morphine are so good at controlling pain.

In spite of morphine's great effectiveness as an analgesic, the problem of its addictive potential is still with us. This is still a problem, which even the greatest minds have not solved. Non-opiate drugs do exist for the treatment of chronic pain, but compared to opiates their effects are not impressive. There are numerous situations in which effective pain-suppressing drugs with nonaddictive properties would be of great use. Might a κ receptor agonist or some completely different type of molecule fit the bill? Research into this problem is one of the most active areas in all of the great pharmaceutical houses around the world. It is the Holy Grail. The search goes on!

> O soft embalmer of the still midnight!
> Shutting, with careful fingers and benign,
> Our gloom-pleased eyes, embowered from the light,
> Enshaded in forgetfulness divine;
> O soothest Sleep! if so it please thee, close,
> In midst of this thine hymn, my willing eyes,
> Or wait the amen, ere thy poppy throws
> Around my bed its lulling charities;
> Then save me, or the passed day will shine
> Upon my pillow, breeding many woes;
> Save me from curious conscience, that still lords
> Its strength, for darkness burrowing like a mole;
> Turn the key deftly in the oiled wards,
> And seal the hushed casket of my soul. (John Keats[45])

NOTES

1. Wilkie Collins (1824–1829) was one of the most famous authors of the Victorian era. A close friend of Charles Dickens, Collins was responsible for several innovations. In particular his novel *The Moonstone* is considered to be the first and one of the greatest detective novels and *The Woman in White* one of the first "sensation novels." Collins suffered from gout and used laudanum for relief of his pain. He became a lifelong laudanum addict. Although he certainly suffered from many of the symptoms associated with this condition (e.g., hallucinations) he had a very productive and successful career as a novelist and essayist.

2. A small pedestrian-only street in central London, which is home to several used bookstores.

3. Bezique is a card game also known as pinochle. Both Wilkie Collins and Christina Rossetti were enthusiasts.

4. Laudanum—tincture of opium (see text).

5. Christina Rossetti. "Listening" from *Poems and Prose*. Ed. Jan Marsh. 1994, p. 40.

6. John Everett Millais (1829–1896). English painter and a founding member of the Pre-Raphaelite brotherhood.

7. Charles Allston Collins (1828–1873). English painter and associate of the Pre-Raphaelites was the younger brother of Wilkie Collins.

8. Christina Rossetti. *"In an artist's studio."* See ref 5, p. 52.

9. Algernon Charles Swinburne (1837–1909). English poet, he was a major figure in the Aesthetic movement in nineteenth-century England.

10. John Anster Fitzgerald (1823–1906). English painter and major figure in the Victorian fairy painting movement.

11. John Anster Fitzgerald. *The nightmare*. See "Victorian Fairy Painting." Royal Academy of Arts. 1994, p. 115.

12. Henry Fuseli (1741–1825). Swiss born English painter was particularly fond of supernatural subjects. *The Nightmare* was painted in 1781 (Detroit Institute of Arts).

13. See ref 11, p. 114.

14. "Goblin Market" by Christina Rossetti (published 1862) in *Goblin Market and other poems* and illustrated by her brother Dante Gabriel Rossetti. A long narrative poem, "Goblin Market" tells of two sisters Laura and Lizzie and their meeting with goblins who try to tempt them into buying their seductive but evil fruits. The poem contains surprisingly highly charged language and overt sexual imagery for the time. Rossetti was extremely religious and the poem's themes clearly encompass the concept of the "fallen woman" and possibly drug addiction as suggested here. See ref 5, p. 162.

15. Christina Rossetti (1830–1894). English poet and sister of the painter Dante Gabriel Rossetti. Christina never married and was a very devout Christian. See *Learning not to be first; the life of Christina Rossetti* by Kathleen Jones. St Martins Press. 1992.

    For further information on Elizabeth Siddal and other women in the Pre-Raphaelite circle see *The Pre-Raphaelite Sisterhood* by Jan Marsh. Quartet Books. 1995.

    Lucinda Hawksley. *Lizzie Siddal: Face of the Pre-Raphaelites*. Walker and Co, NY. 2004.

16. Walter Sneader. *Drug Discovery: A history*. John Wiley. 2005.

    Martin Booth. *Opium: a history*. St. Martins Press, NY. 1996.

    Mike Jay. *High Society*. Park Street Press. 2010.

Barbara Hodgson. *Opium: A portrait of the heavenly demon.* Chronicle Books. 1999

17. *Poppy: the genus papaver.* Edited by Jeno Bernath. Harwood academic publishers. 1998.

18. Krikorian AD. Were the opium poppy and opium known in the ancient near east? *J Hist Biol.* 1975, 8:96–114.

19. Roy Porter, Mikulas Teich. *Drugs and narcotics in history.* Cambridge University Press. 1995.

20. *The Devil's Doctor: Paracelsus and the World of Renaissance Magic and Science.* By Ball P. Farrar, Straus and Giroux. 2006.

21. John Jones. *The Mysteries of Opium Revealed.* London. 1700.

22. Overmier JA. John Brown's Elementa Medicinae: An introductory bibliographical essay. *Bull Med Libr Assoc.* 1982, 70:310–317.

23. Alethea Hayter. *Opium and the Romantic Imagination.* University of California Press. 1968.

24. Thomas De Quincey. *Confessions of an English Opium Eater.* Oxford World Classics. 1996.

25. Mike Jay. *High Society.* Park Street Press. 2010.

26. Charles Baudelaire. *Artificial Paradises: Baudelaire's masterpiece on hashish.* Citadel Press. 1998.

27. Miller RJ, Tran PB. More mysteries of opium revealed: 300 years of opiates. *Trends Pharmacol Sci.* 2000, 21:299–304.

28. A netsuke is a miniature sculpture used by the Japanese of the 17th–19th centuries to secure the sash that was tied around their kimonos.

29. Walter Sneader. *The discovery of heroin.* Lancet. 1998, 352:1697–1699.
    Walter Sneader. *Drug Discovery: A history.* Wiley. 2005.
    Higby GJ. Heroin and medical reasoning: the power of analogy. *N Y State J Med.* 1986, 86:137–142.

30. Alan F. Casy, Robert T. Parfitt. *Opioid analgesics: chemistry and receptors.* Plenum Press. 1986.
    Goodman and Gilman's The Pharmacological Basis of Therapeutics, 9th edition. Edited by Joel Griffith Hardman, Lee E. Limbird, Alfred G. Gilman. McGraw-Hill. 1996.

31. Diarmuid Jeffreys. *Aspirin: The remarkable story of a wonder drug.* Bloomsbury Press. 2004.

32. Eddy NB, May EL. Analgesic. *Science.* 1973, 181:407–414.

33. Michaelis M, Schölkens B, Rudolphi K. An anthology from Naunyn-Schmiedeberg's archives of pharmacology. *Naunyn Schmiedebergs Arch Pharmacol.* 2007, 375:81–84.

34. Walter Sneader. *Drug Discovery: A history.* Wiley. 2005.
    Alan F. Casy, Robert T. Parfitt. *Opioid analgesics: chemistry and receptors.* Plenum Press. 1986.

35. Paton WD. The action of morphine and related substances on contraction and on acetylcholine output of coaxially stimulated guinea-pig ileum. *Br J Pharmacol Chemother.* 1957, 12:119–127.

36. Henderson G, Hughes J, Kosterlitz HW. A new example of a morphine-sensitive neuro-effector junction: adrenergic transmission in the mouse vas deferens. *Br J Pharmacol.* 1972, 46:764–766.

37. Snyder SH, Pasternak GW. Historical review: Opioid receptors. *Trends Pharmacol Sci.* 2003, 24:198–205.

38. Pert CB, Snyder SH. Opiate receptor: demonstration in nervous tissue. *Science.* 1973, 179:1011–1014.

39. Corbett AD, Henderson G, McKnight AT, Paterson SJ. 75 years of opioid research: the exciting but vain quest for the Holy Grail. *Br J Pharmacol.* 2006, 147 (Suppl 1):S153–162.

40. Hughes J. Isolation of an endogenous compound from the brain with pharmaco-logical properties similar to morphine. *Brain Res.* 1975, 88:295–308.
Hughes J, Smith TW, Kosterlitz HW, Fothergill LA, Morgan BA, Morris HR. Identification of two related pentapeptides from the brain with potent opiate agonist activity. *Nature.* 1975, 258:577–580.

41. Akil H, Owens C, Gutstein H, Taylor L, Curran E, Watson S. Endogenous opi-oids: overview and current issues. *Drug Alcohol Depend.* 1998, 51:127–140.

42. Okada Y, Tsuda Y, Bryant SD, Lazarus LH. Endomorphins and related opioid peptides. *Vitam Horm.* 2002, 65:257–279.

43. Vortherms TA, Roth BL. Salvinorin A: from natural product to human therapeu-tics. *Mol Interv.* 2006, 6:257–265.

44. Evans CJ. Secrets of the opium poppy revealed. *Neuropharmacology.* 2004, 47 (Suppl 1):293–299.s

45. John Keats. *Sonnet To Sleep.* 1815.

CHAPTER 6

Divertimento

"Profits substantial will always be made by Switzerland engaged in the drug making trade..."

Anonymous

June 1940. A dark cloud hung over Europe. The Nazi war machine had overrun much of Western Europe including France, Poland, Norway, Denmark, and The Netherlands, while Germany's allies controlled Italy and Spain. In May of 1940 the German army had reached the coast of the English Channel, the British Expeditionary Force fleeing from Dunkirk back to England with its proverbial tail between its legs. Now the Germans were poised to enter Paris and nobody was going to stop them. From the North Sea to the Mediterranean, Western Europe was a vast sea of fascism with only one exception—Switzerland.

The Nazis got very little support from the Swiss, whose multicultural heritage and strong democratic history were generally not in sympathy with their fascist neighbors. Attempts by the tiny Swiss Nazi party to engineer an Austrian style Anschluss were a total fiasco. Nevertheless, many people in Switzerland thought that their days were numbered, as it was known that the Germans had drawn up detailed plans for the invasion of their country. Whispers concerning Germany's "Operation Tannenbaum" were everywhere.

But the Swiss weren't going to be pushed around. Perhaps nothing illustrated this attitude better than something that was going on in Basel, just a few hundred yards from the German border, on the evening of June 11, 1940: a concert by the Basel Chamber Orchestra (BCO). The program was of note for several reasons. First, the programmatic choice of the Symphonic Piece for String Orchestra by Ernst Krenek. This would offend the Nazis for numerous reasons; Krenek was not exactly a Jew, but as far as the Germans were concerned he might just as well have been. His 1927 opera "Jonny Spielt Auf" had caused a considerable sensation and celebrated, of all things, a "negro" jazz musician and "negro music." If ever an opera fitted the Nazi's description of *entartete Kunst*—this was it.[1] Secondly, Krenek's teacher had been Franz Schrecker, who was half Jewish. Finally, Krenek's ex-wife, albeit briefly, had been Anna Mahler, the daughter of the composer and again half Jewish. So Krenek and his music were anything but popular just across the border. Next on the program that night was "Genug is nicht genug" by the Swiss composer Willy Burkhard. Burkhard was a composer with modernist leanings, again something unappreciated by the Nazis. Finally the orchestra played a world premier that had been specially commissioned for them—the Divertimento by the Hungarian Bela Bartok, one of Europe's greatest contemporary composers and a stalwart anti-fascist.

The conductor that night was also the orchestra's founder Dr. Paul Sacher. In 1926, after finishing his conducting studies with Felix Weingartner,[2] the 20-year-old Paul Sacher founded the BCO and since that time it had become one of the world's leading ensembles specializing in avant garde and contemporary music. Sacher and the BCO not only performed such music but also commissioned composers to write new works.

Sacher was a man of excellent taste. He helped to develop the careers of several important Swiss composers including Arthur Honegger, later a member of the influential Parisian group "Les Six," as well as Frank Martin, Burkhard, and others. In addition to the Swiss composers, he also supported the likes of Stravinsky, Hindemith, Martinu, and Bartok. Four years previously, to commemorate the tenth anniversary of the orchestra, he had commissioned Bartok to write his Music for Strings, Percussion and Celesta, one of the twentieth century's greatest and most enduring masterpieces.

This time he had requested something a little lighter of Bartok, perhaps because he felt that given the dark nature of the times, the audience needed to able to relax and just enjoy themselves. So while residing in Sacher's house Bartok had dashed off the Divertimento in just a couple of weeks. The result—another masterpiece in Bartok's now highly recognizable mature style. The concert was a great success. When the Bartok piece finished, Paul Sacher turned and bowed deeply to the audience. The conductor had a smile on his face. Naturally he was happy with the way the evening had gone. But there was another reason for Paul Sacher to smile. He was, after all, the wealthiest man in Europe.

Paul Sacher was not born into a rich family, quite the opposite. He was born in Basel; his mother was a farmer's daughter and his father was a gardener. However, in 1934 he married Maja Hoffmann-Stehlin, the widow of Emanuel Hoffmann and heir to the Hoffmann-La Roche drug company. In 1938 he joined the board of directors to represent his wife's underage children from her first marriage. Paul Sacher's marriage and his place on the board of directors of Hoffman-La Roche brought with it immense wealth. In 1940 Hoffmann-La Roche was already one of the world's largest drug companies. However, over the next year Sacher and his colleagues were to make a decision which would result in the company becoming the largest and most successful drug company in the world by the late 1970s, and to play a major role in the revolution in psychopharmacology that took place in the second half of the twentieth century. The decision they made concerned a familiar problem for the Swiss at that time—how to best protect their Jewish employees from the Nazis.

MR. HOFFMANN MEETS MS. LAROCHE

Basel is the center of the Swiss pharmaceutical industry, one of the largest and most sophisticated in the world. Although there are fewer companies these days owing to mergers, in addition to Roche, companies like Geigy, Ciba, and Sandoz had originated there in the nineteenth century. Prior to the development of the pharmaceutical industry, Basel was not famous for making drugs but for making silk ribbons and related materials, a business that started back in the sixteenth century.

Since that time the government and organization of the town had been under the control of several powerful "silk ribbon" families. However, with the coming of the railroad and the industrial revolution in the nineteenth century things began to change. The population of the city rose from 78,000 in 1890 to 112,000 in 1900. The silk ribbon business declined. However, Basel's advantageous patent laws, together with its excellent geographic location, encouraged the development of related industries, particularly those dealing with dyestuffs.

As we have seen in the case of many other countries, these dyestuff businesses became the seeds of fledgling chemical and drug companies (Chapter 3). The use and sale of different kinds of medicines had undergone a significant change in the nineteenth century. People's general attitude toward disease and its treatment was rapidly becoming more sophisticated. Many new medicines, elixirs, and tonics were being sold to an ever more demanding public. The use of advertising and attractive packaging also encouraged people to believe that they could actually effectively treat the various ailments that afflicted them. An increasing public demand for such products made pharmaceuticals an attractive area for business investment.

In 1894 Fritz Hoffmann, a member of one of Basel's oldest silk ribbon families, and Max Carl Traub, an experienced pharmacist from Munich, founded Hoffmann, Traub and Company, a small company to trade in chemicals and pharmaceuticals.[3] They owned a small factory on the north bank of the river Rhine, and began by selling medicines mostly supplied by other firms. Hoffmann was not a chemist or a pharmacist but a business-man, and he was to be responsible for finances and sales, whereas Traub was responsible for production.

Soon after founding the company in 1894, they built a small factory across the German border in the village of Grenzach. In addition, in the same year Fritz married Adele La Roche, and so his name became Fritz Hoffmann-La Roche, reflecting the usual Swiss convention of composing and hyphenating surnames. For several reasons Hoffmann and Traub soon decided to go their separate ways and the company was relaunched in 1896 as F. Hoffmann-La Roche and Co., frequently just referred to as "Roche."

Fritz Hoffmann was an excellent businessman and was able to appoint sev-eral talented people to help him run the company, which soon began to pros-per. In 1899 Hoffmann-La Roche recorded its last overall loss—a grand total of 181 Swiss francs. The company's turnover was 630,000 francs in 1897 and 19 million in 1914. In 1894 Hoffmann-La Roche had less than 50 employees, but by 1914 this total had grown to greater than 700, of which 145 were in Basel and the rest were in offices around the world including Milan, Paris, Berlin, Vienna, St. Petersburg, London, New York, and Yokohama.

Much of this growth was due to Fritz Hoffmann's considerable business acumen and energy. He traveled constantly, establishing contacts for the company all over the world, and was extremely successful in promoting and advertising his products. For example, a cough syrup named Sirolin was the subject of an intense advertising campaign and was enormously successful.

When he died in 1920, his two sons Emmanuel and Alfred were consid-ered to be too young and inexperienced to run the company and so the job of managing director went to Dr. Emil Barell. Barell was a chemist who was one of the company's original employees but had soon started to take an interest in organizational matters outside the laboratory, ending up being Hoffmann's right-hand man.[3,4] Here again Roche was fortunate, as Barell proved to be a visionary businessman and was responsible for successfully guiding the company through the turbulent times of the Second World War.

As it turned out, Fritz's elder son Emmanuel did join the company in 1921 and began to work his way up the corporate ladder. In 1921

Emmanuel married Maja Stehlin, the daughter of a well known local archi-tect. Emmanuel and Maja moved to Brussels, where Emmanuel became the head of Roche's Belgian subsidiary, and then eventually returned to Basel where in 1932 he was killed in a traffic accident. His widow Maja had wanted to become an architect like her father, but this was not a profession open to women at that time so she had turned to sculpture. Her wealth and interests had made her a prominent patron of the arts in Basel, and so it was little wonder that her path soon crossed with that of Paul Sacher, whom she married in 1934.

THE NEW WORLD BECKONS

Switzerland was not a country that was particularly well known for its anti-Semitism, at least in modern times. The outbreak of the Second World War, however, had presented the Swiss with a considerable dilemma. Although the Swiss were determined to show their independence from their Nazi neighbors, they certainly had to take German attitudes into account when considering trade and other activities. One question was, how many Jewish refugees to admit to the country? Another was, how should Swiss businesses treat Jewish employees or, indeed, should they employ Jews at all?

Several Swiss companies did reduce their number of Jewish employees in an attempt to "Aryanize" their image; however, Roche was not one of them. Considering the situation, the treatment of Jewish employees by Roche was unusually enlightened. One reason for this was clearly the atti-tude of Emil Barell, whose wife Collette Sachs was Jewish.[4]

In 1941, Barell, Sacher, and the Roche board of directors made a signifi-cant decision. They would move the headquarters of Roche to the site of their subsidiary in Nutley, New Jersey, in the United States. Moreover, they would also send Roche's Jewish employees to the United States as a safety measure. Barell's decision turned out to be extremely prescient. Among the Jewish scientists who Roche transferred to Nutley was a young chemist named Leo Sternbach, who will always be remembered as the man who invented Valium, one of the greatest and most important "blockbuster" drugs of all time.

THE EDUCATION OF LEO

Leo Sternbach was born in 1908 into a middle class Jewish family in Abbazia (modern Opatija) on the Istrian Peninsula in what is now Croatia.[5]

His father was Polish and his mother Hungarian. They had moved to Abbazia when a business opportunity arose so that they could open a pharmacy, this being the elder Sternbach's profession. The young Leo Sternbach would often help out in his father's shop mixing and preparing different orders. During the First World War, when Leo was between 6 and 10 years old, Abbazia was occupied by Italian troops who freely distributed carbine cartridges to the local boys who emptied them out to make fireworks of various kinds. Perhaps these different kinds of activities influenced his later decision to become a chemist? At any rate it makes a nice story.

Following the war, Abbazia became part of Italy. There was a good deal of pressure on the inhabitants to speak Italian, which was not the Sternbachs' native language. The Sternbachs sent Leo away to be schooled in Graz in Austria. However, there, for the first time in his life, he encountered serious anti-Semitism. Due to this and diverse other reasons the family moved to back to Poland, settling in Krakow. In 1926 Leo enrolled in the university to study pharmacy. This was what his father wanted, as he expected that his son would eventually take over his business. However, by this time Leo had decided that chemistry was what he wanted to study and, once he had obtained his pharmacy degree, he was able to complete a PhD in organic chemistry, after which he found a junior faculty position at the University. The subject of his PhD research was an attempt to develop a group of new dyes or dyestuff intermediates. At some point he came across a group of substances known as *4,5-benzo-(hept-1,2,6-oxdiazines)* or *benzoheptoxdiazines* and began working with them.[6] Unfortunately Sternbach didn't have much luck turning them into dyes, and he dropped the project so that he could turn to other things. Nevertheless, he never forgot these chemical structures and, as we shall see, they were to play a central role in the future of twentieth-century drug development.

Once his PhD was finished he then obtained a fellowship financed by a wealthy Jewish textile magnate, which allowed him to study abroad. Sternbach chose to go to Vienna. However, in 1937 Vienna was anything but a welcoming environment for a Jewish student, and so he eventually moved on to the laboratory of Professor Leopold Ruzicka in Zurich.

Ruzicka had been born in Croatia like Leo Sternbach, and he was also known for his willingness to help young Jewish scientists. This time the atmosphere of the laboratory was much more welcoming, and Sternbach was able to get on with his work. Socially things also went well. He rented lodgings a few minutes' walk from the laboratory, and a couple of years later in 1940 had married his landlady's daughter, Herta Kreuzer. When his fellowship was finished, Sternbach interviewed for a job advertised at Roche and within a year he was in the United States as a result of Barell's decision to reorganize the company and send its Jewish employees to America. Sternbach's work for Roche went well. In 1949 he developed a new synthesis for the vitamin Biotin, which Roche was able to patent. However, the work that was truly to change the world started a few years later when Roche decided to make a concerted effort to enter the newly developing field of psychopharmacology.

ANXIOUS MOMENTS

As we have seen in previous chapters, starting in the 1950s a great revolution in psychopharmacology completely changed the way mental patients were viewed and treated. The development of drugs like chlorpromazine and haloperidol (Chapter 3) had enabled the vast majority of patients suffering from psychotic illness to leave mental hospitals and to be treated as outpatients. Similarly, antidepressant drugs (Chapter 4) developed around the same time revolutionized the treatment of clinical depression. Suddenly psychopharmacology was becoming an extremely attractive area for drug company research and investment. However, in order to develop a successful drug one first needs to have an officially recognized target for it, one that is sanctioned by the medical community.

As the nineteenth century turned into the twentieth century, our increasingly sophisticated appreciation of psychopathology resulted in a parallel increase in the number of officially recognized psychiatric disorders. Many of these things would not have previously been considered as disease entities at all, and so there would have been no reason to develop drugs for treating them. In 1900 nobody knew that they might be suffering from attention deficit disorder, post-traumatic stress disorder, or fibromyalgia. Modern life brought with it the arrival of several new types of mental disorders that ultimately turned out to afflict a very large portion of the human race, and would provide billions of new customers for the drug industry. In particular, it seems that we were all becoming increasingly anxious.

Of course this had been coming for some time. In the eighteenth century Newton had set the world on a completely deterministic course. One thing led precisely to another—something that could be proved by science. We knew exactly where we were going. The subject of a portrait by Gainsborough or Reynolds might actually look like somebody you knew. Music and architecture reflected classical proportions. However, when Romantic perceptions took over as the driving force of the ninteenth century, many of these things began to unravel, so slowly that it's hard to put

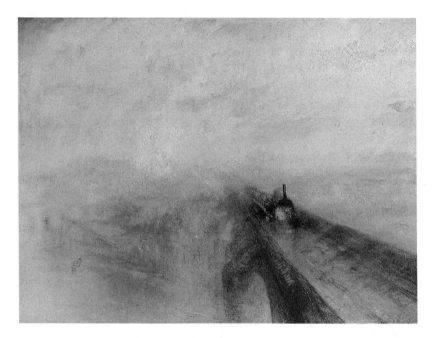

Figure 6.1:
Turner, Joseph Mallord William (1775–1851). Rain Steam and Speed, The Great Western Railway, painted before 1844 (oil on canvas).
National Gallery, London, UK / The Bridgeman Art Library.

your finger on precisely when it began. Many have argued that the opening chord of Wagner's opera *Tristan and Isolde* defined the opening of the door to the modern world—perhaps that is one way to look at it. A great painting like Turner's 1844 "Rain, Steam and Speed" clearly shows us that our perceptions of reality are certainly changing—what exactly are we looking at (Figure 6.1)?

By 1872 Whistler's "Nocturne in Black and Gold" had taken us to the verge of complete abstraction (Figure 6.2), and by the early years of the twentieth century Impressionism and artists like Kandinsky and Mondrian had completed the job. And in the world of music, what Wagner had begun was finished by the likes of Schoenberg. By the last movement of his second string quartet, tonality had been abandoned altogether. A new kind of music had arrived, one that Thomas Mann thought could only have come about through a pact with the devil.[7] People, like music, had lost their tonal center. Now, what we were looking at or listening to was no longer clear.

At the start of the twentieth century the ideas of Einstein, Heisenberg, and Godel[8] pulled the rug out from under Newton's deterministic universe. Relativity, Uncertainty, and Incompleteness opened the door to "the Age of Anxiety." And things only got worse. The senseless massacres of two world

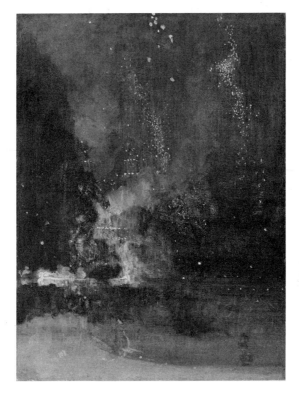

Figure 6.2:
Whistler, James Abbott McNeill (1834–1903). Nocturne in Black and Gold, the Falling Rocket, c.1875 (oil on panel).
Detroit Institute of Arts, USA / Gift of Dexter M. Ferry Jr. / The Bridgeman Art Library.

wars, the Bomb, the Cold War—small wonder people were nervous and filled with apprehension. After the First World War, a Dadaist manifesto encapsulated people's feelings this way:

> *"No more painters, no more writers, no more musicians, no more sculptors, no more religions, no more republicans, no more royalists, no more imperialists, no more anarchists, no more socialists, no more Bolsheviks, no more politicians, no more proletarians, no more democrats, no more armies, no more police, no more nations, no more of these idiocies, no more, no more, NOTHING, NOTHING, NOTHING."*[9]

The idea that anxiety might actually be classed as a clinical entity, rather than merely as a defect in somebody's character, had its roots in the nineteenth century when patients began to be diagnosed with syndromes such as "nervous exhaustion" or "neurasthenia." The industrial revolution had created a burgeoning middle class who had more time for this kind of thing, along with time to get in touch with their "inner feelings." Subsequently, through the work of Freud and his colleagues, anxiety became a symptom associated with neurosis.

Generally speaking these were the kinds of mental disorders that, unlike florid psychotic illness, did not require being committed to an institution such as an asylum but might instead require a rest cure in a comfortable spa, or perhaps psychoanalysis. Such things were much more likely to afflict members of the middle and upper classes than millworkers in Lancashire. Treatments for these symptoms developed hand in hand with treatments for other clinical entities such as epilepsy and insomnia, with which, as we shall see, they share strong mechanistic links.

In the mid nineteenth century, potassium bromide was noted to have a beneficial effect in epilepsy and it was really the first effective treatment to be introduced for this disorder. At the time seizures were thought to be the result of excessive sexual excitement and masturbation, and the effectiveness of bromides was thought to derive from their suppression of this kind of behavior. Ultimately bromides became widely used to calm people thought to be suffering from diverse kinds of overexcitement and of "nervous disorders" in general. Chloral hydrate, the first real sedative hypnotic drug, was discovered in 1831 by Justus von Liebig, although its hypnotic and anesthetic effects were not understood until around 1860 when it became widely used for such purposes.[10] Drugs of this type became generally known as "sedatives," exhibiting a spectrum of activities which included antianxiety (anxiolytic), sedative, hypnotic (sleep inducing), anesthetic, and anticonvulsant effects. These were properties that clearly had considerable potential for the treatment of a variety of disorders. Indeed, the gradual refinement of these activities by pharmacologists in the twentieth century as represented by the barbiturates, meprobamate, and the benzodiazepines are reflective of a common molecular mechanism of action. All of these drugs possess these different activities to some degree, but they are all represented to different extents giving each type of drug its particular utility.

BARBARA'S BREAKTHROUGH

The first real modern breakthrough in the pharmacology of sedatives came in 1903 when the great Nobel Prize winning chemist Emil Fischer and his colleague Josef von Mering published their findings on the compound diethyl barbituric acid, the first widely marketed barbiturate drug.[11]

The same substance became known as *barbital* in the United States and *barbitone* in the United Kingdom. The barbiturates had an extremely distinguished chemical heritage. They originated with the work of Fischer's teacher Johan Adolf von Baeyer, himself a Nobel laureate (1905) and a student of the great chemists Bunsen and Kekule (Chapter 3). Von Baeyer synthesized the compound malonylurea in 1863 by reacting malonic acid with urea. It is said that he made the discovery on December 4 of that year, which is the feast day of St. Barbara, and so named the new substance *barbituric acid* (Figure 6.3), a neologism being part Barbara and part urea (Figure 6.3).

Actually barbituric acid itself is free of sedative/hypnotic properties. However, its diethyl derivative, barbital, proved to be a potent hypnotic or sleep-inducing agent (Chapter 1). It is said that the news of the discovery of this activity was sent by Fischer to von Mering when the latter was on vacation in Verona. Thus, the compound that was then marketed by the German companies of E. Merck and F. Bayer and Company was named "Veronal." Veronal proved to possess marked hypnotic, sedative, and anticonvulsant properties and was much more effective than previous drugs such as chloral hydrate. Barbiturates were so successful that some 2500 of them were synthesized and patented by 1950, although only a few of these became widely used.

Different classes of barbiturates were developed for different indications. One of the first and most successful was phenobarbital—sold under the name of Luminal in 1911. In 1923 and 1929, Eli Lilly developed amobarbital (Amytal) and secobarbital (Seconal). Pentobarbital (Nembutal) and thiopental (Pentothal) followed in 1930 and 1935 respectively. These various derivatives revolutionized the treatment of several types of patients. Many were widely used as hypnotics for treating insomnia. Drugs like phenobarbital were found to have great effectiveness in the treatment of epilepsy, whereas fast-onset, shorter acting compounds such as thiopental became the drugs of choice in anesthesiology.

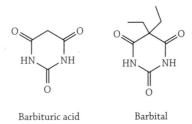

Barbituric acid   Barbital

Figure 6.3:
Barbital, the first barbiturate drug, was derived from barbituric acid.

Barbiturates were also utilized to treat a variety of psychiatric conditions including agitated schizophrenics, delirium tremens, and morphine withdrawal. Further applications included "prolonged sleep therapies" or "sleep cures" for patients with acute psychotic illness, where the patient was put into a deep barbiturate-induced sleep for several days in an effort to outlast and overcome the psychotic episode. Although such treatments were superseded by much more effective and specific antipsychotics in the 1950s, they were at least an initial attempt to utilize pharmacology in the treatment of previously intractable disorders of this type, and in the 1920s and 1930s were considered to be a considerable advance on previous attempts.

As we have also seen, advances in the sphere of psychopharmacology always pique the interest of the CIA, and the development of barbiturates was no exception. The CIA experimented with the use of barbiturates to develop an early form of "brainwashing." Of course the use of sodium pentothal as a "truth serum" is well known in fiction and the cinema, and is obviously based on these experiments. Different doses and types of barbiturates were administered to subjects in attempts to loosen their tongues in answering questions or to allow them to absorb various forms of propaganda played unknowingly to them while they were in states of barbiturate-induced deep sleep.

By the 1940s the use of barbiturates was extremely widespread. It was estimated that some 70 tons of barbiturates were manufactured in 1936, and enough were produced to treat about 11 million people a year by 1955. However, although barbiturates were certainly enormously successful in many areas of medicine, there were two major problems with them. Indeed, the same problems were present with their nineteenth-century precursor, chloral hydrate. The first problem was that they were highly addictive, and the second problem was that they were dangerous to use. By this I mean that the there was not a large difference between the clinically effective dose—meaning how much you need to take in order to get some sleep—and the lethal dose, meaning how much does it take to kill you. This being the case, it is relatively easy to take a fatal overdose.

The addictive properties of the drugs had actually been observed early on, and a report on "the Veronal habit" was published only a year after the drug was first marketed. Eventually, the mounting tide of evidence pointing out the addictive properties of barbiturates resulted in a conference on "the regulation of use and distribution of barbiturates" in Washington in 1945, and in 1952 the World Health Organization recommended that barbiturates should only be available by prescription. Nevertheless, by the early 1960s it was estimated that there were around a quarter of a million barbiturate addicts in the United States alone. Barbiturates were also widely abused as street drugs in mixtures such as "goofballs," where they were used together with amphetamines. Deaths from barbiturate overdosing were a widespread problem.

Ironically this included the death of Emil Fischer. The death of two of Fischer's three sons and his diagnosis with incurable cancer had thrown him into a deep depression. He had been addicted to barbiturates for many years. Perhaps taking a slightly higher dose was just the final step? However, nothing focused the public's attention on these problems like the news that broke on August 28, 1962. "Marilyn Dead" read the headlines of the *New York Daily News* (Figure 6.4).

Marilyn Monroe, the famous actress and movie star, was found dead as a result of acute barbiturate poisoning. Exactly why and how the overdose was administered has become the stuff of conspiracy theorists ever since. Nevertheless, the role of barbiturates was clear and they would never be looked at in quite the same way again.

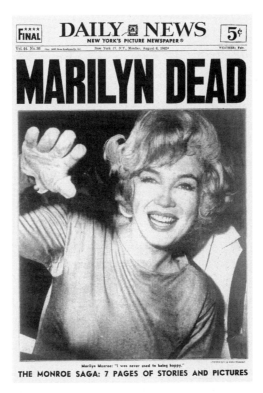

Figure 6.4:
The front page of the *New York Daily News* August 6, 1962, announcing the death of Marilyn Monroe from an overdose of barbiturates.
(Getty Images)

One small advance in the use of barbiturates was the development of barbiturate antagonist drugs such as bemegride, which can be used to reverse the effects of barbiturates and so are used in cases of barbiturate overdoses.[12] Indeed, such agents were involved in one very high profile legal case. Between the years 1946 and 1956, around 150 patients of the British doctor John Bodkin Adams died under suspicious circumstances. Usually the deaths occurred shortly after the patient had given Adams a large cash gift or had added him as a significant beneficiary to their will. He was suspected of being involved in these deaths, although he was acquitted of murder after a sensational trial. Nevertheless, subsequent information has made it abundantly clear that he was indeed the culprit. In one instance a patient of his named Gertrude Hullett somehow took an overdose of sodium barbitone two days after leaving Adams her Rolls-Royce Silver Dawn in her will. Adams was given bemegride to administer to Hullett but only gave her a minute dose which was ineffective, and she died. The coroner concluded that Hullett had committed suicide and criticized Adams for his treatment of the patient and his misuse of the bemegride. Nevertheless, Adams received the Rolls and sold it for a tidy sum.

There were several attempts to produce drugs that had the same spectrum of activities as barbiturates but were free of their abuse potential and had less risk associated with their use. This would include drugs like methaqualone, which are certainly effective clinically. Nevertheless, such drugs did not prove to be free of the problems associated with barbiturate use, and "Quaaludes" also became a widely abused drug in the 1950s.

Today barbiturates are still used in specific areas of medicine including epilepsy and anesthesia. However, they are not generally employed for the treatment of insomnia or anxiety. Benzodiazepines and their derivatives soon became the most widely used drugs for these purposes. However, before Leo Sternbach and his colleagues introduced benzodiazepines to the world, another important drug development was to occur that would set the stage for their arrival.

TRANQUILIZERS IN A MINOR KEY

Miltown was the drug that changed everything.[13] "Miltown" looks and sounds a lot like "Milltown." Indeed, this is hardly surprising since that is how the drug got its name. Milltown is an idyllic hamlet in New Jersey, seemingly far away from the toil and strife of modern life. A mill and a babbling brook conjure up images like those in one of Constable's canvases.

However, Milltown is not that far from New Brunswick, the site of the Carter-Wallace research laboratories.

In the 1950s Carter-Wallace was not what we would think of as a large drug company, having survived for many years on the sales of Carter's Little Liver Pills, a laxative concoction dating back to the Civil War. However, in the years following WWII, the way medicine was practiced in the United States was rapidly changing.

Increasing restrictions on the manner in which medicines were dispensed had led to a rise in the percentage of drugs only available by prescription, and drug companies were becoming more interested in creating unique patentable products that could be sold in this way at high prices. Carter-Wallace decided that they would attempt to move the company in this direction. In order to do this they needed to refurbish their research laboratories and put resources into drug development. They also needed somebody to head up this new enterprise. Here they made an inspired choice by hiring Dr. Fred Berger, a recent immigrant.

The story of Fred Berger and his development of Miltown is a fascinating one and has an enormous number of parallels to the story of Leo Sternbach and the development of benzodiazepines. Like Sternbach, Berger was a European Jew who fled the Nazi tyranny with his young wife. And like Sternbach, Berger's path to his new tranquilizer started with studies that were very far afield. Berger was a native of Czechoslovakia, where he had studied medicine. His flight from the Germans landed him in Britain and a job in Wakefield, Yorkshire, in a Public Health laboratory performing research on the purification of penicillin (the big medical question of the time). He actually made several important advances in the field.

Berger was an extremely egalitarian person and published his findings in the general scientific literature where they would be available to all, rather than trying to patent them for personal gain. He was involved in testing different substances as preservatives for penicillin. At some point he tried a substance called *mephenesin*. To his surprise, when he injected mephenesin into mice they appeared extremely relaxed, although apparently still awake. Indeed, when he reported his findings in 1946 he actually described mephenesin's effect as "tranquilizing."

Berger's findings attracted a reasonable amount of attention, and mephenesin was brought to the market in the United Kingdom and United States basically as a muscle relaxant for use in patients with multiple sclerosis and similar diseases, where it was certainly very effective. Berger's career took him from the UK to the United States in an effort to improve his professional situation. He had an excellent research career behind him at this point, and a growing reputation. After a short period of time spent in academia he was offered the job at Carter-Wallace at a much higher salary, and it proved to be irresistible.

What kind of new drugs should Carter-Wallace develop? In 1950 Berger decided to see if he could make a better version of mephenesin, and together with a medicinal chemist produced several hundred analogues. One called *meprobamate* proved to be particularly effective, producing marked muscle relaxant and sedative effects in both mice and monkeys (Figure 6.5).

Moreover, it appeared that meprobamate was relatively safe. As opposed to barbiturates, the clinically effective dose of meprobamate was many orders of magnitude separated from the lethal dose, providing the drug with a larger safety window. Around this time a limited number of small studies started to appear in the literature suggesting that mephenesin might be a useful drug in the context of psychiatric illness. It was suggested that the fact that mephenesin relaxed people without actually sending them off to sleep might make them much more amenable to psychotherapy or psychoanalysis.

Noting these studies, Berger tested meprobamate in a series of subjects suffering from various psychiatric and neurological disorders such as epilepsy. Meprobamate proved to be extremely effective and free from worrying side effects. More extensive trials carried out by several reputable psychiatrists followed, and it became clear that meprobamate was particularly good at alleviating a patient's anxiety rather than having specifically antipsychotic effects.

Berger's idea was that meprobamate might be a drug that could be used by the general public as an anxiolytic, but this was rather a novel proposal at the time. Nevertheless, Berger and his colleagues at Carter-Wallace presented their data to both the FDA and also several large drug companies. All were impressed. The FDA granted Carter-Wallace the authorization to sell meprobamate, and the Wyeth drug company made Carter-Wallace an offer to codevelop it. In the end it was decided that Carter-Wallace would sell meprobamate under the name Miltown, whereas Wyeth would sell it under the name Equanil. This, of course, is a ploy often used by the

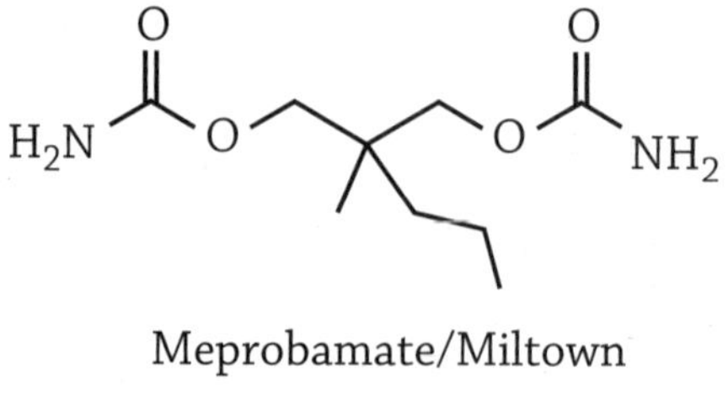

Meprobamate/Miltown

Figure 6.5:
Structure of Miltown (meprobamate).

pharmaceutical industry. Think about how many different companies sell aspirin, given that it's still the same aspirin and it really does the same thing whomever you buy it from. It is also interesting to relate how Miltown came to be categorized. Apparently, Berger was having dinner with two of the leading lights in psychopharmacology of the time: Nathan Kline, who had a key role in the development of antidepressants among other things (Chapter 4), and Paul Janssen, whose Janssen Pharmaceuticals developed haloperidol, one of the world's most successful and important antipsychotic drugs (Chapter 3). Berger described the properties of his new drug and declared that he would market it as a new type of sedative. However, Kline took exception to this. "The world doesn't need another sedative," he said. "If it tranquilizes people, why don't you call it a tranquilizer?" Berger took the advice and the rest, as they say, is history.[13]

MILTOWN HITS HOLLYWOOD

When Carter-Wallace launched Miltown they worried that the public would not be interested in it and that doctors wouldn't prescribe it. Was anxiety something that was really worth medical attention, or was it just part of the fabric of everyday life? They needn't have worried. Within a year Miltown proved to be a sensation. As with many things, good publicity was a key factor and it turned out Miltown got the best one could imagine. The drug was taken up by the Hollywood tastemakers and soon it was seen as a fashionable accessory. Miltown was just the drug for the high-pressure environment of the Los Angeles entertainment industry.

And it wasn't just the denizens of Hollywood that got on board. Artists from other disciplines, such as Aldous Huxley and even Salvador Dali, helped to push the Miltown bandwagon. Dali was commissioned to design an advertisement for Miltown, which he called "Crisalida" and which depicted the progress of an individual as he escaped from the chrysalis of crippling anxiety and gradually attained tranquility and peace. The Miltown fad spread from the West Coast to the rest of the United States, making it the most in-demand drug of all time.

However, it would be wrong to attribute Miltown's success to being just the result of a fashion trend. Another important factor was the fact that the entire way in which the medical community and the public viewed mental disease was undergoing a sea change. It should be remembered that the development of Miltown happened at approximately the same time that the major antipsychotic drugs like chlorpromazine were also developed, and moreover it was coming right on the heels of the development of penicillin.

Penicillin had strengthened the idea that if you had a terrible disease it really could be cured if you just had the right pill to take. The antibiotic revolution had demonstrated that fatal diseases that had plagued mankind from the beginning of time could be dealt with most effectively by the right drug. Inhibit the right enzyme, or block the right receptor, and "hey presto"—you were cured! It was becoming clear in the field of psychiatric illness that enzymes and receptors were at the basis of psychiatric disease as well. Logically, therefore, one didn't need to spend 5 days a week lying on an analyst's couch if you could identify the right drug target.

Hand in hand with this development was the way in which drugs like Miltown/Equanil were actually marketed. Drug companies such as Wyeth started to invest considerably more resources into courting doctors who, after all, were the people who were going to actually write the drug scripts. Teams of young, drug company-trained, attractive and energetic sales people armed with eye-catching literature, movies, and samples were dispatched throughout the country to "inform" doctors as to the virtues of their products.

All of this, however, ignores one other important fact about Miltown—it actually worked! It was just the thing for relieving "everyday" anxieties, thus allowing one to engage in life's activities more effectively. And, unlike barbiturates, Miltown wasn't nearly so likely to result in a fatal overdose. It was initially believed that Miltown wasn't addictive, although this ultimately did not prove to be the case. It was hardly surprising, therefore, that Miltown/Equanil proved to be the most commercially successful drug ever produced at that point in time, and it is also hardly surprising that this came to the attention of all of the other major drug companies. It certainly came to the attention of Hoffmann-La Roche.

LEO STERNBACH'S HOME RUN

It is with all of this in mind that in the mid-1950s Roche made a decision to try to come up with a new tranquilizer that would be superior to meprobamate, and enable them to take a good share of the burgeoning tranquilizer market. One possibility was to just play around with the structure of meprobamate and so arrive at an analogue that wasn't covered in the existing patent literature. If the compound had properties that were as good or better than meprobamate then, with Roche's experienced marketing expertise, the new drug might well be a great success. In fact this type of strategy is frequently successfully employed by pharmaceutical companies wishing to rapidly establish themselves in a hot market area.

Typically, however, the new drugs possess both the same virtues and also the same problems as the parent drug. Such a drug is commonly known as a "me too" drug. For example, "me too" versions of meprobamate have been made and brought to the market. Currently one of these analogues (carisoprodol) with the unlikely trade name of "Soma" is available on the market.[14] This substance was originally developed by Carter-Wallace when they examined possible analogues of meprobamate.

On the other hand, one may decide to attempt to make a drug with the requisite properties from an entirely different chemical starting point. This, of course, is a much riskier enterprise. However, if it is successful it is much more likely that the new drug will have genuinely novel properties. Moreover, if a judicious choice of potential chemical structures is made, it is also likely that the patent position will be favorable.

In the mid 1950s, impressed with the success of Miltown, Roche decided to let Leo Sternbach proceed with a program for the development of minor tranquilizers. "Minor tranquilizer" means a drug like meprobamate as opposed to an antipsychotic drug like chlorpromazine, which was referred to as a "major tranquilizer." Although there was a lot of goal-directed thinking and excellent science involved in the ultimate success of this project, there was a good deal of serendipity as well.[5,6]

In 1955 Sternbach decided not to pursue the "me too" route but to attempt something more original. But where to start? Sternbach recalled the chemical structures he had explored in Poland as a graduate student when he had investigated the series of substances known as benzoheptoxdiazines in an effort to synthesize new dyestuffs. Sternbach's original work on this series of compounds had not yielded anything interesting with respect to new dyes. However, the chemical potential of the series remained relatively unexplored. Moreover, to a medicinal chemist they had the "look" of substances that might be biologically active at some point—several rings, nitrogen atoms, and so forth. Sternbach decided to give them another try.

However, by 1957 the lack of progress of the project in terms of yielding anything of pharmacological interest ultimately led to the decision to stop the research and move on to something else. Prior to that, a major lab cleanup was required. Dirty flasks and beakers filled with diverse chemical products needed to be cleaned, along with the benches and all of the equipment. While doing this, Sternbach's colleague Reeder came across one compound that had been made but never tested. Although it was assumed that, like its relatives, this compound would be similarly inactive, Sternbach and Reeder sent the compound off for testing. Little did they know that the compound was not what they had predicted. The reaction they had used in this case had inadvertently produced a different chemical structure—a benzodiazepine.

This compound, which was originally called *methaminochlordiazepoxide,* proved to have a highly promising profile of pharmacological effects. It was run through a battery of tests where it was compared head-to-head with meprobamate, and in every case it proved to be more effective. The Roche pharmacology laboratory was run by Dr. Lowell Randall, a man with great experience who utilized a series of tests to examine the properties of the new molecule.[15] The first test was one in which mice were observed trying to hang on to an inclined screen. When they were given the new drug they slid off much more easily, demonstrating that the new compound had muscle relaxant activity. This was confirmed in cats. In another important test, the new compound was shown to effectively block the generation of seizures. A third test was of particular interest: brain lesions in the septal area produced rats or mice that were extremely irritable. Just poking them with a pencil would cause them to attack aggressively. However, if animals with such lesions were given the new drug, they didn't do this at all but appeared tame and friendly. Similarly, monkeys that were normally extremely aggressive became very nice monkeys when given the new drug. Importantly, the new drug didn't appear to produce any obvious problematic side effects and was relatively safe, its effective dose being much lower than its lethal dose.

Roche rushed the drug into clinical trials. After testing it in a large number of human subjects, all of their hopes were confirmed. The drug appeared to be an absolute winner. By 1960 the drug was through the FDA and on the market. The name had been changed to chlordiazepoxide and the drug was sold under the name Librium—the first benzodiazepine tranquilizer (Figure 6.6).[10] Even as Librium was being brought to the market, the Roche chemists worked feverishly to produce even better derivatives, and many compounds were produced. One named *diazepam* proved to be a

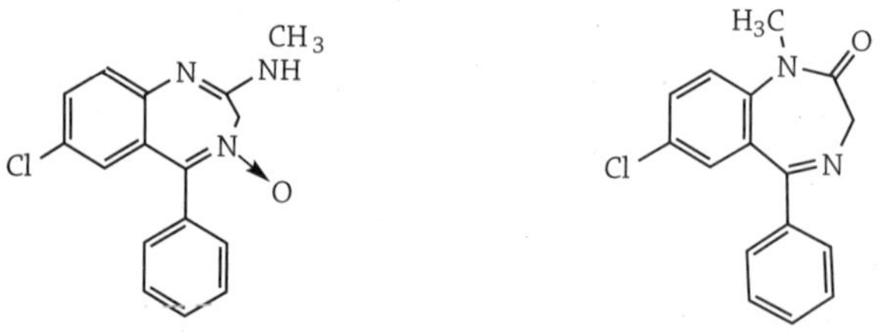

Librium/Chlordiazepoxide   Valium/Diazepam

Figure 6.6:
Librium and Valium, the first benzodiazepine anxiolytic drugs.

considerable advance on Librium, and so it too was brought to the market in 1963 under the trade name Valium (Figure 6.6).

Roche's new benzodiazepine tranquilizers were an immediate success. Not only did they work extremely well, but also they were backed by a highly professional advertising team and soon doctors were completely infatuated with them. The use of Miltown and other tranquilizers was eclipsed. Miltown had been the John the Baptist of tranquilizers, a prophet for the coming age, and now with the benzodiazepines we had the real thing. In the years following the launch of Librium and Valium, Roche filled literally billions of prescriptions for the drugs and became the largest and most profitable drug company in the world. In 1977 alone, 54 million prescriptions were written for diazepam and 13 million for chlordiazepoxide. A conservative estimate suggested that some 8000 tons of benzodiazepines were consumed by Americans in that year.

Naturally Roche and all its competitors proceeded to work intensively on the benzodiazepines, producing numerous new molecules each with slightly different properties designed to fill a niche in the market—tranquilizers, hypnotics, anticonvulsant drugs, drugs for panic disorder, and so on. The list is endless and new possibilities are still emerging. Drugs like Xanax, Klonopin, Dalmane and others, many of which were not developed by Roche, have all had extraordinary success.

Furthermore, as we shall discuss, understanding precisely how benzodiazepines work has allowed the development of newer non-benzodiazepine drugs that have similar or more selective activities, designed to be free of the problems that are associated with benzodiazepines. Because, of course, it ultimately proved to be the case that there were problems associated with benzodiazepines just as there were problems with Miltown, barbiturates, and chloral hydrate. Not the least of these was the fact that benzodiazepines proved to have their own addictive liabilities. They became so widely used that these problems eventually saw the light of day, and something of a backlash to their use kicked in. Nevertheless, they remain some of the world's most widely used drugs and have proved to be extremely useful for numerous purposes.

BENZODIAZEPINES AND RECEPTORS

The path to understanding exactly how benzodiazepines work began in the late 1970s. The research done in this area is some of the most insightful and elegant ever to have been performed in molecular neuroscience. Moreover, much of the work, including many of the key observations, was performed by scientists at Roche. Hence in this instance, the company not only discovered this class of drugs but also successfully engaged in the research elucidating their mechanisms of action.

Two observations were made in the 1970s that were the underpinnings of our understanding of benzodiazepines' mechanism of action. The first was the identification of the "benzodiazepine receptor." As we have discussed in previous chapters, the receptor-binding assays pioneered by Solomon Snyder and his colleagues were used time and time again to make important breakthroughs in the field of molecular pharmacology. Originally developed to identify the molecular nature of opiate receptors (Chapter 6), scientists at Roche as well as other labs took the same approach in an attempt to identify the molecular site of action for benzodiazepines.

Using radioactive drugs such as radioactive diazepam (that is, diazepam synthesized to contain radioactive tritium) it was demonstrated that high affinity binding sites for these drugs could be observed in brain tissue.[16] These binding sites had the properties expected if they really represented the authentic sites of drug action. For example, there were some benzodiazepine drugs that existed as stereoisomers—that is, the two molecules possessed exactly the same atoms but were mirror images of one another, as discussed previously in the case of morphine (Chapter 5). It was found that one isomer acted as a benzodiazepine when given to animals, whereas the other isomer was inactive. This observation tells us that the site of action for benzodiazepines in the brain must be able to distinguish between these two stereoisomers even though they are structurally so similar. When the high affinity binding sites in the brain labeled by tritiated diazepam were examined, it was found that they could indeed distinguish between the stereoisomers of benzodiazepines. Thus, the active isomer bound to the same site as the radioactive diazepam but the inactive isomer didn't.

Another type of experiment investigators performed was to detect the binding sites using autoradiography. In this method the radioactive drug is applied to a slice of the brain under the appropriate conditions so that it will bind to its receptors. A film is then applied to the slice and the radioactive decay from the drug is detected as silver grains on the film. Using this method one can see exactly where the drug binding sites are localized in comparison to the anatomy of structures in the brain. The benzodiazepine binding sites turned out to be very widely distributed in the brain, although this distribution exhibited a marked heterogeneity so that some areas had a lot of binding sites, whereas others had relatively few. Biochemical studies demonstrated that the drug binding sites appeared to be protein molecules, which is the case for receptors such as GPCRs and ligand gated ion channels (Chapters 1 and 2).

However, as in the previous case of the opiate receptor, investigators then asked themselves what the normal physiological function of these binding sites might be? After all, why should the brain possess binding sites for a synthetic drug? This was the same question that had been asked following the discovery of the opiate receptors (Chapter 5). Perhaps these binding sites were normally used for something else? Maybe they were actually the receptors for a naturally occurring molecule in the brain that had an important physiological function? Answering this question was also made easier from some observations using electrophysiology.

THE GABA CONNECTION

When benzodiazepines were discovered, neuroscientists started to perform experiments to see if they would influence the actions of different known neurotransmitter substances. They rapidly demonstrated that drugs like diazepam could enhance the effects of the inhibitory neurotransmitter GABA (Chapter 1). Indeed, these effects were very specific, as the benzodiazepines failed to influence the actions of any other neurotransmitter. It was then demonstrated that the way benzodiazepines seemed to work was not to influence the metabolism of GABA in the brain but to actually influence its effects upon its synaptic receptors.[17]

As discussed in Chapter 1, there are two kinds of GABA receptors: the GABA-A receptors which are ligand gated ion channels, and the GABA-B receptors which are GPCRs. It was observed that the effects of benzodiazepines could be blocked by drugs that blocked GABA-A receptors such as bicuculline and picrotoxin. Hence, it was concluded that the ultimate site of action of benzodiazepine drugs must be the GABA-A receptors.

The next question to answer was exactly how this happened. For example, were the drug binding sites observed using radioactive benzodiazepines actually the GABA-A receptors, or was the observed interaction due to some more indirect effect? Initial studies indicated that it looked like benzodiazepines and GABA didn't bind to the same sites in the brain. Soon. However. things became clearer. It was observed that although GABA didn't directly interact with the binding sites for benzodiazepine drugs, it could influence the binding of drugs to these sites. Further experiments were also carried out labeling the brain GABA-A receptors with radioactive GABA or with drugs like radioactive bicuculline. Again it was observed that drugs like diazepam didn't directly interact with the binding site for GABA but were able to influence the binding of GABA. In fact, the binding of diazepam allowed GABA to interact with its receptors more strongly and hence to activate them more efficiently. This seemed to explain why the electro-physiological studies had shown that benzodiazepines could enhance the ability of GABA to inhibit neurons. Ultimately it became clear that GABA and benzodiazepines did both bind to GABA-A receptors, but to different, non-overlapping sites on these receptors. As we have discussed when we considered the mechanism of action of Gaboxadol (Chapter 1), the GABA-A receptor is a large ion channel consisting of five separate protein subunits. Compared to the size of this protein complex, the size of GABA or a benzo-diazepine drug is very small, and so there is plenty of room on the GABA-A receptor for many different kinds of binding sites.

What we imagine happens is the following. When a drug like diazepam binds to its specific site on the GABA-A receptor complex, the energy imparted by its binding causes a slight conformational change in the recep-tor, resulting in an increase in the affinity of the receptor for GABA. In other words, unlike GABA, benzodiazepines don't actually activate GABA-A receptors directly. Instead, they allow GABA to do its job of opening the channel more effectively. They are facilitators of the action of GABA. If GABA is the key that opens the GABA-A receptor lock, then benzodiaz-epines are the oil that helps the key turn more easily. The kind of effect that benzodiazepines produce is known as an *allosteric* mechanism. With this basic mechanism in mind we can now explore the details of benzodiazepine action further.

We know that GABA-A receptors are very common in the brain. GABA is the brain's major inhibitory neurotransmitter, and so virtually every neu-ron expresses GABA-A receptors. We also know that benzodiazepines have many different effects. As we might expect, these include hypnosis (sleep) and sedation (Chapter 1). In addition, benzodiazepines have significant anticonvulsive effects, they act as muscle relaxants, decrease anxiety, and also produce retrograde amnesia. We also know that GABA-A receptors are made up of five separate protein subunits (Chapter 1). In fact, there is a good deal of heterogeneity in the construction of GABA-A receptors in the brain. As it turns out there are 19 different subunits encoded by different gene families, including α, β, γ, δ, ϵ, and σ subunits which can potentially make up GABA-A receptor channels. Altogether some 150,000 GABA-A receptor subtypes might theoretically exist. In practice, however, the avail-able subunits assemble into a limited number of pentameric receptors with the general stoichiometry of 2 α, 2 β and 1 γ subunits; δ and ϵ subunits may substitute for the γ subunit, and the σ subunit may substitute for the β subunit.[18]

So, one question we might be interested in would be—"do benzodiaz-epines bind to every subtype of GABA-A receptor, or is some selectivity involved?" We could also ask the question, "Is it the case that the different effects of benzodiazepines like Valium are mediated by different subclasses of GABA-A receptors?" If that turned out to be the case, then perhaps we could find types of benzodiazepines or other types of drugs that only activated one subclass, and so only produced selective effects, rather than all of the different effects produced by a drug like Valium. This could be very useful in some instances. For example, we know that consistent use of benzodiazepines results in a significant degree of drug dependence. If the anxiolytic and addictive properties of these drugs resulted from interactions with different subclasses of GABA-A receptors, then could they perhaps be separated?

Studies using molecular biology to make selective mutations to different amino acids have demonstrated that GABA binds to the receptor at a site near the junction between subunits α and β, whereas benzodiazepines bind at the interface between certain α subunits and γ2. So, whereas GABA will bind to all versions of GABA-A receptors, benzodiazepines will only bind to those that contain a γ2-subunit together with certain α subunits. Hence the facilitatory effect of benzodiazepines is only observed on a particular subgroup of GABA-A receptors. These receptors must contain a γ2 subunit.

With such information in hand, molecular pharmacologists at Roche and other drug companies could set about trying to perfect new drugs that specifically targeted different benzodiazepine binding sites on GABA-A receptor subtypes with the expectation that they would produce relatively specific effects. Following a series of experiments using genetically modified mice, they concluded that a drug that selectively activated GABA-A receptors containing α1/γ2 subunits might be a sedative/hypnotic without producing the anxiolytic effects of benzodiazepines. Indeed, the widely used hypnotic drug zolpidem (Ambien) follows this logic and exhibits selectivity for α1/γ2 containing GABA-A receptors.[18] Literally tens of thousands of new chemical compounds have now been produced representing a large number of benzodiazepine and non-benzodiazepine chemical classes, all of which interact with benzodiazepine binding sites in one way or another and produce a bewildering spectrum of different effects.

As we have seen, many of the drugs discussed in this chapter produce inhibitory effects on the brain which can be considered along a continuum starting with sedation and proceeding through hypnosis (sleep) to anesthesia and eventually death. All of these effects are the result of activation of GABA-A receptors by these different types of drugs, which include the benzodiazepines, barbiturates, many anesthetics, meprobamate, chloral hydrate, and others that we will discuss below, including the neurosteroids and alcohol (Figure 6.7). However, even though there are many similarities

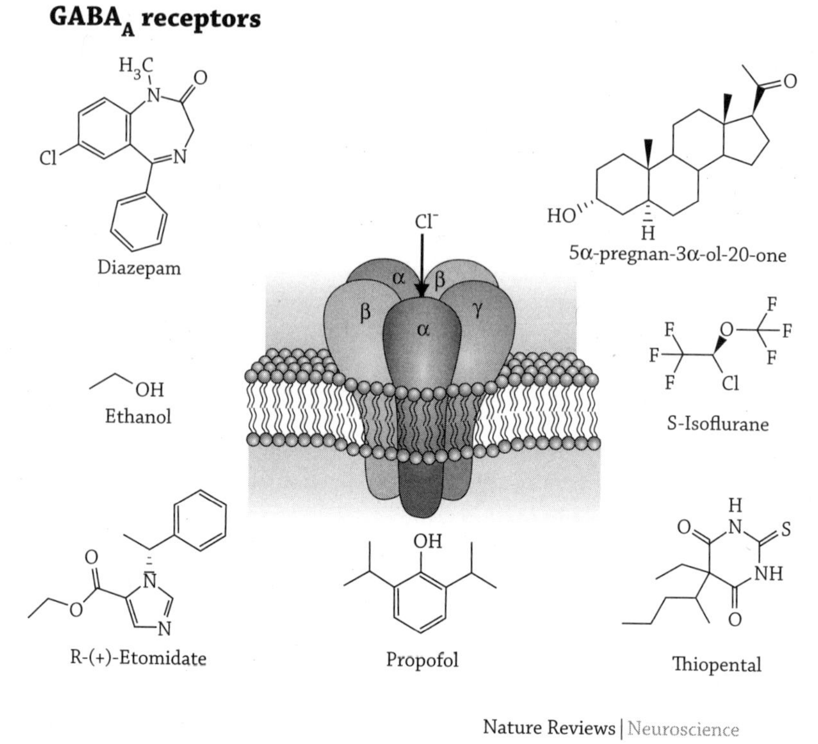

GABA$_A$ receptors

Diazepam

Ethanol

R-(+)-Etomidate

5α-pregnan-3α-ol-20-one

S-Isoflurane

Propofol

Thiopental

Nature Reviews | Neuroscience

Figure 6.7:
The structures of different types of drugs that all act by enhancing the activity of the GABA-A receptor, a five subunit ligand gated ion channel that is permeable to Cl ions.[22]
(Reproduced with permission from *Nature*)

in the effects produced by each of these classes of drugs, each type produces a unique spectrum of actions which gives them their particular clinical utility. Presumably this is because each type of drugs interacts with the GABA-A receptor in a unique fashion.

THE BRAIN ON STEROIDS

Although many types of drugs modulate the action of GABA-A receptors, the natural activator of the receptor is the neurotransmitter GABA. However, it turns out that the situation is a little more complicated, because there is at least one other naturally occurring set of brain chemicals that activate the same receptor. Interest in these substances really began with the observation in 1927 that the lipid molecule cholesterol could have an inhibitory effect on the brain. Now, cholesterol is an extraordinarily important substance for numerous reasons, as it participates in the construction of cell membranes and it is also involved as an intermediate in cell signaling. For example, cholesterol is the basic chemical starting point for the biosynthesis of steroid hormones.

In the 1940s, Selye demonstrated that several steroid molecules that could be derived from cholesterol produced rapid sedation and anesthesia.[19] Indeed, these effects were impressive enough that synthetic steroid derivatives such as alphaxalone were developed as anesthetics. It should be noted that steroid hormones have an enormous number of effects in virtually every tissue in the body. However, these effects usually develop rather slowly. The reason for this is that it is generally accepted that steroid hormones act through binding to a family of receptors within the cytoplasm of cells, which then control the expression of different genes. This type of effect typically takes many minutes or hours to develop. On the other hand, the inhibitory effects of agents like alphaxalone on brain activity were observed to be quite different and occurred almost immediately.

In 1984, Harrison and Simmonds demonstrated that alphaxalone could activate GABA-A receptors, providing a mechanism for its observed rapid inhibitory effects.[19] It was subsequently suggested that perhaps naturally occurring steroid hormone derivatives synthesized locally in the brain might also produce such effects. Although the production of steroid hormones has traditionally been associated with peripheral glands like the adrenal and ovaries, it turned out that all of the enzymatic machinery required for their biosynthesis can also be found within the brain. There is now compelling evidence that various bioactive steroids can be formed directly within the brain. These substances have become known as *neurosteroids*. Moreover, some of these substances, such as 5α-pregnan-3α-ol-20-one (5α3α-THPROG) and 5β-pregnan-3α-ol-20-one (5β3α-THPROG), and the deoxycorticosterone metabolite 5α-pregnan-3α,21-diol-20-one (5α3α-THDOC), which are metabolites of progesterone, have been shown to activate GABA-A receptors through an allosteric mechanism. Consistent with this observation, neuroactive steroids have been shown to exhibit anticonvulsant, antianxiety/sedative, and anesthetic activities, and these molecules are being developed for such purposes. Currently a neurosteroid activator of GABA-A receptors named *ganaxolone* is under development for use in epilepsy and other indications.

One thing to note about the effects of neurosteroids is their potency. Generally speaking they are effective in nanomolar (10^{-9}M) concentrations, whereas we imagine the effective concentrations of GABA are in the micro/millimolar range (10^{-6}-10^{-3}M), meaning that neurosteroids are hundreds or thousands of times more potent than GABA. Indeed, such an observation is consistent with the concentrations of these substances that have been shown to exist in the brain. It is considered likely that neurosteroids may normally be involved in the regulation of synaptic inhibition in the brain and so may be key factors in numerous types of brain pathology. This might include things like premenstrual syndrome (PMS), premenstrual dysphoric disorder (PMDD), catamenial epilepsy (seizures related to the menstrual cycle), and postpartum depression, as well as many psychiatric and neurological disorders. Moreover, given the key role we now know that GABA plays in the development of the nervous system, a role for neurosteroids in brain development has also been suggested.[19]

The discovery of the neurosteroids and their actions is clearly surprising, fascinating, and highly important. It also demonstrates that the GABA-A receptor complex may yet yield further surprises and that new classes of drugs may yet be developed that utilize these receptors in unique ways. However, GABA-A receptors do not only offer us an understanding of the actions of some of our newest drugs but also of one of our oldest.

ALCOHOL AND GABA

Alcohol is one of the most ancient drugs known to man.[20] Alcohol is mentioned in the earliest written records of the Sumerians, but its use clearly precedes this time and archaeological evidence has demonstrated that fermented drinks of various kinds were used in the Neolithic period and earlier. Few preliterate people failed to discover or learn how to utilize fermentation to produce wine or beer from sugar- or starch-containing fruits, berries, flowers, cactuses, tree saps, honey, milk, and every sort of tuber and grain. Such a universal phenomenon can be explained by ethanol's combined analgesic, disinfectant, and profound psychological effects. Indeed alcohol, like certain other ancient drugs such as opium and cannabis, can be used for both recreational and medical purposes. The medical use of alcohol advanced with the development of distilled spirits, first prepared from wine in southern Italy in the twelfth century, where they were named "aqua vita" or "water of life." The use of distilled spirits spread through the grape growing regions of southern Europe, where they became known as brandy—from the Dutch *brandewijn* or "burned wine"—and eventually to Northern Europe, where they were prepared from alternative sources such as mashed grains, leading to the production of beverages such as whiskey and vodka. However, in general these were not of the same quality as brandy imported from southern Europe.

In the mid seventeenth century, however, Dr. Franciscus de la Boe (aka Dr. Sylvius) of the University of Leyden invented a new drink obtained from distilling pure malt spirits with juniper berries. This resulted in a much more palatable drink, which could actually rival real French Brandy. The new drink, which was initially known as Genever, rapidly became extremely popular, particularly in England, where it became known as Geneva, subsequently shortened to Gin.[21]

Gin became a tremendous fad and was widely drunk along with the traditional drinks such as ale, and often in the same quantities. Clearly, however, a pint of gin was likely to have far more profound effects on the consumer than a pint of ale. The associated drunkenness prompted some of the earliest legislation restricting the use of alcohol. Indeed, issues related to the use and abuse of alcohol and the laws associated with this are still very much with us today.

However, if we consider some of the beneficial medical effects of alcohol, these would include anticonvulsant, sedative, and hypnotic effects clearly reminiscent of the effects of the different types of drugs that we have discussed acting at the GABA-A receptors, and suggesting that this might also be a target for the effects of alcohol.[22] But, we should first understand that as a drug, ethanol is not very potent—that is, it does not produce its effects at low concentrations. If we consider that the effects of neurosteroids are observed in the nanomolar range ($nM, 10^{-9}$), and the benzodiazepines in the nanomolar to micromolar range ($nM 10^{-9}$-$\mu M 10^{-6}$), the effects of ethanol are only observed in the millimolar range ($mM 10^{-3}$), meaning that it is tens of thousands of times less potent than other types of drugs that act on GABA-A receptors. Most people who drink for social reasons attain blood alcohol levels of between 5 and 20mM, which produces a mellow relaxed feeling and a reduction in anxiety. Heavier bouts of drinking, resulting in blood alcohol levels of 20–50 mM, produce profound sedation, a loss of coordination, amnesia, and impairment of cognitive functions. If blood alcohol reaches 100 mM it will normally produce anesthesia in most people and could be fatal.[22] The fact that ethanol acts at such elevated concentrations makes it unlikely that it has a highly selective locus of action. Indeed, actions at a variety of ion channels and receptors are probably responsible for the entire spectrum of effects produced by ethanol.

Nevertheless, it is clear that GABA-A receptors are one important site of action. Indeed, there may well be a degree of selectivity associated with its effects. At relatively low concentrations of ethanol, it appears that GABA-A receptors that contain α4 and δ subunits may be the preferred site of action. GABA-A receptors with this composition are highly expressed in the thalamocortical neurons, whose activity is highly correlated with states of sleep and wakefulness. Low concentrations of ethanol produce tonic inhibition of these neurons, an effect which is not observed in lines of mice in which the α4 subunit has been deleted.

The GABA-A receptor is a wonderful molecular machine. It is without doubt the most important locus of drug action in the brain and, as we have seen, mediates the action of a very large number of drugs that have many useful effects. Moreover, it is also clear that many further classes of drugs with novel mechanisms of action at the GABA-A receptor can be envisaged. The experiments that have resulted in our present sophisticated understanding of the structure and function of the GABA-A receptor complex are some of the most elegant carried out in the history of molecular pharmacology. Scientists from industry and academia have contributed extensively to this work, and it is certainly a spectacular success story. Paul Sacher would have smiled.

NOTES

1. *Entartete Kunst*—literally "degenerate art." This was part of a Nazi campaign to control culture. Works of art of a nontraditional, modernist nature were deemed to have Jewish or Bolshevik influence and were banned. An *Entartete Kunst* exhibition was put on in Munich and then traveled to other German cities. In this exhibition the works of Jewish and other artists was displayed together with slogans indicating how they insulted the German Reich and its "volk" and how the nefarious influence of Jews could be documented. Works associated with negroes, particularly jazz, were also considered degenerate. The Nazis sanctioned traditional "heroic" types of painting and music that was basically tonal.
2. Felix Weingartner (1863–1942) was a famous Austrian conductor. He was Gustav Mahler's successor as conductor of the Vienna opera.
3. Hans Conrad Peyer. *Roche, a company history: 1896-1996*. Editiones Roche. 1996.
4. "Roche, traditionally ahead of our time." See www.roche.com/histb2008_e.pdf.
5. Alex Baenninger. *Good Chemistry: The Life and Legacy of Valium Inventor Leo Sternbach*. McGraw-Hill Professional. 2004.
   Leo H. Sternbach. *The Benzodiazepine Story*. Editiones Roche. 1980.
6. Leo H. Sternbach. *The discovery of librium*. Agents Actions. 1972, 2:193–196.
   Leo H. Sternbach. The benzodiazepine story. *J Med Chem*. 1979, 22:1–7.
7. Thomas Mann. *Doktor Faustus*: A bildungsroman describing the life of the composer Adrian Leverkuhn, who is clearly a literary metaphor for the composer Arnold Schoenberg. Leverkuhn writes brilliant music for a period of 24 years, possibly due to the influence of satanic forces.
8. Albert Einstein was the developer of the theory of Relativity. Werner Heisenberg developed important aspects of quantum mechanics, particularly the Uncertainty Principle. Kurt Godel was an important mathematician/logician who devcloped theories of Incompleteness. All these theories put new limits on what things one may actually know and how these things might be determined.
9. The Age of Anxiety: Europe in the 1920s. See http://www.historyguide.org/europe/lecture8.html

10. Sourkes TL. Early clinical neurochemistry of CNS active drugs: chloral hydrate. *Molecular and Chemical Neuropathology*. 1992, 17:21–30.

11. López-Muñoz F, Ucha Udabe R, Alamo C. The history of barbiturates a century after their clinical introduction. *Neuropsychiatr Dis Treat*. 2005, 1:329–343.
    Sans RG, Chozas MG. Historic aspects and application of barbituric acid derivatives: a review. *Die Pharmazie*. 1988, 43:827–829.
    Matthew H. Barbiturates. *Clinical Toxicol*. 1975, 8:495–513.
    Dundee JW, McIroy PDA. The history of barbiturates. *Anaesthesia*. 1982, 37:726–734.
    Cozanitis DA. One hundred years of barbiturates and their saint. *J Royal Soc Med*. 2004, 97: 594–598.

12. Mistry DK, Cottrell GA. Actions of steroids and bemegride on the GABA-A receptor of mouse spinal neurons in culture. *Exp Physiol*. 1990, 75:199–209.

13. Andrea Tone. *The Age of Anxiety; a history of America's turbulent affair with tranquilizers*. Basic Books. 2009.

14. Gonzalez LA, Gatch MB, Forster MJ, Dillon GH. Abuse Potential of Soma: the GABA(A) Receptor as a Target. *Mol Cell Pharmacol*. 2009 1:180–186.
    Gonzalez LA, Gatch MB, Taylor CM, Bell-Horner CL, Forster MJ, Dillon GH. Carisoprodol-mediated modulation of GABA$_A$ receptors: in vitro and in vivo studies. *J Pharmacol Exp Ther*. 2009, 329:827–837.

15. Randall LO, Schallek W, Heise GA, Keith EF, Bagdon RE. The psychosedative properties of methaminodiazepoxide. *J Pharmacol Exp Ther*. 1960, 129:163–171.

16. Möhler H, Okada T. Benzodiazepine receptor: demonstration in the central nervous system. *Science*. 1977, 198:849–851.

17. Tallman JF, Paul SM, Skolnick P, Gallager DW. Receptors for the age of anxiety: pharmacology of the benzodiazepines. *Science*. 1980, 207:274–281.

18. Sieghart W. Structure and pharmacology of gamma-aminobutyric acid A receptor subtypes. *Pharmacol Rev*. 1995, 47:181–234.
    Nutt D. GABA-A receptors: subtypes, regional distribution, and function. *J Clin Sleep Med*. 2006, 2:S7–11.
    D'Hulst C, Atack JR, Kooy RF. The complexity of the GABA-A receptor shapes unique pharmacological profiles. *Drug Discov Today*. 2009, 14:866–875.
    Da Settimo F, Taliani S, Trincavelli ML, Montali M, Martini C. GABA A/Bz receptor subtypes as targets for selective drugs. *Curr Med Chem*. 2007, 14:2680–2701.

19. Belelli D, Lambert JJ. Neurosteroids: endogenous regulators of the GABA(A) receptor. *Nat Rev Neurosci*. 2005, 6:565–575.
    Lambert JJ, Cooper MA, Simmons RD, Weir CJ, Belelli D. Neurosteroids: endogenous allosteric modulators of GABA(A) receptors. *Psychoneuroendocrinology*. 2009, 34 Suppl 1:S48–58.
    Mitchell EA, Herd MB, Gunn BG, Lambert JJ, Belelli D. Neurosteroid modulation of GABA-A receptors: molecular determinants and significance in health and disease. *Neurochem Int*. 2008, 52:588–595.
    Ahboucha S, Butterworth RF. The neurosteroid system: an emerging therapeutic target for hepatic encephalopathy. *Metab Brain Dis*. 2007, 22:291–308.
    Reddy DS. The role of neurosteroids in the pathophysiology and treatment of catamenial epilepsy. *Epilepsy Res*. 2009, 85:1–30.

20. McGovern PE, Zhang J, Tang J, Zhang Z, Hall GR, Moreau RA, Nuñez A, Butrym ED, Richards MP, Wang CS, Cheng G, Zhao Z, Wang C. Fermented beverages of pre- and proto-historic China. *Proc Natl Acad Sci U S A*. 2004, 101:17593–17598.

Keller M. A historical overview of alcohol and alcoholism. *Cancer Res.* 1979, 39 (7 Pt 2):2822–2829.

21. Jessica Warner. *Craze: Gin and Debauchery in an Age of Reason.* Profile Books. 2004.

22. Lobo IA, Harris RA. GABA(A) receptors and alcohol. *Pharmacol Biochem Behav.* 2008, 90:90–94.

Jia F, Chandra D, Homanics GE, Harrison NL. Ethanol modulates synaptic and extrasynaptic GABA$_A$ receptors in the thalamus. *J Pharmacol Exp Ther.* 2008, 326:475–482.

Korpi ER, Debus F, Linden AM, Malécot C, Leppä E, Vekovischeva O, Rabe H, Böhme I, Aller MI, Wisden W, Lüddens H. Does ethanol act preferentially via selected brain GABA$_A$ receptor subtypes? the current evidence is ambiguous. *Alcohol.* 2007, 41:163–176.

Belelli D, Harrison NL, Maguire J, Macdonald RL, Walker MC, Cope DW. Extrasynaptic GABA$_A$ receptors: form, pharmacology, and function. *J Neurosci.* 2009, 29:12757–12763.

CHAPTER 7

ᴄᴠᴐ

Harry and Tonto

"Reefers make darkies think they're as good as white men."

Harry Anslinger

Harry Anslinger was a man who knew his own mind. He knew what was right and what was wrong; he was not afflicted by self-doubt. Sometimes people would present him with "facts" to try and make him change his mind about this or that. But usually Harry wasn't interested. Harry knew what he knew. Harry worked hard, and when he came home in the evening he liked to relax by listening to the radio. Tonight, like millions of other Americans, he was listening to one of his favorites—The Lone Ranger. Harry identified somewhat with the masked lawman. Like the Lone Ranger, Harry was concerned with protecting the American people from evil. Often it was a lonely business. Yes, in some ways Harry thought of himself as a bit of a "lone ranger." Although Harry liked the Lone Ranger, he had some doubts about his supposed sidekick. Who was this guy anyway? Some degenerate Indian? Who knew what he was talking about—"Kemo Sabe?" What was that all about? Probably Indian for "White Sucker!" Harry also had a good idea as to how and where Mr. Tonto got his supposed wisdom. Sneaking off and smoking Mr. Muggles like all the other degenerates. Oh yes, Harry knew a thing or two about that!

Harry was patriotic and knew that the United States was the greatest country in the world. But now it was under attack. The original inhabitants of the country (not counting Indians like Tonto, who simply didn't count) were white folks from Northern and Central Europe like his own ancestors, fine upstanding folk who had immigrated here from Switzerland. Harry knew, because it had been demonstrated scientifically, that white folks had the best genes. White races were superior to others and it was their destiny to run things. Mixing white people up by intermarrying with other races was an abomination and would only weaken the gene pool, ultimately leading to an overall decline in the quality of the US population.

These things were being vigorously debated at the time. Correct breeding of gene pools would lead to the preservation of pure American stock. However, now there were all the niggers, kikes, spics, chinks, and God knows who else who had come to this country as slaves and laborers and who were attempting to seduce young white women and breed some kind of genetically inferior progeny. Not only did they want to intermarry with whites, but the birth rate of these degenerates was far higher than that of people of pure "Nordic" stock. Basically the United States of America was committing "race suicide." Harry also knew that there were forces in the United States that were trying to reverse these trends and to limit the immigration of genetically undesirable individuals into the country. Laws had been passed encouraging the sterilization of those individuals who should not be bearing children on the basis of their weak genes. This included epileptics, morons, imbeciles, and people from undesirable races like niggers.

These laws, which allowed forced sterilization of people who were genetically undesirable, had been supported by the great Supreme Court judge Oliver Wendell Holmes. Harry could repeat his closing argument from the 1927 case of Buck v Bell word for word—

> "We have seen more than once that the public welfare may call upon the best citizens for their lives. It would be strange if it could not call upon those who already sap the strength of the State for these lesser sacrifices, often not felt to be such by those concerned, to prevent our being swamped with incompetence. It is better for all the world, if instead of waiting to execute degenerate offspring for crime, or to let them starve for their imbecility, society can prevent those who are manifestly unfit from continuing their kind. The principle that sustains compulsory vaccination is broad enough to cover cutting the Fallopian tubes. Three generations of imbeciles are enough."

Some people had heeded his warning. In particular there was the Eugenics Records Office at Cold Spring Harbor. Everybody knew that Cold Spring Harbor was a place where they did real cutting edge science on race and genes in particular. Professor Charles Davenport had founded the laboratory on an idyllic site on Long Island and had established the scientific basis which supported legal use of eugenics in the United States. Indeed, the United States led the world as far as these things were concerned. The eugenics office within Cold Spring Harbor was now trying to give its scientific findings on race and genes some legal muscle. These attempts were headed by Harry Laughlin, one of Professor Davenport's most trusted assistants. Harry had heard Laughlin lecture and had been completely convinced by what he had to say. And it had just been announced that Laughlin had been awarded an honorary degree by the University of Heidelberg for his work on racial hygiene. Even more to the point, the German chancellor Herr Hitler had based his own eugenic and racial laws and the use of forced sterilization on the laws of the United States. Yes, the USA was the world leader in the practice of racial hygiene. Harry was proud of that.[1]

By this time Harry had been around the block a few times. As a young fellow growing up in Altoona, Pennsylvania, his Dad had got him a job with the railroad.[2] After college he had risen to the rank of head of railroad police. During and after the First World War he had continued serving his country in the police force, and was stationed in various parts of the world including Germany, Japan, South America, and the Bahamas. Harry was now fluent in several languages. In the Bahamas he had played a major role in the control of "rum running" during Prohibition and had eventually been given the job of assistant commissioner in the Prohibition Bureau (which at the time was part of the Bureau of Internal Revenue). Unfortunately the agency had fallen foul of a scandal and had been reconstituted in 1930 as the Federal Bureau of Narcotics (FBN), with Harry as its first Commissioner.

Harry knew he could do his bit to help the American people win two important wars—the race war and the drug war. In Harry's mind these two aims were frequently closely connected. As head of the FBN, Harry had a vital role to play in guarding Americans against the terrible menace of dope peddling. Of course in the beginning there had been the heroin problem, and that was still with us. But laws had been passed to start bringing heroin use under control, and Harry and his agents had made great strides in destroying the underworld gangs that were responsible for all of this. But once in a while, even with something like heroin, things got a little murky from the political point of view. For example, Harry knew very well that one of the world's largest heroin rackets was run by that despicable little chink, Chiang Kai-shek. Harry had evidence on this that would fill a hundred volumes. But he also knew it was hands off. Chiang used his heroin sales to finance his Kuomintang army, who were the only buffer between the Chinese and the Japanese army, and perhaps even worse, the nascent Chinese communist party. So, from the political point of view, Chiang was a US ally and his interests and the those of the United States were the same. So Harry had to turn a blind eye. Anyway, there were more than enough other punks to take up Harry's time. And now there was a new menace, something that Harry had correctly surmised would put his stamp on the face of American politics for a very long time.

THE VILIFICATION OF HEMP

The new problem had started with the immigrant Mexican laborers who had come across the border to get work in Texas and the Southwest of the United States.[3] This immigration had begun at the turn of the century and, initially, had seemed like a great benefit to the country. The Mexicans worked for low wages and were basically kept on large farms segregated from the rest of the US population. So, who cared? Gradually, however, they spread north and east and, of course, their birth rate was astronomically high. By the time the Great Depression kicked in around 1929, the Mexicans weren't so welcome anymore. They were just foreigners, who had no right to keep real American citizens out of the job market.

However, it wasn't just on the economic front that the Mexicans were objectionable. There were also moral considerations. The main one of these was the fact that the Mexicans had a national drug habit—a habit called marijuana. Well, it wasn't originally called marijuana in the United States, if anything it was called "hemp" or possibly "Indian Hemp." In fact, the hemp plant had been grown in the United States and all over the world since time immemorial as a source of hemp fibers for making cloth and paper. The seeds of the plant could be used to make hemp oil, which was also an extremely useful product. In the early days of the United States, all citizens were actually *required by law* to grow hemp for the national good. This included George Washington, who had a large hemp plantation at Mount Vernon. A little known fact is that the initial drafts of the American Declaration of Independence were actually copied on paper made from hemp! The fact was, however, that useful things like hemp fiber and oil weren't the only thing you could make from the hemp plant. It was known that if you smoked or ate parts of the plant it would produce what seemed to Harry to be a powerful psychological effect.

The drugs obtained from hemp were generally known by the term *cannabis*. Although cannabis had been around in the United States for a long time, it hadn't been any sort of a problem until the Mexican workers had brought it with them. Harry had discovered that the Mexicans called what they smoked "marihuana" or marijuana. He thought that this Spanish-sounding name was to be preferred, as people would associate its use with Spanish-speaking people like the Mexicans. Now that the

Mexicans had settled in large cities like Chicago and New York, something else had happened. The use of marijuana had spread to other degenerate types, particularly darkies who played jazz music. During Prohibition, posh white folks who could be found slumming it in speakeasies could not only obtain alcohol but also marijuana from the black musicians and other low-lifes that frequented such places. It should be remembered that from 1919 until 1933, Prohibition had been in effect in the United States. This legis-lation reflected the powerful political clout of the American temperance movement in general. In spite of the fact that Prohibition was ultimately a failure, there were clearly a very large number of people in the United States who wished to see tight controls on drugs of any type.

As a topic demanding Harry's attention, the spread of marijuana use from the Mexican community, to the black, and ultimately the white communities, had a lot to recommend it. First of all it seemed to Harry that this could be played up as a major problem facing American society. Unfortunately, America was as yet unaware of the problem but Harry would fix that. Harry had also determined from sources known "only to him" that marijuana was in fact one of the most dangerous, if not the most dangerous drug on the planet. This was particularly true when it was used by people from degenerate races, where the drug served to strip away any semblance of civilization revealing the savages for what they truly were. If Harry and the FBN could (a) bring the problem to the attention of the American people and then (b) solve the problem, this would be publicity of the greatest possible value. It would serve to illustrate the value of the FBN and it would also serve to illustrate the value of one Harry Anslinger. All this at the expense of some racially undesirable degenerates.

It seemed to Harry that these aims would be relatively easy to achieve. For a start, the trafficking of marijuana didn't involve enormous interna-tional drug cartels with important political connections, as was the case with heroin and cocaine. This meant that the people who trafficked the drug would generally be easier to deal with. The people that traded mari-juana were generally Mexicans and Blacks, and frankly nobody cared what happened to people like that. Also, again unlike heroin and cocaine, it was not on the FBI's radar, which meant it could be dealt with solely by the FBN and Harry wouldn't have to cross swords with his archenemy, J. Edgar Hoover, the head of the FBI.

Harry also had a lot of other important support for his crusade against marijuana. There were several extremely powerful people in the United States who would be delighted to see the end of the hemp industry in gen-eral. These included William Randolph Hearst, Andrew Mellon, and mem-bers of the DuPont family, all of whom Harry knew very well and all of whom were prepared to back him in every way. Indeed, Harry was actually related to Andrew Mellon's family through his wife, who was Mellon's niece. The three financial giants had interests in industries making paper and synthetics like nylon, and didn't need any competition from the hemp industry, which was a distinct possibility that was now on the horizon. Although fiber isolated from hemp plants was clearly tremendously useful for numerous reasons, treating the stems of the plants in order to obtain this material was labor intensive and difficult. Now the decorticator had been invented, a little machine which would make such operations infinitely easier. It was predicted that hemp-related products might be America's next great growth industry. These developments posed a direct threat to the financial interests of Hearst and the others. Moreover, Mellon, Hearst, and the DuPonts were extremely conservative and certainly supported current views on the supremacy of the white race and the importance of race hygiene in the United States. Clearly, therefore, the idea of a campaign to discredit hemp/marijuana and put pressure on racial minorities at the same time was an ideal project for both Anslinger and his powerful supporters.

Harry Anslinger had not climbed the ladder of bureaucratic success so rapidly for no reason. He was energetic, tough, intelligent, and a shrewd politician. Harry went after marijuana with the typical zeal that he brought to bear on all of his projects. For the campaign to work, Harry needed the support of the press, and this was provided unreservedly by Hearst. Harry collected newspaper stories in what he called his "Gore file." Every so often he would take one of these and dress it up a bit for his own purposes. Harry's attacks on marijuana and its users in the press made scintillating reading. Harry blamed marijuana for just about everything. He claimed that the merest puff would send even the mildest man raving mad. A particular feature of marijuana was that the madness it induced was often associated with terrible sex crimes. Young men who smoked marijuana frequently became sex maniacs and rapists. These were usually portrayed as young Mexicans and Blacks whose lust for innocent white girls was inflamed by marijuana, frequently leading to brutal rapes. If young white women could be induced to smoke marijuana, they were likely to become crazy nymphomaniacs who abandoned their middle class suburban upbringing to indulge themselves in a life of wild orgies with members of degenerate races, while listening to the sounds of jazz. Another thing that marijuana was likely to do was to turn people into mass murderers. According to Harry, if young men on marijuana couldn't find anybody to rape, they would murder whoever was at hand instead. Reading these reports nowadays it is difficult to take them seriously, but at the time they were taken very seriously indeed.

According to Harry[3,4]—

"There are 100,000 total marijuana smokers in the USA, and most are Negroes, Hispanics, Filipinos and entertainers. Their Satanic music, jazz and swing, result from marijuana usage. This marijuana causes white women to seek sexual relations with Negroes, entertainers and any others."

And if that wasn't enough—

"Colored students at the Univ. of Minn. partying with (white) female students, smoking [marijuana] and getting their sympathy with stories of racial persecution. Result: pregnancy." ... "Two Negros took a girl fourteen years old and kept her for two days under the influence of hemp. Upon recovery she was found to be suffering from syphilis."

As far as marijuana's ability to produce violent crime was concerned—

"An entire family was murdered by a youthful addict in Florida. When officers arrived at the home, they found the youth staggering about in a human slaughterhouse. With an axe he had killed his father, mother, two brothers, and a sister. He seemed to be in a daze. He had no recollection of having committed the multiple crimes. The officers knew him ordinarily as a sane, rather quiet young man; now he was pitifully crazed. They sought the reason. The boy said that he had been in the habit of smoking something which youthful friends called 'muggles', a childish name for marijuana."

Not only did Harry carry out his attacks on marijuana in the press, but in other media as well. Special movies were made which were to be shown by teachers and parents to students in which the horrors of marijuana induced madness were vividly displayed. The classic of this type was the movie "Reefer Madness" (the title tells you everything), but there were several others as well.

The plain fact was, however, that in the early 1930s outside of the world of migrant workers, jazz musicians, and the like, marijuana simply wasn't an issue in the United States. Most people who didn't move in these circles wouldn't have come across it. Unlike alcohol or subsequent marijuana use in the 1960s, smoking marijuana at that time wasn't a middle class phenomenon. There simply wasn't an epidemic of marijuana use in the United States as Harry wanted people to believe. In order for it to become an issue, Harry had to make into one. In fact, there wasn't really any scientific information at the time suggesting that marijuana was the "evil weed" that Harry made it out to be. He had to manufacture or embellish countless stories about the drug, and to make sure the press presented these to the public in a convincing manner. Here the collaboration with the Hearst publishing empire was a key element, and the use of sensational "yellow journalism" helped to fan the flames.

At the same time it was in his interest to suppress any information that might run counter to his arguments. He also did this very effectively. As a result, Harry's efforts were successful. Marijuana became the issue that he wanted it to be, a drug that was deemed as dangerous as anything on earth. Ultimately this led to the first real attempts to legally restrict the use of marijuana in the United States at a federal level. This was the Marijuana Tax Act of 1937. This law made using marijuana for any purpose prohibitively expensive. It was necessary to pay a tax of $100 per ounce every time marijuana changed hands for any purpose, including growing, selling, or prescribing it. Moreover, the Act also made medical use of the drug virtually impossible because of extensive bureaucracy involved if doctors wanted to prescribe it. The overall result was that the extreme bureaucratic and financial obstacles completely eliminated all legal trade in hemp or medical use its of products, however reasonable these might have been.

During the debates that preceded enacting this law, Anslinger stacked the deck effectively so that any dissenting voices were either not heard or discredited. The vote to ratify the act was brought to the floor late one Friday afternoon when nearly everybody had gone home for the weekend, and it stimulated virtually no debate whatsoever. So, on the basis of a carefully organized scare campaign based on no credible data, Harry had made marijuana one of America's most "dangerous" drugs, a substance with no redeeming features and certainly no place in medicine and therapeutics. Because of the enormous tax burden imposed by the Marijuana Tax Act, Harry had also simultaneously destroyed the American hemp industry, and so it was no longer financially possible to manufacture hemp cloth, oil, or other products.[5]

In the years following the Marijuana Tax Act, marijuana's pariah status grew to the point where it was removed from the *American Pharmacopeia*. A brief hiatus in all of this took place during the Second World War, during which time the US population was actually encouraged to grow hemp once again for the purposes of hemp fiber and hemp oil production. However, this ceased again after the war. Anslinger actually initiated a campaign to try and free the country of wild hemp plants (it grew in the wild as a weed), but wasn't successful in doing this. Arrests started to become more common for selling marijuana and related crimes. Indeed, there were also some unexpected turns of events, such as people using things like "temporary marijuana-induced insanity" as a defense in homicide and murder trials. In one trial a doctor who was testifying for the defense described his own "scientific" tests with the drug. "After two puffs on a marijuana cigarette,

I was turned into a bat!" he declared. It was difficult to be too hard on murderers who were suffering from self-delusions of this type. Needless to say the accused escaped the ultimate punishment.

In fact, Harry's campaign to demonize marijuana wasn't the only voice to be heard at that time. Frank LaGuardia, the mayor of New York, actually set up a commission to determine the truth about marijuana in spite of all Harry Anslinger's proselytizing pronouncements and Hearst's yellow journalism. Indeed, this was one of the first truly well controlled studies on this subject. The results of these investigations were published between 1942 and 1944. The LaGuardia study concluded, "From the study as a whole it is concluded that marihuana is not a drug of addiction, comparable to morphine, and that if tolerance is acquired, this is of a very limited degree. Furthermore, those who have been smoking marihuana for a period of years showed no mental or physical deterioration which may be attributed to the drug." Anslinger immediately moved to suppress the results of the report, and it ultimately had little influence on the immediate policy of the US government. Indeed, the public attitude to marijuana in the United States (and in much of Europe as well) had been set for many years to come. In the early 1950s following the passage of the Boggs Act, the penalties for even first-time possession of marijuana became increasingly severe, including several years on prison and thousands of dollars in fines.[3,5]

The idea that marijuana was a dangerous "narcotic" with no redeeming medical properties ultimately had an influence on its status as a category Schedule 1 drug when new legislation was eventually drafted in the 1960s and 1970s. Because, of course, it was in the 1960s that marijuana use became truly popular as a middle class activity. Challenges to the Marihuana Tax Act led to it being found unconstitutional in 1969, and it was replaced by the Controlled Substances Act of 1970.[5] According to this law, all controlled substances were to be placed into a particular "Schedule." There were five Schedules, with Schedule 1 being the most restrictive reserved for drugs with the highest potential for abuse. However, the decisions about which drugs should end up in which Schedule were left to politicians rather than to scientists and doctors. As a result, marijuana was placed in Schedule I together with heroin and LSD. Drugs placed in this category were considered to have such a high potential for abuse that they could not be used under any circumstances, even with a physician's prescription. In other words it was concluded that they didn't have any medical utility. As we shall discuss, opposition to this view began to gain momentum in the 1970s. However, even today the laws concerning marijuana use in the United States are clearly incomprehensible, with state and federal laws frequently being completely at odds with one another.

THE MANY USES OF HEMP

These events raise some important basic questions. The first of these being what is the real truth about the medical potential of marijuana? Also, just how dangerous a drug is it in our contemporary environment? Currently the government's attitude toward marijuana still reflects the influence of Harry Anslinger. However, since the time when Harry was at the peak of his power and influence, a great deal of important new information has been obtained about exactly what marijuana is and how it works. So we are now in a much better position to provide some detailed answers to these questions, and we shall certainly return to them. One thing we can say for sure is that understanding the mechanism of action of marijuana has led to the discovery of one of the most important biochemical signaling systems in the entire body—a system whose influence is arguably more prevalent than any of the other neurotransmitter systems we have discussed. To understand how this all occurred and what it means, we should first take a step back and consider some of the history of marijuana and exactly how scientists solved the puzzle of its mechanism of action.

All of the drugs discussed here, such as cannabis and marijuana, are derived from the same source, the hemp plant, or as it is often known the "Indian" hemp plant. As we have seen, psychoactive drug use aside, hemp is one of the great natural resources for the production of fibers when making cloth and other products.[3] Hemp rope and canvas have always been vital for the shipping industry, and indeed the word *canvas* is derived from the word *cannabis*. The hemp plant really looks like a tall, ungainly, gangling weed and can attain heights of well over 10 feet (Figure 7.1). Indeed, it does still grow wild as a weed, although it was also one of mankind's earliest cultivated plants. In the United States, for example, wild hemp is known as "ditch weed." Hemp is a very hardy plant and can grow in virtually any kind of environment, and at altitudes up to several thousand feet. It needs some water, but not a great deal, and prefers strong sunlight and warm Mediterranean temperatures if possible. Such beneficial conditions certainly make a great deal of difference to its content of psychoactive chemicals. Indeed, because the production of psychoactive drugs has been one of the main reasons for growing the plant, there have been an enormous number of investigations, many of these carried out by "amateurs," as how to optimize its psychoactive characteristics. What is the best way to grow the plants outdoors and under what conditions? How best to grow the plants indoors? Should hydroponic techniques be used to improve drug content and related issues? A huge bibliography, both in the form of

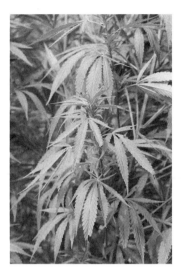
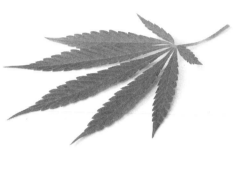

Figure 7.1:
Cannabis sativa, the cannabis plant.
(Heike Kampe © Photoscom and Sukharevskyy Dmytro Shutterstock)

the printed word and on line, now offers the potential hemp grower more advice than the cook who wants to make something like an apple pie.[6]

The hemp plant belongs to the genus *Cannabis.* There has been some discussion as to exactly how many types of *Cannabis* plants exist. The original type, as described by the great botanist Linnaeus in 1753, is known as *Cannabis sativa.* Linnaeus named the plant after the Greek word for hemp (*kannabis*). It is somewhat related to the hop plant which, of course, has a primary role in the production of beer. More recently it has been suggested that two other varieties of cannabis, known as *Cannabis indica* and *Cannabis ruderalis,* also exist. *C. indica* grows to an intermediate height and has a more bushy appearance than the tall, gangly *C. sativa,* whereas *C. ruderalis* only grows to a height of about 3 feet or less. Whether these are really different types of plants or just represent adaptations of *C. sativa* to different environments is still unclear. All of these types contain psychoactive chemicals to some degree, and it was originally claimed that *C. sativa* was a better source of hemp fiber whereas *C. indica* was a better source of psychoactive substances. In truth, however, the content of these chemical constituents varies so widely according to diverse growing conditions that it would be difficult to come to such a general conclusion.

The *C. sativa* plant is characterized by the presence of widely spaced branches bearing highly recognizable leaves with serrated edges (Figure 7.1). The stem is very tough due to the high concentration of fibers and is often hollow. It is this stem which is the source of hemp fiber. As we have discussed, obtaining hemp fiber is a very labor intensive process. The traditional procedure, known as *retting*, involves soaking the stems in water or dew, which produces swelling and eventual decay of the nonfibrous material. The remaining bast fibers can then be removed, dried, and turned into rope or cloth. The seeds of the hemp plant are also useful for a number of purposes. Primarily they can be processed to yield a rich oil, something akin to linseed oil. Hemp seeds can be eaten or ground up and reconstituted into a type of porridge. They are also widely used in feed for domestic animals and birds like budgerigars/parakeets. Sometimes this can lead to unexpected outcomes. The birdseed is irradiated so that no germination occurs, but the process isn't necessarily 100% effective, leaving a small residue of seeds that can actively germinate. Some years ago the British tabloid press reported one related incident. "Busted!!" screamed the headline above a picture of a granny complete with blue rinse, in handcuffs, standing in her garden by the side of a towering hemp plant. A copper stood next to her. "It's the budgie wot did it!" protested the granny, and indeed she didn't look the type. But I suppose you never know.

MARIJUANA, CANNABIS, AND HASH

Finally, there is the use of hemp for the production of its psychoactive chemical constituents. These occur in most parts of the plant but are concentrated in a sticky resinous material secreted by small hair-like glands known as *trichomes*. The biological reason for this resin production is unclear. However, hemp plants are dioecious; that is to say, they exist as male and female plants, the former producing seeds and the latter producing pollen. It is possible that a covering of sticky resin helps pollen to stick, but that is only one possibility. A commonly used trick when growing hemp plants for the purpose of drug production is to remove all of the male plants so that the female plants remain unpollenated. Under these conditions, the empty seed pods fill with resin with a very high drug content. This technique is known as *sensimilla* (Spanish for "without seeds"). Such plants are highly prized by aficionados of the psychoactive cannabis experience.

The fact is that there are an enormous number of ways in which hemp plants can be prepared for drug use. Because of the widespread use of cannabis as a drug, the names and exact nature of these preparations vary a great deal. Basically, the most common way to use the plant is to dry the leaves or flowering tops of female plants and to smoke them. The preparation of leaves, perhaps with some dried flower material added, is what is normally referred to as marijuana, or as "bhang" in India. Bhang may also be made into a drink such as bhang lassi. Marijuana is also commonly referred to as *grass, weed* or *pot*. In African countries such as Morocco, it is often mixed with tobacco and referred to as *kif*. In Western countries a marijuana cigarette is usually referred to as a *joint* or a *blunt*. The word *reefer* is also used, but would be considered somewhat retro at this point.

Preparations of dried female flowering tops have an increased drug content and are usually referred to as *ganja* in India. In truth, however, the exact composition of a marijuana cigarette can vary according to what is available and might even contain the addition of other drugs such as opium under some circumstances. The crème de la crème of cannabis preparations, however, is the pure resin which can be dried into blocks of crumbly material and is referred to as *hashish* or *charas* in India. Hashish has by far the highest psychoactive drug content and can also be smoked by crumbling some material into the contents of a cigarette or joint. The advantage of smoking cannabis preparations is that the smoke directly enters the lungs, which are very highly vascularized, and so the drug can easily enter the bloodstream and travel directly to the brain. Hashish can also been eaten in a variety of guises, and when consumed in this manner will enter the bloodstream more slowly, producing a somewhat different type of experience. One popular way of eating hashish is to cook it into brownies. In Eastern countries, it is included in delicious candies with other ingredients such as marzipan, sugar, and spices known as *majoon* (majoun). Actually, not only in Eastern countries—in the nineteenth century, prior to cannabis becoming the bête noir of the US drug administration, hashish candies were openly available in the United States. As advertised in *Vanity Fair*:

"A most wonderful Medicinal Agent for the cure of Nervousness, Weakness, Melancholy, confusion of thoughts, etc. A pleasurable and harmless stimulant. Under its influence all classes seem to gather new inspiration and energy. Price, 25c. and 8 per box, Beware of imitations. Imported only by the Gunjah-Wallah Company 476 Broadway. On sale by druggists generally."

Around the same time Louisa May Alcott of *Little Women* fame published her story "Perilous Play," which begins[7]—

"If someone does not propose a new and interesting amusement, I shall die of ennui!" said pretty Belle Daventry, in a tone of despair. "I have read all my books, used up all my Berlin wools, and it's too warm to go to town for more. No one can go sailing yet, as the tide is out; we are all nearly tired to death of cards, croquet, and gossip, so what shall we do to while away this endless afternoon? Dr. Meredith, I command you to invent and propose a new game in five minutes."

Dr. Meredith has been spending his time "surveying Belle's piquant figure," and guess what? Dr. Meredith does indeed have an "interesting new amusement" in form of heart-shaped hashish candies: "Eat six of these despised bonbons, and you will be amused in a new, delicious, and wonderful manner," said the young doctor, laying half a dozen on a green leaf and offering them to her." Belle and Dr. Meredith eat lots of the candies and get really stoned. In the end love conquers all. The story concludes, "He stretched his hand to her with his heart in his face, and she gave him hers with a look of tender submission, as he said ardently, 'Heaven bless hashish, if its dreams end like this!'"

CHINA, INDIA AND PERSIA

Like many of the other substances discussed in this book, the hemp plant from which cannabis-related drugs are derived has clearly been used by humans since the beginnings of recorded time.[3] As in the case of the poppy, a good question would be: what were these original uses? As we have seen there are certainly many possibilities in the case of the hemp plant, the majority of which have got nothing to do with its psychotropic effects. It seems clear that hemp was one of the earliest plants to make the transition from a weed to an actively cultivated plant. As with other plants of this type we don't exactly know when and where this occurred, but it seems likely to have been in China. Remains discovered on Taiwan dating to around 10,000 BC include crude pottery, which has been decorated by pressing hempen cloth and rope into its surface. On mainland China, remains of hemp cloth and rope dating to around 4000 BC have been discovered. Chinese texts from the Warring States period (475–221 BC) categorize hemp along with rice, barley, millet, and soy as the most important crops. Most likely the major use of *C. sativa* at that time was for the production of cloth and the use of hemp seeds as a food and a source of oil. In addition, however, it is also clear that from relatively early times the Chinese were aware of the psychotropic effects of the plant. In what is probably the world's oldest pharmacopoeia, written around 2000 BC, Shen Nung, the "father of Chinese medicine" recommended a tea or decoction of *C. sativa* leaves and flowers for the treatment of numerous disorders including malaria, and also noted that its use in large quantities could lead to visions of demons. The use of cannabis was also associated with the rise of Taoism from around 600 BC. It was originally viewed as a bad influence, although attitudes changed over the years so that by the first century AD it was employed to assist magical ceremonies. Moreover, Chinese doctors were also clearly using tincture of cannabis (i.e., cannabis in alcohol) as an aid to anesthesia and surgery.

The use of cannabis was ultimately to have its greatest impact in India, China's giant neighbor. Here again, the early use of the drug in some form is recorded in the Vedas which, as we have previously discussed (Chapter 1), date from around 1500 BC. Several Vedic legends refer to the use of cannabis. One tells of how the god Shiva was resting in a field of C. *sativa* for shade. Being hungry, he ate some of the leaves and found them to be absolutely scrumptious. Hence he is often referred to as "the Lord of Bhang." It is said that use of cannabis allows one to commune with Shiva. Cannabis also features in the related traditions of Buddhism, Zoroastrianism, and Tantrism. Legend has it that while waiting for enlightenment the Buddha Siddhartha Gautama lived on nothing but hemp seed for years. The fact that he is said to have only eaten one hemp seed per day certainly supports stories about their great nutritional value (!). The Avesta, the sacred text of Zoroaster and the ancient Persians, lists cannabis as the most important of 10,000 medicinal herbs and plants. Thus, it can be seen that cannabis was widely used in Southern Asia from China to Persia from the earliest times. Its use was completely integrated into various aspects of society. As we shall see, this is the situation the British found when they first arrived in India at the beginning of the seventeenth century. In the nineteenth century the British Raj was to make a careful study of the situation, and we will return to this topic later.

How and when did the use of cannabis begin in Europe? Ancient remains of hemp seeds excavated from Neolithic graves in different parts of the continent attest to the fact that its use in some form was very ancient. However, it is not clear what it was being used for and there is no reason to think that the plant was being actively cultivated as it was in China. One strong influence in bringing cannabis use to Europe may have been the ancient Scythians, a nomadic Indo-Aryan people who originated in the area of the Altai mountains and Mongolia, and who swept across the Asian Steppes as far as the Black Sea and the fringes of Eastern Europe around 600 BC. Not surprisingly they appear to have utilized cannabis in their religious ceremonies, these being along the same lines as those associated with Zoroastrianism. The major source of literary information concerning the Scythians and their habits was the Greek historian Herodotus, writing around the fifth century BC. Herodotus describes observing a Scythian funeral in Macedonia in which the participants threw hemp seeds (perhaps other parts of the plant as well) into a pit containing red hot stones. The participants then breathed the smoke that was produced, and this made them "howl with joy" and generally carry on in an inebriated manner.

Archaeological excavations have tended to confirm Herodotus' descriptions and have suggested the widespread use of cannabis by the Scythians, perhaps in a recreational as well as a religious context. Both Dioscorides and Galen also mention cannabis in their writings—Galen clearly referring to its psychoactive properties. The Romans certainly did use hemp products widely, including for cloth and rope, and so spread its use throughout the Roman Empire. Nevertheless, it seems as if cannabis was not widely used for its psychoactive properties in Europe at this time, at least to the same extent that it was used in southern and eastern Asia.

Things started to change when European explorers began to make regular contact and trade with the peoples of Asia and to bring back stories about their use of cannabis. Of course the best known of these is the legend associated with Marco Polo concerning the Old Man of the Mountains and the Assassins. According to Marco Polo there was an Islamic leader who was head of a sect known as the Ismailis. The Ismailis claimed to be descended from the prophet Mohammed's daughter Fatima, and so to be the true guardians of Islamic tradition.

The head of the Ismaili movement was Hassan ibn-Sabah, who was born in Qum in 1050. He gathered a group of acolytes around him and established a base for his sect in the mountains of northern Persia in the castle of Alamut, situated high above a valley many hundreds of feet below. Gradually his power spread to include other fortified sites in northern Persia. According to Marco Polo, Hassan ibn-Sabah trained his men to act as terrorist shock troops who would do anything they were commanded to, even if it meant their death. It was also said that at Alamut, Hassan ibn-Sabah had cultivated a fabulous secret pleasure garden. At the appropriate time a young soldier would be drugged and taken to these gardens, where his every whim would be cared for by hordes of gorgeous *houris*. Then after a few days he was drugged again and removed. Hassan ibn-Sabah would then tell the young man that what he had seen was a glimpse of Paradise, and that if he obeyed all orders, no matter what, he would return there after death. In this way he trained a group of fanatical followers.

The speculation has been that the drug used by ibn-Sabah was hashish, and so his followers became known as *Hashshashin*—ultimately corrupted to "Assassins." Indeed, it is clear that ibn-Sabah used his followers to carry out political assassinations on a wide scale. The legend of the Assassins was also spread throughout Europe by the Crusaders who had encountered ferocious Ismaili troops while in the Middle East. They spread the rumor that these troops had been driven into a frenzy by drugs—presumably again hashish. Most of this speculation is unlikely to be true, and a great deal of ink has been expended attempting to debunk the historical faults in these legends. Nevertheless, the Romantic tales of the use of hashish by the Assassins have persisted to this day. Indeed, even Harry Anslinger used these stories in court to support his arguments that cannabis makes people "act crazy."

CANNABIS AND THE WEST

The use of cannabis in Europe, however, basically remained the equivalent of folklore and witchcraft. It wasn't until Europeans began to make significant contact with Asian societies where hashish was widely used that real information about the drug and its properties began to make its way back to Europe. The British and travelers from Portugal and Spain were primarily responsible for this. For example, Garcia Da Orta was a Portuguese Marrano Jewish doctor who went to Goa in 1534, where he spent the remainder of his life. Da Orta's *Colloquies on the Simples and Drugs and Medicinal Matters of India and of a Few Fruits* is a model of scientific observation and include detailed information about the use and effects of hashish and other psychoactive plants such as opium and Datura. He accurately reported the fact that the effects of "bangue" (in the Portuguese) induced what we now call "fatuous euphoria"; that is, laughter prompted by the smallest thing, as well as its use as an aphrodisiac, sleeping aid, and in producing psychoactive effects. Da Orta's book was published in Europe and became what might be described as a best-seller, prompting widespread experimentation with cannabis products. Unfortunately, the Inquisition got wind of the fact that he had continued to practice Judaism in secret (clearly you never do know when to expect the Spanish Inquisition!) and had all copies of his book destroyed. Incredibly, one copy survived and was translated into several languages, thus maintaining its influence. Although Da Orta is a major example, he was certainly not the only writer who sent back this kind of information.

Another important influence on the subsequent use of cannabis was the discovery of tobacco in the New World and the practice of smoking. When this was introduced into Europe, smoking became a craze (Chapter 8). It was a small step before smoking the dried leaves of the hemp plant, or hashish crumbled into a cigarette with tobacco, became an easy way to enjoy cannabis. This practice became widely employed in those areas of the world such as the Middle East, where cannabis was already used for its psychoactive effects.

By the middle of the eighteenth century, the recreational use of cannabis was very widespread throughout Asia, the Middle East, and Africa.

Europeans such as the British were also well aware of its existence. Indeed, the British taxed "hemp" products in India but did not trade in it. However, the "idea" of recreational use of cannabis was not yet widespread in Europe and North America. With the dawn of the nineteenth century, however, this situation was to change forever.

As we have seen, the late eighteenth and early nineteenth century ushered in the Romantic movement. One aspect of this was an increasing European fascination with oriental arts and culture. Eventually this would contribute greatly to the development of the late Romantic movement known as *Art Nouveau.* There were certainly many other examples of such oriental influences; one thinks for instance of Debussy's discovery of the gamelan when a Javanese group visited Paris, or of the influence of a similar exhibition in London on Gilbert and Sullivan's operetta "The Mikado." In painting, Whistler's work is an obvious example of Japanese influence, and the exoticism of many popular Victorian painters also clearly echoes the influence of Asian themes. In the decorative arts, Arthur Lazenby Liberty founded Liberty's in London's Regent Street as an emporium for the import of Asian products into England, and it later became an important source of ideas for the Arts and Crafts and Art Nouveau movements.

One particularly important influence derived from the conquest of Egypt by Napoleon in 1798. Following the defeat of his navy by the British at the battle of the Nile, Napoleon's army was basically trapped in Egypt. The troops did not have access to alcohol, Egypt being a Moslem country. However, cannabis was widely available even though the French authorities tried to ban it. Of course some of this cannabis found its way back to France and, along with the growing interest in Asian cultures, became an important atmospheric accompaniment to Romantic fantasies of the Assassins or the stories of Scheherazade and *The Thousand and One Nights.*

At this point cannabis came to the attention of a highly significant figure in the history of psychopharmacology. Jacques Joseph Moreau was a Parisian doctor who was extremely interested in diseases of the "mind." He was a student of Esquirol, one of the key figures of what was eventually to develop into the science of psychiatry. Moreau experimented with cannabis and other psychoactive drugs, and came to the conclusion that in some respects the mental states produced by such drugs mimicked the abnormal mental states observed in psychiatric patients. He discussed his theories in his book *Of Hashish and Mental Derangement.* Thus, rather than attributing mental illness to the realm of demons and the supernatural, Moreau favored a model in which mental illnesses represented dysfunctions of the brain which could be mimicked by the actions of psychotropic drugs. Here we can see the first clear suggestions of a modern neurochemical theory for the basis of psychiatric disorders.

Moreau was anxious to have others experiment with psychoactive drugs so that he could observe their reactions. In this way the "Club des Hashichins" was founded by Moreau and his friend, the author Theophile Gautier. Gautier was an important figure in bohemian Paris and his credo was "L'art pour L'art" ("art for art's sake"). We have introduced this group when we discussed opiates (Chapter 6). However, in addition to opium the members of the group actively experimented with cannabis. One of the forms of taking the drug that they favored was *dawamesk*—imported from North Africa. This was a green paste made of hashish and marzipan with other spices added, as well as a little "Spanish Fly" to act as an aphrodisiac. One member of this circle of writers was Alexander Dumas, and one may recall that the Count of Monte Cristo was apt to offer dawamesk served from a silver chalice when people visited his secret island abode. Basically, all the members of the club playacted and experimented with cannabis in their dark, romantic hideaway on the Isle St. Louis, and all of them wrote about their experiences to some extent. However, it was Charles Baudelaire whose writings in his *Paradis Artificial* were the most extensive.[8] Actually, Baudelaire probably didn't use cannabis all that often as he wasn't very keen on it, concluding that getting stoned was quite an inferior experience to getting really drunk. His descriptions of the results of cannabis ingestion, however, were very much on the mark and were widely disseminated. Originally greatly influenced by De Quincey, Baudelaire's writings then returned the compliment and were very influential back across the channel in England. Artists and bohemians in England also began to cultivate interest in the orient and Middle East, as well as the lifestyles that went along with this. Some of the responses were quite remarkable—the famous Arab hall built for the painter Lord Leighton in his house in Holland Park being one of the world's greatest examples of High Victorian design (Figure 7.2).

Other developments in the United Kingdom concerned the medical use of cannabis. The first figure of importance in this regard was an Irish doctor named William Brooke O'Shaughnessy, who worked in India for the East India Company. An excellent scientist, O'Shaughnessy became extremely interested in the therapeutic potential of cannabis and performed several series of well controlled experiments on humans and animals. He concluded that use of cannabis was not dangerous and that it had promising anticonvulsant, analgesic, and sedative properties. He presented scientific papers on his research and investigated all aspects of the subject including the properties of the hemp plant, the effects of cannabis-taking on the Indian population, different ways of preparing the drug, and other topics.

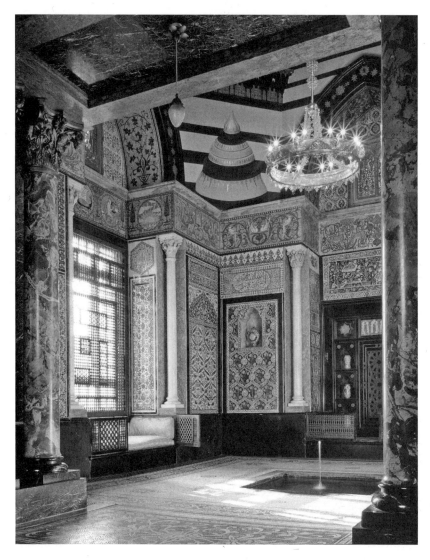

Figure 7.2:
The famous Arab hall of the Leighton House in London's Holland Park.
(Arcaid Images / Alamy)

A polymath, O'Shaughnessy was also interested in other topics and was influential in building India's first telegraphic communication system, for which he was subsequently knighted. O'Shaughnessy's work with cannabis was widely disseminated both in the United Kingdom and the United States, and interest in the medical use of cannabis was greatly stimulated.

O'Shaughnessy returned to England from India in 1842, bringing a large supply of cannabis with him which was then marketed as a tincture known as "Squire's Extract" by Peter Squire, a pharmacist friend of O'Shaughnessy's. At the time, drugs of all types were freely available and so were very easy to market. As with laudanum, tinctures of cannabis started to appear more frequently on the market. The medicinal uses of cannabis were taken very seriously and endorsed by authorities such as the *Lancet,* the most prestigious British medical journal. Even Queen Victoria was prescribed tincture of cannabis. It is believed she was amused (perhaps very amused). Many patent medicines included tincture of cannabis. For example, it was mixed with laudanum and sold as Chlorodyne. In the United States, tincture of cannabis was sold by Eli Lilly, Parke-Davis, and Squibb among others, and was listed in the *US Pharmacopeia* (see Chapter 4, Figure 4.3). Indeed, as cannabis was viewed as being nonaddictive, it was often used instead of opium/morphine because it was thought of as being safer. It is interesting how the medical fortunes of cannabis have gone up and down over the years. By the dawn of the twentieth century, cannabis tinctures were somewhat out of fashion owing to the arrival of new synthetic drugs supplied by the burgeoning pharmaceutical industry (Chapter 3). The drug was mostly used during the twentieth century for recreational purposes. Today, however, there is once again enormous interest in the medical potential of cannabis and its derivatives, as we shall discuss below.

THE KID FROM POUGHKEEPSIE

The availability of cannabis tinctures in Europe and the United States had some interesting consequences. One of the most famous of these was the case of Fitzhugh Ludlow from Poughkeepsie, New York. Fitzhugh was not a conventional kind of young man. He befriended the local pharmacist in town, and by his own admission liked to "make a trial of the effects of every strange drug that the laboratory could produce." One day in 1854, when he was 16 years old, while visiting the pharmacy he noted the delivery of some bottles of tincture of cannabis. He had read a little about the drug and, in keeping with his hobby, Ludlow decided to give the tincture a try. He probably took rather a high dose, and anyway he was a very imaginative and creative fellow who had already made his mark at school as an author. At any rate, Ludlow experienced what he described as radical changes in his perception accompanied by vivid hallucinations and visions. Ludlow had never experienced anything quite like this and was very impressed. He continued to experiment secretly with cannabis all the way through high school and college. He then spent some time as a teacher and started to submit and publish articles in various magazines. One of these was "The Apocalypse of Hasheesh," which discussed the possibility, among other things, that Pythagoras and his students had experimented with cannabis.

This article, however, was only a dry run for an autobiographical book which he subsequently authored entitled *The Hasheesh Eater: being passages from the life of a Pythagorean*. The book was published in 1857 by Harper Brothers, a very respectable publisher in New York, and was also published in the United Kingdom. The book was clearly influenced by De Quincey, and Ludlow had obviously set out to accomplish for cannabis what De Quincey had accomplished for opium. Ludlow's book was an extensive meditation on the uses and abuses of cannabis, and became a best-seller on both sides of the Atlantic. As for Ludlow, his literary star had risen and he became part of the New York literati, including the likes of Walt Whitman among his friends and colleagues. His most important meeting, however, was with the painter Albert Bierstadt, a member of the Hudson River School. Together with Bierstadt, Ludlow traveled to the Wild West and West Coast writing articles to go along with Bierstadt's romantic, idealized canvases. These descriptions of their journey were a great critical success. Unfortunately it also led to an affair between Bierstadt and Ludlow's young wife, who divorced him and married Bierstadt instead. Ludlow's health, which had always been somewhat precarious, declined after that. Eventually his family took him to Switzerland for a "cure" but he died there in 1870 at the age of 36. Nevertheless, Ludlow's book proved to be extremely influential on both sides of the Atlantic.

As we have seen, the arrival of cannabis in Europe and its influence on the bohemians of Paris had produced repercussions in England, where the drug was taken up by members of the Aesthetic Movement, the British proponents of art for art's sake and the decadent lifestyle of the time. This included people like the now older Rossetti, Algernon Swinburne, Oscar Wilde, Whistler, and the poet William Butler Yeats, as well as the prodigiously talented Aubrey Beardsley. The members of the movement were certainly aware of Ludlow's writings, and Beardsley provided illustrations for an edition of his book (Figure 7.3).

In addition to all of the different artistic media, spiritualism was also becoming wildly popular at the time with séances being held at social events hosted by the rich and famous. The fad for spiritualism attracted many reputable people, including Sir Arthur Conan Doyle. In addition, organizations that centered on the use of magic and all kinds of ridiculous nonsense also flourished. This included organizations such as The Hermetic Order

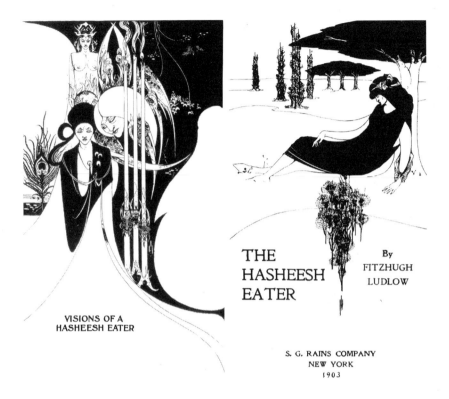

Figure 7.3:
The 1903 edition of *The Hasheesh Eater* by Fitzhugh Ludlow used illustrations by Aubrey Beardsley.[24]

of the Golden Dawn, which included Yeats as a member as well as Aleister Crowley, the self-styled "Great Beast" and prophet of the New Age widely known as a proponent of cannabis use. This heady mix of artistic bohemianism, spiritualism, neopaganism, pantheism, witchcraft, and other occult type influences were fertile ground for the use of different psychotropic drugs such as cannabis as part of various ritual practices. These things were really rediscovered by the hippies in the 1960s, who took up the writings of people like Crowley once again.

In summary, by the start of the twentieth century the recreational use of cannabis was widespread over much of Asia and Africa. It had also been discovered by Europe and the United States but was not nearly so widely used in these countries, being mostly taken up by bohemian elements rather than the *hoi polloi*. Cannabis was also widely appreciated for its medical uses, although these were on the wane as new synthetic drugs started to appear on the market.

THE PURIFICATION OF THE CANNABINOIDS

It will be recalled that the chemical secret of opium had been revealed as early as 1805 with the isolation of morphine (Chapter 5). Following this, many other alkaloids including strychnine, quinine, cocaine, and nicotine were soon isolated from natural sources. The question therefore arose as to what constituted the active principle of cannabis? It turned out that this was a much more difficult problem from the chemical point of view and, although attempts were made to solve it in the nineteenth century, it wasn't really until well into the twentieth century that the problem was effectively put to rest.[9,10] When the first attempts to purify the active constituents of cannabis were made in the middle of the nineteenth century, the prejudice at that time was that by comparison with just about everything else, these active constituents would be alkaloids. Indeed, there are alkaloids that occur in C. sativa, but it turns out that these are not what are responsible for its psychotropic activity. Some attempts were made in the 1840s to purify the active principles from C. sativa, and alcoholic extracts were prepared which were then evaporated to give a resinous material. These resins certainly had biological activity and were assumed to be pure agents, being given names such as "cannabin" or "hashishin." In one report the authors noted that "two-thirds of a grain of this resin acts upon ourselves as a powerful narcotic, and one grain produces complete intoxication." Clearly, however, although these resins contained the active principles from the plant, they were not pure preparations. Interestingly, they were found to be neutral in character, giving an initial indication that the active components were not alkaloids.

Little further progress was made until the last decade of the nineteenth century when a group of researchers at Cambridge University prepared ether extracts of potent *charas*. Using distillation they obtained different fractions, one of which was a "ruby red oil" that appeared to be associated with psychotropic effects. From this oil they then prepared what they deemed to be a pure substance that they named *cannabinol*. Their further analysis indicated cannabinol had the formula $C_{21}H_{28}O_2$, the absence of nitrogen further indicating that it wasn't an alkaloid. Unfortunately they also assumed that cannabinol was what was responsible for the psychotropic activity of the red oil, and didn't actually test it. Although they had indeed purified cannabinol, this turned out not to be the active component everyone was looking for. Nevertheless, cannabinol was the first of the class of compounds generally known as "cannabinoids" that are uniquely produced by C. sativa, C. indica, and C. ruderalis. Generally speaking, however, the chemical analytic techniques available at that time were not up to separating what turned out to be a highly complex mixture of these substances, together with their numerous biosynthetic intermediates and metabolites.

Although cannabinol did not ultimately prove to possess the required psychotropic activity, it did set the scene for the subsequent isolation of structurally similar cannabinoid molecules that did prove to be the active constituents of the plant. Following the isolation of cannabinol, work by Adams in the United States and Lord Todd in the United Kingdom elucidated its structure and a complete synthesis of the molecule. Of particular interest was the observation that one of the intermediates in the synthesis $\Delta^{6a,\ 10a}$-tetrahydrocannabinol, did indeed have powerful psychotropic effects and so was used in investigations of the effects of cannabis prior to the isolation of the genuine active principle (Figure 7.4). This was ultimately achieved in 1964 by the Israeli chemist Rafael Mechoulam, who isolated Δ^{9}-tetrahydrocannabinol (Δ^{9}-THC) from C. sativa as well as several other cannabinoid molecules, including cannabidiol, which was also found to be another major constituent (Figure 7.4). Solving the chemical structures of all of these molecules was greatly aided by the use of Nuclear Magnetic Resonance (NMR) techniques, which were just starting to be widely employed at that time.

At any rate, it was clear that the major problem had been solved and the major psychoactive principle of C. sativa had at last been identified. As it turns out, C. sativa contains a very large number of cannabinoid-related substances,[11] and many of these produce their own pharmacological effects which may contribute to the overall experience of smoking marijuana. This would include substances like cannabidiol. Nevertheless, the psychoactive actions of the plant are certainly mostly associated with Δ^{9}-THC.

THE CANNABINOID RECEPTORS AND THEIR AGONISTS

Although there have been many incredible surprises along the way, the intellectual development of the cannabinoid field closely followed the path laid out by the previous research into the mechanism of action of the opiates which we have already discussed (Chapter 5). First—purify the active constituent drug. Second—identify its receptor. Third—identify the natural ligand for the receptor. In the case of opium this line of reasoning had proceeded along the lines of morphine – opiate receptor –endorphin. Indeed, the results of the opiate field were certainly in the minds of researchers in the cannabinoid field when they went about their own investigations. Because of the prior success in the search for the opiate receptor and the

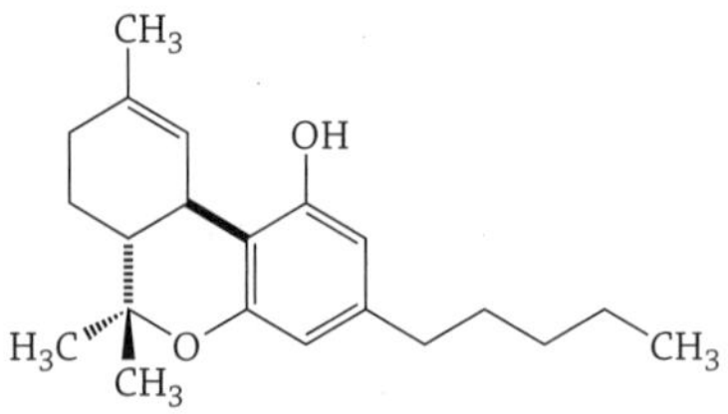

Δ^9-tetrahydrocannabinol (THC)

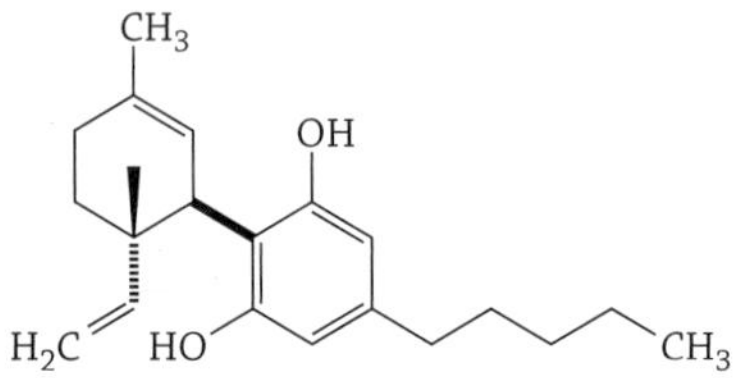

Cannabidiol (CBD)

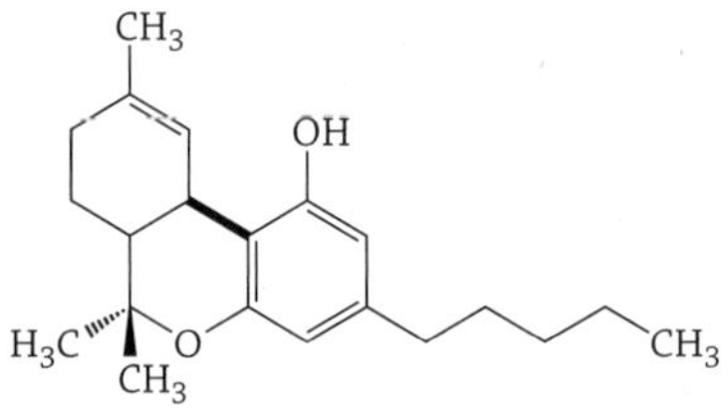

Cannabinol (CBN)

Figure 7.4:
The structure of Δ^9-Tetrahydrocannabinol, the psychoactive principle of cannabis and related molecules.

endorphins, researchers in the cannabinoid field could adopt the same strategies with confidence and with considerable hope for success. This is indeed what happened.

Following the identification of Δ^9-THC, numerous synthetic and semi-synthetic analogues of this molecule were synthesized in the hope of producing interesting therapeutic agents that might be free of the psycho-tropic actions of Δ^9-THC, but retain its other useful effects. Let us consider for a moment what kinds of effects these might be.[12] Because of the experiences resulting from many hundreds of years of cannabis use throughout the world, several things are certainly clear. In addition to its psychotropic effects, cannabis has often been used for its analgesic effects. Calming, sed-ative, hypnotic types of effects have also often been reported. Stimulation of appetite is also commonly observed and may be very marked. Other effects such as antiemetic and anti-inflammatory actions have also been regularly observed. A potentially beneficial effect of cannabis in reducing the intraocular pressure associated with glaucoma is also well established. This is only a partial list. It will be obvious from these reports why there is a strong interest in trying to develop novel cannabinoid-related analgesics, anti-inflammatory agents, hypnotics, and appetite stimulants—the latter being of importance for patients with diseases such as AIDS or cancer. However, to put current cannabinoid pharmacology in perspective we should first discuss what is known about the mechanism of the action of the drug.

Once Δ^9-THC was isolated, there was immediate speculation about its mechanism of action. Because of the highly lipophilic (i.e., water insoluble) nature of the compound, it was suggested that it must act by dissolving directly into the membranes of cells and that it wasn't necessary to postulate that a true protein receptor such as a ligand gated ion channel or a GPCR actually existed. However, other scientists did not believe this, particularly after it was demonstrated that some highly potent synthetic cannabinoids exhibited stereoselective properties. This was similar to the differential effects of (+) and (–) morphine, something that had been extremely influential when thinking about the mechanism of action of opiates (Chapter 5). In addition it had been observed that, just like morphine, Δ^9-THC would inhibit the electrically stimulated contraction of the guinea pig ileum. However, unlike morphine this inhibition was not reversed by the opiate antagonist naloxone, indicating that it was likely to be mediated by a non-opiate type of receptor.

The major breakthrough in the search for the cannabinoid receptor came in the 1980s through work by Dr. Allison Howlett and her colleagues.[13,14] Their argument went like this. If there is a real Δ^9-THC receptor, it is most likely to be a GPCR. Now when you activate GPCRs, Gproteins are activated and this can be measured very easily. So, what happens if one takes some neuronal cells and adds Δ^9-THC to them—do you see the activation of Gproteins or their sequelae? If so, this would most likely indicate the expression of a cannabinoid receptor that was a GPCR. The results of these experiments were unequivocal. When Δ^9-THC was added to neuronal cells it clearly produced inhibition of the enzyme adenylate cyclase, the enzyme which produces the molecule cyclic AMP, a typical Gprotein-mediated response. Furthermore, the effect was only produced by biologically active cannabinoid drugs and not inactive ones with closely related structures.

Now in order to demonstrate the existence of the receptor protein, it was necessary to perform a receptor binding assay similar to the one that Pert and Snyder had used to demonstrate the existence of the opiate receptor.

Unfortunately, radioactive Δ^9-THC was not very suitable for this purpose as its high lipid solubility meant that the background, or non–receptor related binding, was just too overwhelming. Fortunately, by this time several pharmaceutical companies had started to come up with synthetic cannabinoids that turned out to be much more suitable. For example, the Pfizer company had come up with a series of very potent compounds typified by the structure CP55940. It was decided to make a radioactive version of this molecule, and in 1990 its use quickly led to identification of the receptor protein itself. Thus one could conclude there was indeed a cannabinoid receptor, and it was a GPCR. Soon the receptor was cloned using molecular biological methods, and so its amino acid sequence was obtained.

A few years later, to everybody's surprise, a second cannabinoid receptor was identified and cloned, the two receptors being designated the CB1 and CB2 receptors. It quickly became apparent that the CB1 receptor was the major receptor expressed in the nervous system. In fact, the CB1 receptor proved to be one of the most widely expressed GPCRs in the entire brain. Additionally, it was observed that CB1 was expressed in several non-neural tissues including the liver, lung, pancreas, and gut. On the other hand, the CB2 was found to be rarely expressed in the nervous system but to be highly expressed in the cells of the immune system. These data suggested that the cannabinoid system represented an extremely widespread and important signaling system throughout the body, particularly in, but not limited to, the nervous system.

Just as had been the case with opiates, the question now arose as to the identity of the normal endogenous signaling molecule(s) that interacted with the cannabinoid receptors. It didn't seem to be any known natural substance, indicating that, as with the endorphins, something new and exciting was waiting to be discovered.

But what could it be? Experience with the endorphins had shown us that the endogenous activator of the cannabis receptors did not necessarily have to have a chemical structure that made it look like Δ^9-THC. In the end, the assay that was used to detect the endogenous cannabis-like molecules, which have become known as *endocannabinoids,* was the receptor binding assay.[10,14] Here again the successful laboratory was that of Rafael Mechoulam and his colleagues in Israel. Using cells in which the CB1 receptor was labeled using the binding of a radioactive agonist, Mechoulam and his colleagues looked to see if they could extract anything from the brain that would displace the radioactive drug by competing with it for the receptor. In 1992 they hit the jackpot. There was something in the brain that did just that. They also found that the presence of this material was enhanced by increasing the levels of Ca ions. As we have seen from their success in isolating Δ^9-THC, the Mechoulam group had outstanding chemical skills and were particularly adept at using the emerging techniques of NMR and mass spectrometry to aid in the determination of the structure of different chemical substances. Soon they had identified the endogenous material as arachidonoylethanolamide (AEA). They sent a minute amount of the new material to be tested by their collaborators in Scotland who, as we have seen, were the most adept scientists in the world in the use of isolated nerve muscle bioassay systems. In the mouse vas deferens bioassay, Mechoulam's newly isolated molecule inhibited the electrically stimulated contractions of the muscle, just like endorphins had done. The difference in this case was that while the effects of the enkephalins were reversed by the selective opiate antagonist naloxone, the effects of AEA were not, indicating that AEA activated a different receptor. In recognition of the cannabis-like effects of AEA, Mechoulam and his group named the new material "anandamide" after the word *ananda,* which is Sanskrit for "bliss." Soon afterward the same group isolated a similar compound named 2-arachidonoyl glycerol (2-AG), which also proved to have genuine CB receptor agonist activity. A number of other compounds followed, indicating that there was a large family of such endogenous substances made by the brain and other tissues.[15,16] (Figure 7.5).

These results were very satisfying for a number of reasons. One was the obvious success in solving the problem of the chemical nature of the

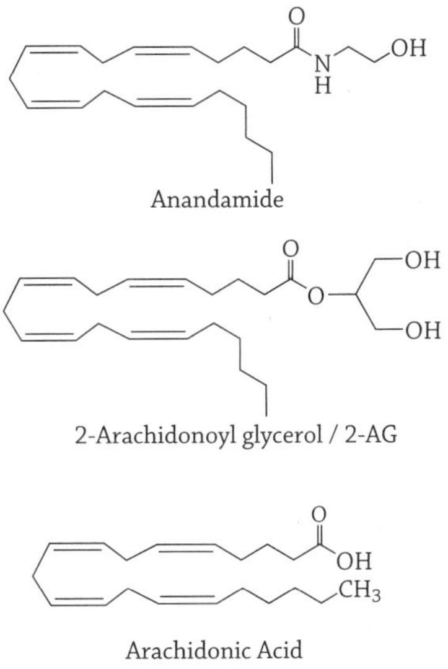

Anandamide

2-Arachidonoyl glycerol / 2-AG

Arachidonic Acid

Figure 7.5:
The endocannabinoids anandamide and 2-acylglycerol are derived from arachidonic acid.

endogenous cannabinoids. However, another was the comfortable feeling that we had been down this road before. In retrospect, the fact that the endocannabinoids were derived from arachidonic acid was not all that surprising, as it was already known that many important biological messenger molecules were derived from this same source. Arachidonic acid (AA) is what is known as a polyunsaturated fatty acid (PUFAs; see Figure 7.5). AA is found as a component of the phospholipids that make up cell membranes attached to the 1 or 2 position of a glycerol molecule. Clearly, membrane phospholipids are of great importance for the structural integrity of the cell membrane. However, when attacked by the enzymes called *phospholipases,* they can release PUFAs such as AA. This AA can then be further transformed into an enormous number of important signaling molecules generally known as *eicosanoids.*

The products of this pathway, which include prostaglandins, prostacyclins, thromboxanes, and leukotrienes, generally act upon unique families of GPCRs or sometimes on other types of receptors such as the nuclear receptor PPAR-γ and related molecules. These are receptors that exist within cells and regulate the transcription of many genes involved in the inflammatory response. It had been very well established that eicosanoids played a vital role in the generation of inflammation. Indeed, the British pharmacologist John Vane had won the Nobel Prize for demonstrating that drugs like aspirin produced their anti-inflammatory effects by inhibiting the synthesis of prostaglandins.[17] Although they were not eicosanoids, anandamide, 2-AG, and other members of the endocannabinoid family could be considered as yet another arm of the extensive repertoire of AA-derived signaling molecules. The wide distribution of CB1 and CB2 receptors not only within the brain but in other tissues as well also suggested that endocannabinoids represented widely utilized signaling molecules.

ENDOCANNABINOIDS AND NEUROTRANSMISSION

In the present instance, however, we are particularly interested in the fact that CB1 receptors are widely distributed in the brain, and that Δ^9-THC is a psychoactive drug. Everybody had expected that endocannabinoids would be neurotransmitters. When the endorphins had been discovered, their peptidergic nature had been a surprise, but at least they clearly behaved like classical neurotransmitters. They obeyed all of the normal rules—they were made in the presynaptic neuron, stored in synaptic vesicles, and released at synapses in response to Ca influx into the presynaptic terminal. So, what about endocannabinoids like anandamide and 2-AG—are they neurotransmitters?

The answer to this question is yes and no, or rather yes but not in the way we normally think about such molecules. A clue to their mechanism of action can be gleaned from what we know about the mechanism of action of prostaglandins and other AA-derived molecules. Generally speaking, these substances are used as "local hormones." That is to say, they are released from one cell and act upon other cells in close proximity, rather than being transported long distances through the blood like classical hormones. Moreover, prostaglandins are produced when they are needed, rather than being preformed and stored in vesicles or other structures waiting to be released.

A model for how endocannabinoids function as "neurotransmitters" was provided by the neurophysiologist Roger Nicoll in 2001.[19] He was able to show that endocannabinoids were actually released by postsynaptic neurons when they were subject to the action of a neurotransmitter that increased the level of Ca in the cell. Although endocannabinoids are not pre-stored in vesicles by postsynaptic neurons, they are synthesized in response to an increase in Ca. Once synthesized they can leave the postsynaptic neuron and diffuse backward across the synapse to act upon CB1 receptors expressed by the presynaptic terminal, inhibiting the release of its neurotransmitter.

So, are endocannabinoids neurotransmitters? Well, it is true that they are released in response to an increase in Ca, which is also true of other neurotransmitters. On the other hand, they aren't stored in synaptic vesicles but are synthesized "on demand" in response to a Ca increase. Secondly, when endocannabinoids are released they travel *backward* across the synapse from the postsynaptic cell to produce effects on the presynaptic nerve terminal. They could therefore be described as "retrograde" neurotransmitters. So, there are plenty of things about endocannabinoids that don't fit the description of any classical neurotransmitter. Nevertheless, they clearly are neurotransmitters and their job is to carry information across synapses. Indeed, continuing research has now clearly demonstrated the endocannabinoid system is a complete neurotransmitter system consisting of receptors (CB1 and CB2), endogenous agonists (e.g., anandamide and 2-AG), as well as the appropriate biosynthetic and degradative enzymes for making and destroying these molecules. Extensive electrophysiological studies have now demonstrated the mechanisms by which endocannabinoids can regulate synaptic function through both rapid and long-lasting actions.

THE PRESCRIPTION OF POT

Given the many important pharmacological effects of Δ^9-THC, there has been tremendous interest in the development of drugs that work through the cannabinoid system for a very large number of disorders.[12,20] Indeed, every conceivable type of cannabinoid drug has been successfully synthesized at this point in time. This includes specific CB1 and CB2 agonists and antagonists, inhibitors of the enzymes responsible for the degradation of AEA and 2-AG (known as *fatty acid amide hydrolase* [FAAH] and *monoacylglycerol lipase* [MAGL] respectively), as well as chemicals that block the movement of endocannabinoids in and out of cells. Prior to discussing these developments, however, one should realize that pure Δ^9-THC is actually a marketed drug in the United States. Synthetic Δ^9-THC is sold under the name dronabinol (Marinol). This reflects the confusion in the laws that govern cannabis use in the United States because, as we have seen, crude cannabis itself is a Schedule 1 drug and cannot be prescribed or used for any purpose whatsoever. On the other hand Marinol, which is a pure preparation of Δ^9-THC, the main psychoactive ingredient of cannabis, can be prescribed and used therapeutically. Confused? You have every right to be. Marinol is employed as an antiemetic for cancer and AIDS patients and also as an appetite stimulant in these patient populations. It is basically Δ^9-THC, dissolved in sesame oil, dispensed as a capsule. Obviously, when taken this way, the effects of the drug will take longer to become apparent than if it were smoked. Also, Marinol is pure Δ^9-THC, so one will not get the effects of any other cannabinoids such as cannabidiol that might normally contribute to the effects of smoking hashish or marijuana. It seems as though Marinol is effective in many patients, although some do report psychoactive side effects—no surprise there. Nabilone (Cesamet), a semisynthetic THC derivative which acts as an agonist at CB1 and CB2 receptors, is also available by prescription as a treatment for nausea associated with chemotherapy, and more recently as an adjunct therapy for chronic (neuropathic) pain. Finally, Sativex, available in Europe and Canada, is an extract of *C. sativa* which contains mostly Δ^9-THC and cannabidiol together with smaller amounts of many minor cannabinoid components found in the hemp plant. It has been approved for the treatment of neuropathic pain and spasticity associated with multiple sclerosis. Clearly Sativex is closer to the composition of "natural" marijuana than Marinol or Nabilone, and this is one of its marketing points.

Generally speaking there are several classes of chemical compounds that have been developed as cannabinoid receptor agonists.[20] These include "classical" structures, by which one means molecules are clearly based on the structure of natural cannabinoids like Δ^9-THC. This would also include drugs like Nabilone and numerous others like HU-210 (HU for Hebrew University), as well as molecules that have been made by many drug companies (Figure 7.6). In addition, there are a variety of chemical structures

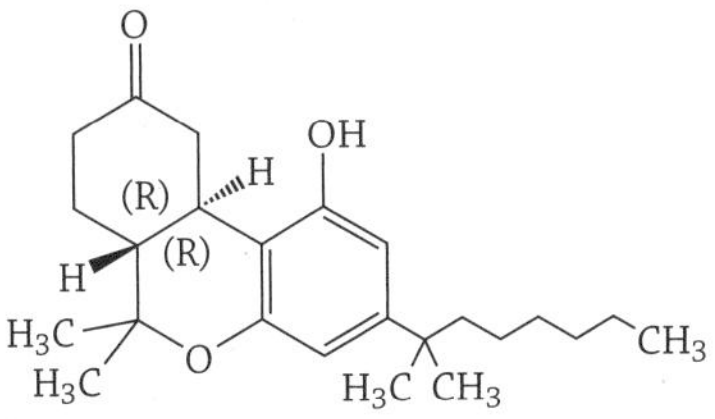

Figure 7.6:
The synthetic cannabinoid agonists Nabilone and HU-210.

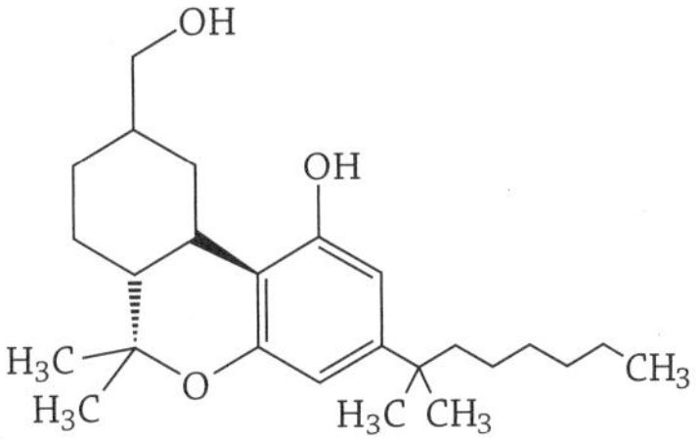

that have been discovered which are not cannabinoids but do act as ago- nists or antagonists at cannabinoid receptors. Finally, there are novel drugs that are based on the endocannabinoid structure.

These different classes of chemical structures exhibit a quite varied spec- trum of actions as agonists at CB1 and CB2 receptors. Some are very selec- tive for CB1 and some for CB2, and so potentially produce very different effects. Another difference with respect to their properties relates to how well they stimulate each receptor. It turns out that nature's own agonists are not full agonists at CB1 and CB2. Δ^9-THC is actually a partial agonist for both of these receptors, particularly the latter. Many of the synthetic compounds noted above are actually more effective receptor agonists than Δ^9-THC. In addition, anandamide, the archetypal endocannabinoid, is also not a full agonist at CB1 or CB2 and, as is the case for Δ^9-THC, acts as a partial agonist at these receptors.

Attempts have already been made to develop some of these substances into drugs, and the results have been most educational. As it is clear that CB1 agonists make people want to eat, it therefore follows that CB1 antag- onists should produce satiety; that is, a decrease in appetite. Such a drug might be a very good drug for treating obesity. That seems like a reason- able idea. So, with this in mind, it was decided to develop the compound SR141716A,which is a very good CB1 antagonist (actually an inverse ago- nist), as a drug of this type.

After the normal amount of appropriate clinical and preclinical testing, the drug was found to be very effective and was put on the market in sev- eral European countries as rimonabant, or Accomplia. "Lose weight, feel great!" trumpeted the ads. Rimonabant's arrival was highly anticipated as a totally new type of weight loss drug. Of course, getting the drug through the FDA in the United States was a major aim as well because, as we have seen, the US market is really the big drug market in the world, and the

United States does not lack people who are overweight. The results started to come in. Many women who were perhaps a little plump managed to lose weight and to fulfill their dreams of getting into a size zero Prada or Comme des Garcons. Unfortunately, although these women "lost weight" they didn't "feel great." Indeed they were very unhappy, some to the point of wanting to kill themselves. The FDA didn't like what they saw and balked at allowing rimonabant to be marketed in the United States. Alarmed at the results, the company also took the drug off the market in Europe.

So, what went wrong?[21] Well, it is clear that rimonabant does cross the blood-brain barrier and so will block CB1 receptors both inside and outside the brain. Now we know that the CB1 receptors that are responsible for the psychoactive effects of Δ^9-THC are in the brain. We know that when you activate these receptors with Δ^9-THC it makes people feel "good." People describe this in different ways—"more relaxed…more mellow…less anxious" and so on. So, what would be the predicted effect of blocking these receptors and endogenous signaling by endocannabinoids? One doesn't have to be a rocket scientist to realize that this would likely make people feel pretty bad, and indeed that is precisely what happens. So, is it therefore the case that all CB1 antagonists that get into the brain will have the same negative effects as rimonabant? Probably so.

However, it turns out that the initial views as to how the endocannabinoid system regulated food intake and its consequences were somewhat naïve. Obesity is only one manifestation of metabolic disease that also includes comorbid syndromes such as diabetes and cardiovascular disease. The appetite/satiety system controlled by the brain is in constant communication with peripheral systems controlling metabolism, adipogenesis, muscle, and gastrointestinal function. Indeed, analysis of the distribution of CB1 receptors outside the brain has indicated that endocannabinoids and CB1 receptors are expressed in tissues that are generally involved in the control of energy homeostasis, including the intestine, the liver, white adipose tissue, skeletal muscle, and the pancreas. In fact, it is now thought that the endocannabinoid system is a key regulatory component involved in the peripheral control of metabolism, lipogenesis, and insulin release, as well as other important factors.[22] Inhibition of these effects using a CB1 antagonist are predicted to be generally beneficial in the treatment of obesity/diabetes spectrum disorders. Hence the development of a peripherally acting CB1 antagonist that doesn't enter the brain might be very useful in this context. Overall, it is clear that there are exciting prospects for the therapeutic development of drugs that act through the endocannabinoid signaling system, particularly agents that don't produce psychoactive effects.

One could, of course, take the opposite view, which would be that it is really great to have all these new psychoactive synthetic cannabinoids. Many street consumers have certainly felt this way and have been quick to take advantage of the situation. Consider the group of compounds synthesized by Dr. John Huffman, a medicinal chemist working at Clemson University who has made important contributions to the field of cannabinoid medicinal chemistry and pharmacology. These include powerful CB1 agonists such as JWH-018 and JWH-073.[23] Over the last decade, certain popular Internet products have been herbal mixtures sold under names such as Spice and K2. These are advertised as producing effects like marijuana but legally; that is, they didn't contain cannabis-related products. This indeed was found to be the case. Some Spice products produced a very profound "high." However, the reason for this soon became clear. Rather than containing marijuana or hashish, these mixtures contained a liberal amount of JWH-018, which is certainly a potent CB1 agonist but which was not covered by the law at that time. Once this was detected in Europe, the authorities quickly moved to make this synthetic cannabinoid illegal. So, of course, the makers of Spice-like products just switched to another synthetic cannabinoid, JWH-073, that could produce similar effects. Once that had been detected, they switched to a compound made by Mechoulam and his colleagues known as HU-210. These synthetic cannabinoids have therefore taken on the status of designer drugs, as previously discussed when we considered hallucinogens (Chapter 2). The object is to keep one step ahead of the law with respect to the introduction of new psychoactive substances. As with Shulgin's synthesis of hallucinogenic tryptamines, there are virtually an infinite number of different chemical changes that could be envisaged as producing synthetic psychoactive cannabinoids. The legal status of such substances is constantly under review. Synthetic cannabinoids represent a new hypertext drug phenomenon whose future is unclear. How exactly legal considerations will keep up with the ingenuity of medicinal chemists remains to be seen.

POT AND THE LAW

Following the Second World War, Harry Anslinger moved to increase the penalties for marijuana use.[3,5,9] Now, in addition to racism he also had a new target: communism. The Boggs Act passed in 1950 imposed extremely severe penalties for marijuana use—2 to 5 years for a first offense, 5–10 years for a second offense, and up to 20 years for a third offense. Second- or third-time offenders also would have no opportunity for parole.

Anslinger at this point was also starting to push the idea that marijuana was a "stepping stone" drug and that its use led inevitably to the use of harder drugs like opiates. Basically Anslinger argued that marijuana was an ideal tool for both racial and political subversion of American youth by inferior races and communists. Nevertheless, the world was starting to change. The late '40s and 1950s saw the rise of a new bohemian element in the United States—the Beats. Artists such as William Burroughs, Jack Kerouac, and Alan Ginsberg started to have an important influence on the lifestyles of young people. The Beats wrote about drugs and also used them extensively. Burroughs wrote about heroin, Burroughs and Ginsberg about yage/ayahuasca, and all of them about marijuana and alcohol. Their drug use constituted a part of their New American Romanticism. Soon what they were doing started to be copied by young people in general—and the Beatniks had arrived.

The scene was set for marijuana use to become a middle class phenomenon. As the 1950s became the 1960s, students and hippies opposed to the Vietnam war coalesced into a radical new pro-peace movement and used marijuana and other drugs as part of their badge of identity. Marijuana use swept through middle class America and Europe like wildfire, and it became virtually impossible for drug use to be controlled by the existing laws. Because of this problem, the Marijuana Tax Act was found to be unconstitutional and, as mentioned above, Congress passed the Controlled Substances Act of 1970 leading to the categorization of abused drugs in one of five Schedules. Marijuana was placed on Schedule I, a completely political decision. As we have discussed, this meant that marijuana could not even be prescribed by physicians and was only available to scientific researchers after the filling out millions of forms with various federal agencies. However, the government's stance was based on politics not on a realistic assessment of marijuana's true characteristics. Inevitably the widespread use of marijuana, and the growing modern awareness of its possible therapeutic uses, produced an extremely "schizophrenic" attitude in Washington.

By this time the FBN had become the DEA (Drug Enforcement Agency). In 1976, at the same time that the DEA was doing everything in its power to persuade everybody that marijuana was a dangerous and useless drug, Congress moved in the completely opposite direction, and between 1976 and 1988 quietly created the "Compassionate IND" program, which provided a small number of patients with government-grown marijuana if they were deemed to require it for medical purposes. Eventually the program was disbanded by the Bush administration, not because they had become convinced that marijuana had no therapeutic value but because they realized that the program was actually undermining their overall anti-drug position.

The fact is that every time the US, British, or other European governments have investigated the recreational and medical use of marijuana through the workings of an official government commission, they have always concluded that the drug was not the "killer weed" described by Anslinger or others. The first commission to investigate marijuana, and still the most complete, was the Indian Hemp Drugs Commission set up by the British in India in 1893 in response to pressures exerted by the temperance movement in England. The commission was charged with investigating every aspect of cannabis use, ranging from its cultivation to its effects on users, its potential taxation, and prohibition. Over 1000 witnesses from every walk of life were called and the result was a report of over 3500 pages! The commission came to several important conclusions. First of all, that cannabis use was extremely widespread and used for both recreational and religious purposes. Second, that cannabis use wasn't particularly dangerous and wasn't associated with increased violent crime or mental disorders. Third, that attempts to ban the use of cannabis or to tax it out of existence would impact the religious practices of a large part of the population and was likely to result in civil unrest.

The British were to revisit these questions in the 1960s, now of course in the context of widespread marijuana use in the United Kingdom. A commission was set up under the leadership of Baroness Wooton, a widely respected social scientist. It is worth quoting some of the commission's conclusions—"Having reviewed all the material available to us we find ourselves in agreement with the conclusion reached by the Indian Hemp Drugs Commission appointed by the government of India (1893–1894) and the New York Mayor's Committee on Marihuana (1944), that the long term consumption of cannabis in 'moderate' doses has no harmful effects." They also commented that, "The evidence before us shows that an increasing number of people, mainly young, in all classes of society are experimenting with the drug, and substantial numbers use it regularly for social pleasure. There is no evidence that this activity is causing violent crime or aggressive anti-social behavior, or is producing in otherwise normal people conditions of dependence or psychosis, requiring medical treatment."

As with the Indian Hemp Drugs Commission and the New York Mayor's Committee, the government in power (Labor at that time) completely ignored the conclusions made by the Wooton Report, instead branding the Wooton Commission as a "cannabis lobby." In fact it wasn't only the New York Mayor's Committee that had come to similar conclusions in the United States. Back in 1929, the US Army had set up an investigation into the smoking of marijuana by soldiers stationed in the Panama Canal zone. Here again, the military committee concluded, "There is no evidence that Marihuana as grown and used in the Canal zone is a habit forming drug or that it has any particular deleterious influence on the individual using it." Indeed, conclusions of this type were subsequently made by a commission set up by President Nixon in his "war against drugs" (he wasn't pleased), as well as commissions set up in other countries such as Canada and Australia. In general the recommendations of all these committees and commissions to revise and reduce their punishments for cannabis possession were in large part ignored.

There was one notable exception, however, and that was the Netherlands. In the early 1970s the Dutch launched their own investigation into drug culture. They concluded that, roughly speaking, drugs could be divided into two categories. Really dangerous drugs, heroin being a good example, and less dangerous drugs like cannabis. In this respect their attitude was the opposite of that of the US government, who had made cannabis a class I restricted drug in the same category as heroin and LSD. The Dutch couldn't make cannabis legal because, like most other countries, they had signed international treaties that made all signatories responsible for keeping many drugs, including cannabis, illegal. Nevertheless, these treaties did provide a certain amount of leeway into how each individual country handled the situation. The Dutch decided that whereas they would maintain a very tough attitude and appropriate penalties for possession of drugs like heroin, they would back off where cannabis was concerned. It was decided that possession of small amounts of cannabis would only be considered a "misdemeanor" and in fact, in most instances, it would be completely ignored. Indeed, cannabis sales were permitted in specifically licensed cafes. So an interesting situation arose where cannabis could be sold in such cafes although cultivation of cannabis was actually illegal. One might therefore wonder where the government of the Netherlands thought that cannabis being sold in the cafes was coming from? Nevertheless, they let things go their own way and did not interfere. The cannabis cafes have become extremely popular, particularly in Amsterdam or close to the German border. One reason for this is "drug tourism" where tourists from less enlightened countries can just slip across the border and can sample one of the café's exotic offerings. This has now become something of a nuisance problem, and some revision of the current laws are in the works.

Nevertheless, the experiment has been carried out. What has happened to the Netherlands since the 1970s? Have the Netherlands descended into a miasma of violent crime and cannabis-induced lassitude? The fact is that the Dutch are now the tallest, most strapping people on the planet. As far as their reputation for physical and mental fitness is concerned, let us not forget that this is the country who gave us Johan Cruyff and Dennis Bergkamp, and whose football team went to the finals of the last World Cup. Heaven knows what the Dutch would have been like if they hadn't been smoking all that cannabis! One has to say that something akin to the Dutch model of moderation is the way of the future. Indeed, in the United States there has been a recent trend for many states to start decriminalizing the possession of small amount of cannabis, a trend that continued in the 2012 presidential election.

The pharmacology of cannabis and the endocannabinoid system remains one of the most fascinating topics for the psychopharmacologist to consider. It is also one of the most untapped in terms of its therapeutic potential. It seems highly likely that useful drugs based on cannabinoid pharmacology will be with us in the not too distant future. Hemp's finest hour is yet to come. 'High-ho Silver!'

NOTES

1. Harry Bruinius. *Better for all the world. The secret history of forced sterilization and America's quest for racial purity*. Alfred A Knopf. 2006.
2. Douglas Valentine. *The strength of the wolf*. Verso Books. 2004.
3. Martin Booth. *Cannabis: A history*. Picador. 2005.
   Leslie L Iversen. *The science of marijuana*. Oxford University Press. 2007.
4. http://www.drugwarrant.com/articles/why-is-marijuana-illegal/
   http://en.wikipedia.org/wiki/Harry_J._Anslinger
   http://dissention.wordpress.com/2010/09/10/harry-anslinger-and-marijuana/
5. http://www.druglibrary.org/schaffer/hemp/history/mustomj1.html
   http://www.leda.law.harvard.edu/leda/data/352/Ransom.pdf
6. Jonathon Green. *Cannabis; a history*. Thunder's Mouth Press. 2002.
7. http://gutenberg.net.au/ebooks06/0603031h.html
8. Charles Baudelaire. *Artificial Paradises* (1996 ed). Citadel Press.
9. Leslie L. Iversen. *The science of marijuana*. Oxford University Press. 2007.
   Raphael Mechoulam. *Marijuana: Chemistry, Pharmacology, Metabolism and Clinical Effects*. Academic Press. 1973.
10. Mechoulam R, Hanus L. A historical overview of chemical research on cannabinoids. *Chem Phys Lipids*. 2000, 108(1-2):1–13.
11. Appendino G, Chianese G, Taglialatela-Scafati O. Cannabinoids: occurrence and medicinal chemistry. *Curr Med Chem*. 2011, 18(7):1085–1099.
12. Pertwee RG. Emerging strategies for exploiting cannabinoid receptor agonists as medicines. *Br J Pharmacol*. 2009, 156(3):397–411.
13. Howlett AC. Cannabinoid receptor signaling. *Handbook of Experimental Pharmacology*. 2005, 168:53–79.
14. Pertwee RG. Cannabinoid Pharmacology: The first 66 years. *Brit J Pharmacol*. 2006, 147:S163–171.
15. Di Marzo V. Endocannabinoid signaling in the brain: biosynthetic mechanisms in the limelight. *Nat Neurosci*. 2011, 14(1):9–15

16. Wang J, Ueda N. Biology of endocannabinoid synthesis system. *Prostaglandins Other Lipid Mediat.* 2009, 89(3-4):112–119.

    De Petrocellis L, Di Marzo V. An introduction to the endocannabinoid system: from the early to the latest concepts. *Best Pract Res Clin Endocrinol Metab.* 2009, 23(1):1–15.

17. Diarmuid Jeffreys. *Aspirin: The remarkable story of a wonder drug.* Bloomsbury Press. 2004.

18. Wilson RI, Nicoll RA. Endogenous cannabinoids mediate retrograde signalling at hippocampal synapses. *Nature.* 2001, 410(6828):588–592.

19. Pertwee RG. Pharmacological actions of cannabinoids. *Handbook of Experimental Pharmacology.* 2004,168:1–51.

20. Clapper JR, Moreno-Sanz G, Russo R, Guijarro A, Vacondio F, Duranti A, Tontini A, Sanchini S, Sciolino NR, Spradley JM, Hohmann AG, Calignano A, Mor M, Tarzia G, Piomelli D. Anandamide suppresses pain initiation through a peripheral endocannabinoid mechanism. *Nat Neurosci.* 2010, 13:1265–1270.

21. Di Marzo V, Després JP. CB1 antagonists for obesity–what lessons have we learned from rimonabant? *Nat Rev Endocrinol.* 2009, 5(11):633–638.

22. Di Marzo V, Piscitelli F, Mechoulam R. Cannabinoids and endocannabinoids in metabolic disorders with focus on diabetes. *Handb Exp Pharmacol.* 2011, (203):75–104.

    Di Marzo V. The endocannabinoid system in obesity and type 2 diabetes. *Diabetologia.* 2008, 51(8):1356–1367.

23. For a discussion of cannabinoids of this type see *Erowid Monthly,* Nov 2010. (Erowid.org)

24. Fitzhugh Ludlow (1903 ed.). *The Hasheesh Eater.* SG Raines Co. New York.

CHAPTER 8

The Man with the Dragon Tattoo

"Salomon saith, there is no new thing upon the earth. So that as Plato had an imagination, that all knowledge was but remembrance; so Salomon giveth his sentence, that all novelty is but oblivion."

Francis Bacon, *Essays* LVIII

The river junk had made its way several hundred miles upriver from the port of Ningbo to an area of countryside of outstanding beauty. In the distance was a range of tall mountains carved by time and weather into extraordinary shapes, their tops covered by a blanket of clouds. And near the river, in the foothills for miles around, were terrace after terrace of bright green tea plants interspersed with peach trees from which hung the most splendid and delectable looking fruit. At this point all further progress upriver had stopped, owing to the great press of boats trying to pass through a giant river lock. These boats were lined up in an orderly manner waiting for their turn. All, that is, except one. A ramshackle looking boat with an unsavory looking man at the helm was barging its way to the front of the line by pushing all of the other boats out of the way, one by one. Now, he was approaching the river junk. At that moment a large man appeared on the deck of the junk.

"And just where do you think you are going?" said the man to the interloper, but the latter just continued his progress without bothering to reply.

"Do you realize this boat is carrying my master, a mandarin?" said the large man.

The interloper bared his yellow teeth and replied:

"The fact is, I don't give a fig about mandarins, so just get out of my way fat boy."

"Is that so?" said the large man; "Well, perhaps you would like to look at this?"

The servant, for that is indeed what he was, stuck his hand deep inside the pocket of his robe and pulled out a small scroll, which he unfolded and exhibited to the interloper. On the scroll was a picture of the imperial dragon of the Chinese court. The effect was immediate and dramatic.

"Aieeeee!" cried the interloper, and immediately fell to his knees on the deck of his boat. At the same time he began to kowtow, repeatedly touching the deck with his head. And not just touching the deck, banging his head into the wood as hard as he could, and groveling as if trying to administer some type of self-punishment. "Please", he whined "Have mercy on me, I didn't understand, please Master I am so sorry."

"Listen, you miserable turd," said the servant, "If you ever attempt to insult my master in this way again, the Emperor's men will take you and, while you are still alive, cut you into tiny bite-size morsels to be fed to the Emperor's dogs!"

The interloper ran to the front of his boat and started to reverse his course as quickly as he could until he was out of sight.

Watching these events from the shadows in the stern of the boat was the mandarin in question. He was dressed in the wide flowing garments which were the appropriate style for a man of his station. But apart from that, he appeared like other Chinese men of the time with his tonsured head and long queue falling halfway down his back. On the other hand, there were some remarkable things about the mandarin. First, on the wrist of his right hand he had a tiny tattoo illustrating the same dragon as depicted on his servant's scroll. He was also very tall and his eyes were extremely round, which was believed by the local people to indicate high intelligence. While on the journey he had left most of the talking to his servant. When he did speak however, he used a strange accent. His servant had explained to the other passengers that his master came from far away, "from north of the great wall." This explanation had assuaged the curiosity of everybody concerned.

The mandarin walked out of the shadows and returned to his cabin. Once settled comfortably in his chair, he opened one of the cases carrying his possessions and took out an old and very worn book. He opened the book and read for a while and then began to speak softly to himself in a broad Scottish accent.

"The Lord is my shepherd, I shall not want. He maketh me lie down in green pastures. He leadeth me beside still waters. He restoreth my soul."

Indeed, this was no Chinese mandarin but Robert Fortune, Esq., currently the director of the Chelsea Physic Garden in London and one of Britain's most eminent botanists.[1] This was his public persona when he was at home in England. But now he had a new role to play, for he was also Robert Fortune—secret agent!

After a while, Fortune closed his Bible and then closed his eyes. He cast his mind back to the day that his present adventure had begun. He had been sitting in his drawing room in Chelsea when his servant had announced that he had a visitor. Fortune immediately recognized the visitor's name, as it was that of another very well respected botanist. The man came in and Fortune made him comfortable. Fortune then asked the man how he could help him.

"Indeed, I believe you could help us a great deal," said the man, "You see I am not here just on my own behalf but on the behalf of others. We should like to ask you for a great favor."

"And who is it that you represent?" asked Fortune.

"The Company," said the man. There was no need for further explanation. There were many companies but only one "Company."

"And what is it that you want to achieve?" asked Fortune.

"That is simple" said the man. "World domination." Again, no further explanation was necessary. Such a goal was certainly consistent with all that Fortune knew about the operations of the Company.

"But how on earth could I be of any help to the Company?" queried Fortune.

"Your mission, should you decide to accept it," said the man, "would be one of the utmost danger and complexity, requiring you to work undercover in the most difficult of circumstances for an extended period of time. In brief, we want you to steal something of the greatest importance."

"And what might that be?" asked Fortune, raising an eyebrow.

"Tea," said the man.

With this single word everything was immediately clear to Fortune. Yes indeed, that would be a task of the greatest difficulty. But was it "mission impossible"? Nobody had ever succeeded. But why him? The two men talked until the early hours of the morning, all of Fortune's questions were answered, and the path for what was to become his life's work was set out before him. It was also why, many months later, Robert Fortune had gone to China and hired a man as his servant who had previously been employed by the emperor and still carried his seal. The man had helped Fortune disguise himself, and now they were headed upriver to the Bohea region around the Wuyi mountains, China's premier tea growing region, in order to carry out their secret mission (Figure 8.1).

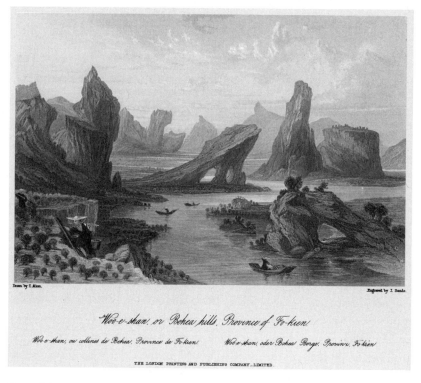

Figure 8.1:
Thomas Allom (1843). A view of the Bohea hills (Wuyi Shan).
(Reproduced with permission from Ancestry Images)

LIQUID JADE

Although there are many varieties of tea on the market today including white, green, oolong and black, all of these are derived from a single source, the tea plant *Camelia sinensis*.[2] As a matter of fact it wasn't until well into the nineteenth century, and in no small part due to the efforts of Robert Fortune, that this became entirely clear. Previously there had been a vigorous debate as to whether these different types of tea all came from one or more plants. When the buds and leaves of the tea plant are picked, they will gradually turn from green to black as their natural chlorophyll is broken down by a process of enzymatic oxidation. However, this process can be halted by heating or "roasting" the leaves at various points, thereby regulating their final color. As this process is also characterized by the production of tannins and other elements, the taste of the resulting tea also changes along with the color. The curing process for tea is continuously creative. Consider something like Lapsang Souchong, with its characteristic smoky aroma and flavor resulting from a fine Bohea tea being cured over smoking pinewood and taking on the character of the smoke, like an Islay malt whiskey takes on the character of peat.

Over the years, different cultivars have been derived from *C. sinensis* that grow under somewhat different conditions and are more or less suitable for the production of different teas. Moreover, flavorings such as jasmine or bergamot can be added to the final tea products to produce even greater varieties. In Robert Fortune's time the most important tea-growing area in the world was in southwest China in and around the province of Fujian. Black and green teas were grown in somewhat different areas, the black teas being from the area known as Bohea around the Wuyi mountains.

The original name for tea as referred to in Chinese texts from around 700 BC was *tu*. Later, around 700 AD, the Chinese ideogram *cha* appeared. This ideogram closely resembles the character *tu*. The word for tea nowadays in most of China and Japan is "*cha*." The exception is in Fujian where *te* (pronounced "tay") is still used. As trading in tea first involved Dutch traders carrying tea from this region, the name "tea" was spread throughout the world. However, where the habit of tea drinking was spread by other means, the word "cha" is used. Sometimes both terms are used. In Britain, for example, the word *tea* is commonly used. However, it is also not unusual to hear somebody asking for "a nice cupp'a cha." Of course these days almost anything that grows can be dried, packaged, and sold as "tea." Indeed, the habit of drinking infusions from many different dried plants is clearly an ancient custom. However, only *C. sinesis* is really tea, and these other products, often called "tisanes," are not.

Tea plants like to grow in subtropical climates with a fair amount of rain. They can certainly be cultivated at higher elevations, where they grow more slowly but are considered to produce teas of superior quality. Typically, in more elevated areas of Fujian or in the Indian Himalaya regions, the weather is moist with frequent rains and foggy misty conditions as well as mild temperatures. This is ideal for producing high quality tea. Although China, India, and Sri Lanka are all generally thought of as major tea growing areas today, the origins of tea as a drink and of tea culture in general are clearly associated with ancient China.

There are many legends as to how the Chinese began drinking "liquid jade." The most common of these involves the mythical emperor Shen Nung, who is supposed to have lived around 2800 BC and is revered as the father of Chinese agriculture. Shen Nung was an altogether remarkable person, as he had the body of a man and the head of a bull. He could speak fluently when only 3 days old, and walk when he was a week. Not only that, but he could plow an entire field by himself when he was 3 years old.

Shen Nung also studied herbs and plants for their potential medicinal purposes. One day he was on an expedition with some of his retinue when they stopped for a rest. Shen Nung's followers boiled some water because he had taught them that it was much safer to drink water that was boiled first. At some point a strong breeze came up and some leaves of *C. sinesis* floated into the boiling water. When Shen Nung drank the resulting infusion he noted that it made him feel energized and refreshed. He also enjoyed the slightly bitter and astringent flavor. He collected some of the leaves and took them home to experiment with.

And so the tradition of drinking tea was born. Shen Nung is supposed to have collected his wisdom in what is considered to be the earliest Chinese pharmacopeia, the *Pen Ts'ao Ching*, traditionally dated to the year 2737 BC to coincide with the period when Shen Nung lived, but in fact probably not written until the time of the Han dynasty (25–221 AD). Myths aside, the *Pen Ts'ao Ching* does contain interesting information concerning the properties of tea. For example, "Tea is better than wine for it leadeth not to intoxication, neither does it cause a man to say foolish things, and repent thereof in his sober moments. It is better than water for it does not carry disease; neither does it act like a poison, as does water when the wells contain foul and rotten matter." Such a description with similar sentiments could certainly have been written today. Indeed, the favorable properties of tea have ensured that, apart from water, it is the most widely consumed beverage in the world, and its popularity shows no signs of abating.

TEA CONQUERS EUROPE

Tea first really arrived in Europe courtesy of the Dutch and Portuguese traders who brought it back with them around 1600 as a curiosity along with their main preoccupation, different kinds of spices. Tea drinking slowly began to catch on in Europe, although it was not particularly common in England. However, after the Glorious Revolution of 1688, which saw British rule being transferred to a Dutch monarch, tea began to be imported into England more frequently and tea drinking began to take off in earnest. Soon the popularity of tea drinking overtook coffee, which was already well established as the major social beverage used by all levels of society at the time. Black tea was favored, together with the use of sugar, owing to its general availability from the British West Indies. The possible addition of milk or cream was another early innovation. Indeed, tea is often drunk with milk in countries that consume dairy products, such as India and Britain, and not in countries such as China where dairy items are rarely used. If, as it is believed, the first introduction of tea into England occurred in 1664 when two pounds and two ounces were given as a gift to the king, the fact that 60 years later England's annual tea import was in the region of a million pounds illustrates that England had rapidly become the tea-mad country that it remains today.

Of course, the great increase in tea drinking was also a wonderful opportunity for making lots of money. Tea imports were heavily taxed by the British government and by the time of Queen Victoria's ascension in the nineteenth century made up a staggering 10% of the government's revenue. Along with tea there grew up an entire world of tea culture and paraphernalia. Tea houses, which also served other stimulating drinks such as coffee and chocolate, became key meeting spots for the entire population to socialize, gossip, and discuss politics. The import of products such sugar were greatly stimulated due to their use as additives to tea. Moreover, the accoutrements of tea drinking such as fine china were also of great importance. To satisfy the demand for Chinese style cups and saucers, the Staffordshire potters began to make and market their ever popular lines of blue and white wares that were meant to resemble the products of the Ming and then Qing Chinese.

Importing tea into Britain was a very profitable affair. In 1600 Queen Elizabeth the first had granted a charter to "the Governor and Company of Merchants of London Trading into the East Indies," giving them a monopoly to trade with the countries of the Orient including the East Indies, India, and China. The company prospered and gradually became known as the East India Company, or "John Company" in common parlance. The interaction between the Company and its different trading partners varied a great deal. In India the Company had gradually expanded its power to the extent that it was actually the de facto government. It printed its own money, raised its own armies, fought its own wars, and basically ran the country on behalf of the British Crown. Indeed, the Company could do more or less as it wished with India. On the other hand, the Company's access to China was highly restricted. For many years the British were only allowed to trade through the port of Canton, and entry into the interior of China for trade or any other purpose was basically impossible. Over the years the Company traded several different products with the Chinese, but by the nineteenth century two of these had the greatest prominence—opium and tea. Trade in tea was particularly important. Then, as now, the British were addicted to tea, and so vast quantities had to be imported so that the average Englishman could have his breakfast or afternoon cup. However, all the tea in the world came from one place, and that place was China.

EUROPE CONQUERS TEA

From the European point of view, the Chinese, and for that matter the Japanese, left a great deal to be desired as trading partners. They were not at all keen on welcoming Europeans with their horrible religious beliefs. Indeed, not only was foreign trade with China restricted to the port of Canton until 1842, but the Japanese were even more restrictive, only allowing trade through the man-made island of Deshima situated in the harbor of the city of Nagasaki.[3] Moreover, by the early years of the nineteenth century, the British trade balance with China was extremely lopsided. Tea arrived in Britain from China, and lots of silver currency (one of the only commodities acceptable to the Chinese) left British coffers moving in the opposite direction. In order to redress this imbalance, the British needed to find something that they could easily provide to the Chinese, something desired even more than silver. To achieve this they came up with the perfect product—opium. As everybody knows, to the opium addict nothing is more important than the next opium pipe—nothing, not even gold or silver. The British had plenty of opium available to them, as it was grown and manufactured under the auspices of a Company monopoly in Bengal. Now all the British had to do was to flood the Chinese market with opium and use it to trade for products such as tea.

In spite of the fact that opium use in China was actually illegal, the British used every kind of connivance to encourage opium smuggling into the country. The result, as predicted, was a precipitous rise in the number of Chinese opium addicts who were, in all respects, the company's perfect customers. By 1839, however, the Chinese had had enough. A high ranking Chinese official in Canton rounded up all the supplies of opium and threw them into the harbor.[4] Perhaps he was inspired by the success of similar actions carried out by the residents of Boston in 1773 as a symbol of resistance to the British when they deposited all of the East India Company's tea into Boston harbor. Unfortunately, the British government thought that the treatment of their stocks of opium by the Chinese just wasn't cricket and sent a fleet of gun boats to teach the "Orientals" a lesson. This they duly did by shooting up several Chinese ports, leading the Chinese to sue for peace at the treaty of Nanking in 1842. The Chinese were charged 21 million silver dollars as compensation for the opium they dumped into Canton harbor, they were forced to open several ports up to "free trade," and to cede the island of Hong Kong to the British.

The East India Company had lost its monopoly to trade with China in 1834, and now events were moving fast. Trade with the newly humiliated Chinese was becoming very lucrative and competitive, and other British and European companies were trying to get into the act. In addition, the Americans, who had built the tea clippers, by far the fastest trading ships in the world, were also becoming a formidable presence. It was time for the East India Company to change tack. However, in spite of the change in the political and trading situation with the Chinese, one thing remained the same. It was the Chinese who grew and processed the tea. Somehow somebody had to put a stop to this and bring tea manufacturing under British and Company control. But how? Virtually all of the tea in the world was in China. In fact, a variety of C. sinensis had been identified in the Indian province of Assam, close to the Chinese border, but this only produced a low grade kind of tea. No, it just wouldn't do. As the Chinese would certainly never give up their precious tea voluntarily, somebody was going to have to steal it. Nevertheless, that would be no easy task. Even though several ports were now open to European trade, that was all that they were open to. Foreigners had to remain within restricted regions of these port towns with highly restricted access to the Chinese interior. So, who was going to sneak into China and how were they going to steal tea? The Company had to identify the right man, and in Robert Fortune they had done just that.

Fortune had impeccable credentials. First of all he was a brilliant botanist. Second, he had already previously sneaked inside China to a limited extent, bringing back a large number of interesting ornamental plants to the delight of British gardeners. However, tea plants and seeds were well known for their delicacy and it was not considered likely that they would normally survive a long sea journey, as would be the case when bringing them from China to Calcutta. If that could be successfully achieved, then the Company had the next step well thought out. The foothills of the Himalayas, the area near Darjeeling on the border with Sikkim, had a climate and elevation that was similar to the Chinese tea growing regions in Fujian. Now there was also a possible solution to the problem of getting the plants out of China in good shape. The solution came in the form of the Wardian case (Figure 8.2).

This had been invented a few years previously by Dr. Nathaniel Bagshaw Ward. A Wardian case was basically an early form of the terrarium in which plants could be kept in an enclosed environment protected from the elements. Prior to this, shipping plants had been a very hazardous affair because, while on the deck of a boat, they were subjected to wind, salt spray, and other factors that were anything but conducive to their survival. As things turned out, Fortune's secret visits to China, particularly his visit to the Wuyi mountain area, were an extraordinary success. As we have seen, Fortune disguised himself as a Chinese and also hired a servant who had previously been employed by the emperor and still carried the royal seal.

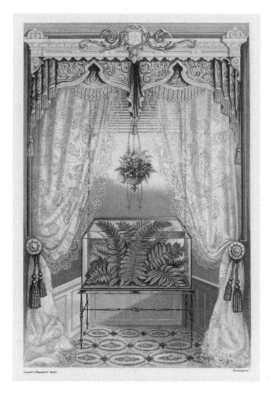

Figure 8.2:
A Wardian case, an early form of the terrarium.
(Mary Evans Picture Library / Alamy)

He managed to leave China with some 20,000 plants and a large number of seeds, and to ship these to Calcutta in excellent shape. These plants were the basis of the subsequent Indian tea enterprise which, as we all know, is now so closely associated with that country. The gradual development of new cultivars produced the wonderful teas of the Darjeeling area, as well as many other types. India, rather than China, became Britain's main source of tea and this has been the case ever since.

THE ARRIVAL OF COFFEE

At the time tea was becoming a national obsession in Britain, Europe was also in the process of adopting two other beverages that played a similar role both from the social and pharmacological points of view, these being coffee and chocolate. As far as we know, the drinking of coffee is not as ancient a practice as that of drinking tea. The practice appears to have had its origins in the area around the Horn of Africa in Ethiopia and Yemen.[5] Although it is true that coffee is mentioned in the *Canon of Medicine* by the Islamic doctor and alchemist Avicenna around 1000 AD, there is no further mention of its use until the Arabic literature of the sixteenth century. This is certainly odd, because it is known that the source of coffee, plants of the genus *Coffea,* which include *C. arabica* and *C. canephora* (also known as Robusta), grow wild throughout many parts of Africa.

As with the "discovery" of tea, coffee also has its own creation myth as first recorded by Antoine Faustus Nairon in his book of 1671 entitled *De Saluberrima Cahue seu Café nuncupata Discurscus,* probably the first real treatise on the topic. This tells of an Ethiopian goatherd called Kaldi, who noticed that when the animals under his care chewed the red berries of the coffee plant they became extremely frisky. So, Kaldi decided to try chewing the berries himself and found that they gave him quite a lift. Excited by his discovery, Kaldi took the berries to an Islamic priest in a monastery. However, equating them with something akin to alcohol, the priest threw them into the fire. The enticing smell of the roasting coffee beans made the priest change his mind. He rescued the roasted beans and ground them up. He then added boiling water and "voila," he had the world's first cup of coffee.

Although the truth of this charming tale is certainly doubtful, we do know that Sufis in and around the Yemenite city of Mocha were using coffee in the sixteenth century and that the habit spread rapidly throughout the Muslim world. In particular it spread to the Ottoman empire, where the Turks picked up the practice and made it the center of an entire social network of coffee shops. These institutions varied from the most humble shacks to the meeting places of high society, and they were also frequently used as venues for various political groups to hold discussions. As these were frequently of a revolutionary nature, there were times in cities like Istanbul and Cairo when the government attempted to close them down. Nevertheless, the coffee houses continued to prosper. Coffee spread from the Arab world to the Venetians, who traded it with the rest of Europe and, of course, the Ottomans also spread the use of coffee to their near neighbors in Vienna. The Dutch began trading in coffee early on, and established plantations for it in Ceylon and Java. By the middle of the seventeenth century, coffeehouses and cafes started to open in cities like London and Paris where they were a great success. As in the Islamic world, cafes became important meeting places for the political and literary intelligentsia, something that is still true today. It would be difficult, for example, to imagine Jean Paul Sartre and Simone de Beauvoir writing anywhere except at Les Deux Magots on the Boulevard St. Germain. The fad for coffee drinking in the eighteenth century is nowhere better described than in the "Coffee Cantata" by J. S. Bach. Consider the following extract:[5]

Father:
You wicked child, you disobedient girl,
oh! when will I get my way;
give up coffee!

Lieschen:
Father, don't be so severe!
If I can't drink
my bowl of coffee three times daily,
then in my torment I will shrivel up
like a piece of roast goat.
Mm! how sweet the coffee tastes,
more delicious than a thousand kisses,
mellower than muscatel wine.
Coffee, coffee I must have,
and if someone wishes to give me a treat,
ah, then pour me out some coffee!

CHOCOLATE, BITTER AND SWEET

While tea and coffee were invading Europe from the Far and Middle East, another drink was extending its influence to Europe from the West.[5] In fact, chocolate was actually the first of the three to arrive. During his fourth visit to the Americas in 1502, Columbus encountered several native vessels off the coast of Honduras. One of the things he found on these boats were "almonds" which were in fact cacao beans, and he brought some back to Spain as a gift for King Ferdinand. He was, however, apparently unaware of how they were used. On the other hand, the secrets of how to use chocolate were readily revealed when Cortes and his conquistadors encountered Montezuma and the Aztecs. When Cortes arrived in central America in 1528, he observed that as the final course for his state ban-quets Montezuma would take golden goblets filled with a thick frothy bit-ter drink that was made by grinding roasted cacao beans, the seeds of the tree *Theobroma* (literally "the food of the Gods") *cacao*. The drink, known as *cacahuatl*, was brewed from the roasted beans and often had other ingredients such as vanilla, honey, and spices added to it. It was said that Montezuma drank vast quantities of cacahuatl and used it as a pick-me-up, particularly prior to visiting his numerous concubines. It is clear that cacao had been widely used by the Mesoamerican population for many years, and it is thought that the word *cacao* derives from an Olmec root word from as early as 1000 BC. The origin of the word *chocolate* is quite obscure, however, but somehow once the drink reached Spain, *cacahuatl* became *chocolatl,* and this name and its close derivatives stuck.

Following its introduction into the Spanish court, drinking chocolate became enormously popular with the aristocracy and clergy. It eventually spread to Italy and then to the rest of Europe, where it took its place alongside tea and coffee as a popular beverage served in tea and coffee houses. One important development occurred in 1828, when a Dutchman named Van Houten developed a process for removing much of the bitter fat from cacao and rendering the remainder more water soluble. This led the way to the production of solid chocolate for eating, which was first made by the company of Fry and Sons who produced the first chocolate bars in England in 1847.

GOETHE'S QUESTION: RUNGE'S REPLY

It is therefore clear that for a considerable time coffee, tea, and chocolate have been grouped together for numerous reasons. For example, the manner in which these drinks were used socially clearly identify them together as a group. However, it is also true that another important common feature is the psychopharmacological effects they produce. All three of the drinks are commonly reported to have a refreshing and energizing effect on consumers, making them feel more alert and awake, and this has always been one of their major attractions. Indeed, we know that they all contain the same group of chemicals that produce these effects. In general we refer the such chemical substances as *stimulants* or *psychostimulants*.

The question as to exactly what produces the stimulant effect of drinks like tea and coffee, like so many other questions concerning the chemistry of natural products, was answered in the nineteenth century with the advent of modern organic chemistry. Indeed, the story of the discovery of caffeine and its close chemical relatives is of considerable interest, as it concerns one of Europe's most prominent artists, the writer Johann Wolfgang von Goethe. Born in 1749, Goethe had contributed to the literature of the nascent Romantic movement with works such as *The Sorrows of Young Werther, Wilhelm Meister,* and poems such as *Faust.* By the early nineteenth century he was perhaps Europe's most celebrated author. However, it should not be forgotten that Goethe was also a passionate natural scientist, contributing to the literature on morphology and evolution as well as to the theories of color. In the year 1819, Goethe, who was then living in Weimar, was visited by a 25-year-old chemist named Friedlieb Runge. Runge was studying with Professor Johann Dobereiner, a distinguished chemist and close friend of Goethe.[6] Runge had stumbled upon the observation that he could cause the pupil of a cat's eye to dilate by adding a drop of extract from the deadly nightshade plant. Dobereiner sent young Runge to visit Goethe with a view to demonstrating this phenomenon to him, which he duly did. Apparently Goethe was impressed with Runge and, when the latter was leaving, he handed him some coffee beans with a request that he should analyze them to see if they contained anything interesting.[5,6] Runge proceeded to do this, and within a few months he had isolated a new alkaloid which was subsequently named *caffeine* after its source *Coffea* (Figure 8.3).

Runge went on to have his own distinguished career, making many contributions to organic chemistry. He was one of the first to isolate quinine and also one of the first to demonstrate the potential of aniline for producing chemical reactions leading to highly colored products, something that as we have seen was later utilized by William Perkin in his discovery of mauve (Chapter 3). Caffeine is one of a family of alkaloid substances that are known as *xanthines*. Several xanthine psychostimulants are found in coffee, tea, and chocolate. Caffeine is found in all three preparations. Additionally, theobromine and theophylline are found in chocolate. Theophylline is also found in tea, but in very small amounts. The structure of caffeine was first elucidated by Emil Fischer in 1881 when he was just 29 years old, and was quoted as one his achievements when he won the Nobel Prize. He concluded that it was a trimethylxanthine (Figure 8.3), and he devised a synthesis for it in 1882. Nowadays caffeine is not only found in the three drinks we have discussed, but also as an additive to many soft drinks. Many over-the-counter drug preparations also contain caffeine. An example would be Excedrin, which is a combination of caffeine and the anti-inflammatory drug acetaminophen.

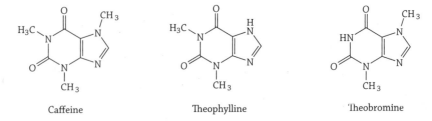

Caffeine   Theophylline   Theobromine

Figure 8.3:
Structures of typical methyxanthines found in tea, coffee, and chocolate.

Today caffeine is the most widely consumed psychoactive drug in the world, and it is so completely integrated into our everyday lives that we hardly consider it as a drug anymore. Nevertheless, it is certainly a psychostimulant and can produce both highly desirable as well as negative effects.[7] Many of us will have inadvertently experienced both sides of the caffeine coin. The uplifting effects of caffeine when we first get up in the morning, the fact that a cup of tea in the afternoon will keep us going when we begin to flag. We may also have experienced those days when we are ready jump through the roof after our tenth espresso. Caffeine produces a wide variety of effects that depend on the dose ingested, as well as the pattern of previous caffeine use in the individual in question.

The typical daily human consumption of caffeine is estimated to be around 70–350 mg, which is equivalent to about 3 cups of tea or coffee. After drinking tea or coffee, the plasma concentration of caffeine (around 0.25mg/ml or between 1 and 10µM) reaches a peak in approximately one hour and produces its stimulant effects, which include a reduction in fatigue and an increased ability to concentrate. As we shall also discuss, there is some evidence that caffeine can enhance what is generally known as "cognition." By this we mean a complex of phenomena that relate to how efficiently we process information, pay attention to relevant stimuli, make appropriate decisions, and carry out complex tasks such as language. These are the kinds of things that are greatly affected in syndromes like Alzheimer's disease, and pharmacological approaches to treating such disorders are the subject of enormous current interest. At elevated doses (above 400–500 mg/day), caffeine can also produce undesirable effects that include increased confusion and anxiety, as well as a rise in blood pressure. All of these effects are the result of the ability of caffeine to act upon both the central and peripheral nervous systems.

ATP: THE "ENERGETIC" NEUROTRANSMITTER

To understand the mechanism of action of caffeine, we need to introduce another unusual neurotransmitter. As we have discussed in previous chapters, the original concept of a neurotransmitter as being a substance like acetylcholine or a biogenic amine has gradually become subverted. Peptides are now okay (Chapter 5). Lipids are now okay (Chapter 7). So, how about ATP? ATP, or adenosine triphosphate, is a molecule with which many of us will be very familiar. To make ATP we must first begin with the purine base, adenine. When we attach a ribose sugar moiety to this, we get the nucleoside adenosine, and when we further attach 3 phosphate groups to

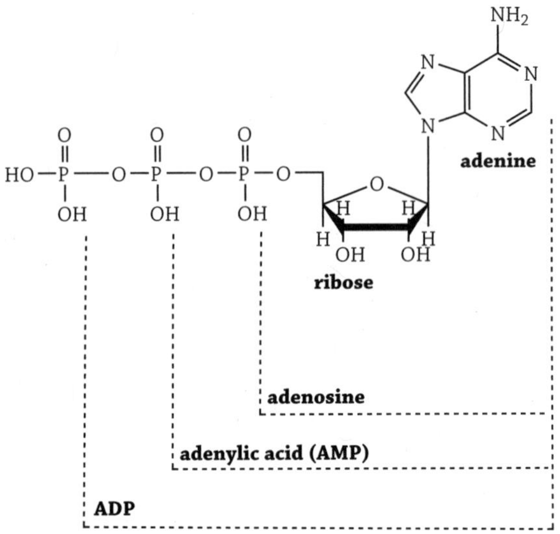

Figure 8.4:
The structure of adenosine triphosphate (ATP).

the ribose sugar, we get the nucleotide known as *adenosine triphosphate* or ATP (Figure 8.4). This molecule has many important functions within cells. Cells make ATP molecules as a way of storing energy, transporting it to different parts of the cell where it can drive important chemical reactions. ATP is also important in the synthesis of messenger molecules like cyclic AMP, which help to coordinate the cell's diverse activities. Of course all of these vital functions take place inside the cell, within the confines of the cell's plasma membrane.

However, it has long been known that ATP also produces effects when added to the outside of cells.[8,9] In 1927 Fiske and Subbarao at Harvard demonstrated that isolated muscle normally released phosphorous into its incubation medium, and in 1929 determined that ATP was the source of this phosphate. That same year, Albert Szent-Györgyi and Alan Drury obtained a sample of ATP isolated by Fiske and Subbarao and injected it intravenously into dogs. They observed that it "disrupted the cardiac rhythm, inhibited the contractility of intestinal smooth muscle and dilated the coronary artery."[30] In the years that followed, it was further observed that ATP could produce effects on the nervous system when injected directly into the brain, as well as on peripheral nerve preparations. Other data indicated that ATP could be released intact from nerves in an activity-dependent manner, just like a neurotransmitter.

The pioneering work of Geoffrey Burnstock and his colleagues, who investigated synapses between nerves and muscles, demonstrated that synaptic transmission at these junctions could sometimes be produced when receptors for acetylcholine and norepinephrine had both been blocked. This phenomenon was described as NANC, or "non adrenergic, non cholinergic" neurotransmission. On the basis of the fact that these synaptic events were mimicked by the addition of ATP, Burnstock and his colleagues suggested that ATP was normally the neurotransmitter used by such neurons. It also became clear that extracellular ATP released from neurons (or possibly by other cell types as well) was metabolized rapidly by a series of enzymes that would remove the phosphate groups to produce adenosine, and then metabolize adenosine to form inosine. Interestingly, it was demonstrated that addition of adenosine to cells could also produce specific effects that were often quite different from those produced by ATP.

An obvious question to answer was exactly how ATP and related substances like adenosine were producing their effects on cells. If they interacted with the cell membrane, did such an interaction involve a specific receptor? In order to test this possibility John Daly, a scientist at the National Institutes of Health in Washington DC, added adenosine to neurons and observed that it greatly increased the levels of cyclic AMP within the cells.[9,10] As we know that increases or decreases in cyclic AMP production are linked to the activation of GPCRs, this result suggested that adenosine acted upon a receptor in the cell membrane that produced an increase in cyclic AMP. In a key experiment it was shown that the effects of adenosine could be blocked by caffeine and other methylxanthines. Indeed, the blocking effects of caffeine occurred at concentrations that were similar to those that occur following the consumption of a cup of coffee. From this kind of data one might hypothesize that there was such as thing as an "adenosine receptor" that could be blocked by caffeine. Furthermore, it would also seem reasonable to suggest that this is how caffeine normally produces its biological effects. Using the cyclic AMP stimulation assay, Daly and his colleagues now began to explore how structural chemical changes of the molecule altered the ability of adenosine to stimulate its putative receptor. Synthetic analogues of adenosine and caffeine were created that acted with great potency and specificity as agonists and antagonists of the effects of adenosine on cyclic AMP production in neurons. To finally demonstrate the existence of an adenosine receptor, Daly collaborated with Solomon Snyder. They prepared radioactive versions of two of the most potent compounds Daly had developed, the agonist N6-cyclohexyl adenosine and the antagonist 1,3-diethyl-8-phenylxanthine, analogues of adenosine and caffeine respectively. They utilized these radioactive derivatives in Snyder's receptor binding assay and were soon able to demonstrate specific binding sites that appeared to have the correct properties of the putative adenosine receptor.

These studies, together with others such as those relating to NANC neurotransmission, were important in the development of an entirely new neurotransmitter concept which has come to be known as *purinergic* neurotransmission. An important subsequent development in this field has been the identification of a very large number of receptors for adenosine and ATP. These receptors are generally referred to as *P1 receptors* for adenosine and *P2 receptors* for ATP.[7-10] Four types of P1 adenosine receptors have been identified and cloned. They are all GPCRs and are named the A1, A2a, A2b, and A3 receptors. In addition, a large family of P2 receptors have been identified which mediate the different effects of ATP. P2Y receptors (there are at least 8 of them) are GPCRs. In addition, there are a variety of ATP receptors classified as P2X, which are ligand gated ion channels; that is to say, they consist of separate subunits which combine together in a manner similar to that we have described for the GABA-A receptors (Chapters 1 and 6). These numerous types of adenosine and ATP receptors are widely distributed in every tissue of the body. Thus it appears that, like arachidonic acid derived lipid signals (Chapter 7), purinergic signaling is one of the most ancient and generally used in regulating the functions of every tissue. In the nervous system in particular, it is thought that ATP can be stored in neurotransmitter vesicles and released from neurons, often together with other neurotransmitters. Once ATP is released it may act on P2 ATP receptors. In addition, it may be metabolized to adenosine, which may then act on P1 adenosine receptors.

From the point of view of the present discussion, it is clear that PI adenosine receptors represent the major sites of action of caffeine and related methylxanthines. Actually caffeine is a fairly nonselective blocker of these receptors.[7,8] However, it is the A1 and A2A receptors that are the most highly expressed in the brain, and so these appear to be the most important targets. As with other types of drugs, the different effects of caffeine can be dissected out by using selective receptor antagonists and mice in which the genes for different receptors have been deleted ("knockout" mice).[11] When this is done with P1 adenosine receptors, the results are very revealing. Caffeine produces no psychomotor stimulation in mice that lack A2A receptors. On the other hand, the effects of caffeine on other mental phenomena such as sleep/arousal and cognition may also depend on A1 receptor activation, this being an issue which is still not completely clear at this time.

The widespread use of caffeine is certainly related to the fact that it is a stimulant, albeit rather a mild one. Both its positive and negative effects can easily be experienced within the requirements of normal everyday life, which is why its use has been so easily integrated into human society throughout the world. However, there are other drugs which, although they produce somewhat similar effects to caffeine, are much more powerful. In particular one thinks of the psychostimulants cocaine and amphetamine. Like caffeine, both of these agents also produce increased arousal, psychomotor stimulation, and other related effects. The former is a very old drug indeed, and the latter rather a new one.

COCAINE REACHES EUROPE

Cocaine is yet another example of an important pharmacological discovery resulting from the collision between the Old World and the New. We have already discussed how visitors to the New World discovered chocolate, quinine, and the powerful hallucinogens psilocybin, mescaline, and ayahuasca (Chapter 2). The modern world's appreciation of the properties of cocaine began shortly after the discovery of the New World when reports began to filter back describing the fact that South American Indians could be frequently observed chewing the leaves of the coca shrub, *Erythroxylum coca*. There appeared to be two main reasons why they did this. Indeed, these are the same two reasons that its products are still used today—stimulation of the nervous system and local anesthesia.

For example, in 1539 Vicente de Valverde, who had accompanied Pizarro during his conquest of the Incas, wrote:

> "...*coca*, which is the leaf of a small tree that resembles the sumac found in our own Castile, is one thing that the Indians are ne'er without in their mouths, that they say sustains them and gives them refreshment, so that, even under the sun they feel not the heat, and it is worth its weight in gold in these parts, accounting for the major portion of the tithes."

And in 1653 the priest Bernabe Cobo wrote:

> "And this happen'd to me once, that I repaired to a barber to have a tooth pull'd, that had work'd loose and ach'd, and the barber told me he would be sorry to pull it because it was sound and healthy; and a monk friend of mine who happen'd to be there and overhearing, advised me to chew for a few days on *Coca*. As I did, indeed, soon to find my toothache gone."[12]

There is every reason to believe that the habit of chewing coca leaves together with lime rapidly became a habit not only among the Indians, but also among their Spanish masters. By the beginning of the nineteenth century, travelers from outside Spain, such as the German biologist Alexander von Humboldt, also began to send back reports about the remarkable properties of coca, particularly about how it allowed Indian workers to allay fatigue and hunger. For example, a report in the *Gentleman's* magazine in London in 1817 observed:

> "The Indians masticate Coca and undergo the greatest fatigue without any injury to health or bodily vigor. They want neither butcher nor baker, nor brewer, nor distiller, nor fuel, nor culinary utensils."[13]

As we have seen, the early part of the nineteenth century was a time of great excitement and achievement in the organic chemistry of natural products. Alkaloids like morphine and caffeine were being isolated at a rapid rate, and it was natural for people to turn their attention to coca. Some progress was initially made demonstrating that the active principle of coca could be extracted into organic solvents. However, coca leaves were indifferent travelers, much worse even than tea, and getting large quantities of fresh leaves to Europe for analysis proved problematic. Nevertheless, in 1859 a German scientist named Carl Scherzer managed to import a large quantity of good quality coca leaves into Germany and gave them to Friedrich Wohler, a chemistry professor at the University of Gottingen. The professor then passed the leaves on to his graduate student Albert Niemann as an appropriate topic of investigation for his doctoral thesis. Niemann duly obliged, and isolated pure cocaine as a white crystalline substance that produced numbness when he placed it on his tongue. Unfortunately, Niemann also discovered mustard gas and died, probably from contact with this substance, the very next year. His colleague Wilhelm Lossen elucidated the chemical formula of cocaine in 1865, and the chemical structure was obtained by Richard Willstatter in 1898.

Cocaine is a tropane alkaloid, which means that it contains the heterocyclic tropane group, making it somewhat similar in structure to atropine, which as we have seen is a commonly used antagonist of muscarinic acetylcholine receptors (Figure 8.5). This interesting substance, also known as "belladonna," is isolated from the deadly nightshade plant and, as we have mentioned, was what Runge used to dilate the pupils of a cat's eye as a demonstration for Goethe. When considering the bipartite structure of the cocaine molecule, a question of immediate interest is whether its psychostimulant and anesthetic properties are derived from the same parts of the molecule?

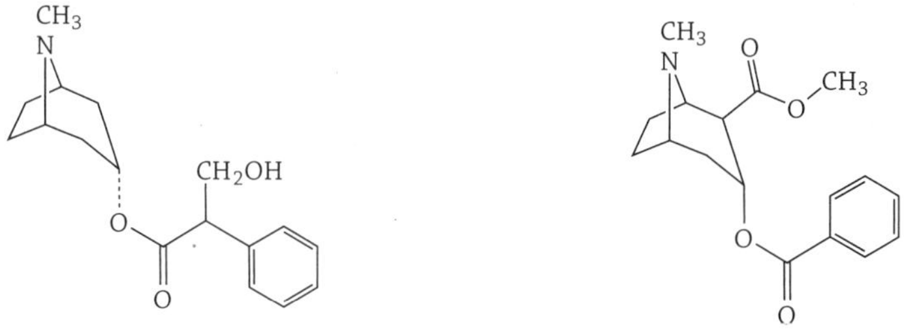

Figure 8.5:
The structure of cocaine and the related structure of atropine.

The use of cocaine as a local anesthetic is itself an interesting story. It was none other than the young Sigmund Freud who developed a strong interest in the drug early in his career.[15] Having acquainted himself with both its psychostimulant and local anesthetic properties, he passed his knowledge along to his colleague the ophthalmologist Karl Koller who, intrigued with the anesthetic properties of the drug, began to investigate its possible use as a topical anesthetic for eye surgery. His efforts were met with considerable success and his results widely disseminated. Eventually they were translated and published in the prestigious British medical journal *The Lancet,* where they were read by the pioneering American surgeon William Halsted. Halsted then attempted to use cocaine as an anesthetic for producing nerve block (i.e., the deadening of sensation due to an entire nerve) and found he could successfully carry out dental surgery on his medical students this way (students are less amenable to this kind of thing nowadays).

Results such as these were quickly followed by widespread adoption of cocaine as an effective local anesthetic in medical practice. However, it also became apparent that the drug produced toxic effects, primarily due to its actions on the cardiovascular system if it reached the systemic circulation, and so enthusiasm for its use gradually waned. Nevertheless, its evident utility encouraged the search for analogues of cocaine that would retain its local anesthetic effects but be free of its psychostimulant and toxic actions. Chemical synthetic efforts quickly demonstrated that it wasn't the tropane portion of the molecule that produced effective anesthesia, and derivatives of the benzoic acid portion of the molecule starting with amino acid and amino ester derivatives were developed. These were mostly produced by the Hoechst company in Germany under the leadership of Dr. Alfred Einhorn, and soon gave rise to drugs such as procaine and lidocaine, and subsequently to a large number of other local anesthetics that are still in

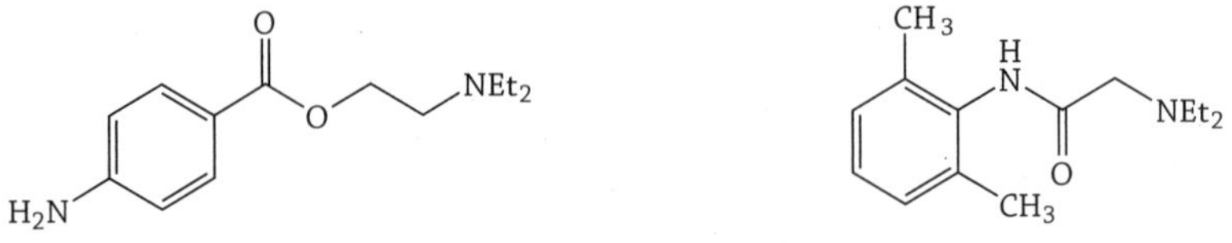

Procaine   Lidocaine

Figure 8.6:
The structures of the local anesthetics procaine and lidocaine, which are related to cocaine.

use today.[14] (Figure 8.6). Actually, cocaine is also still used for this purpose in particular instances, such as some types of ear, nose, and throat surgery due to its unusual ability to combine local anesthesia with vasoconstriction.

FROM COCA TO COKE

It was in the nineteenth century that recreational use of cocaine also began to take off in Europe. In 1859 an Italian neurologist named Paolo Mantegazza visited Peru and performed a great deal of self-experimentation with coca, ranging from low to extremely high doses. He reported his experiences in a paper entitled "On the hygienic and medical values of Coca," which discussed the drug's ability to reduce hunger and fatigue, as well as to produce a mad mental "rush" at higher doses.[13] This kind of literature started to increase interest in using the drug back in Europe. One notable feature over the years has been the development of different ways of taking the drug. To begin with, cocaine was readily available in a variety of drinks and tonics. These helped to cover up the basically bitter taste of the alkaloid. A good example was the Vin Mariani developed by the Corsican Angelo Mariani (Figure 8.7).

Vin Mariani was a concoction of cocaine in claret, which was certainly a very reasonable idea. Not surprisingly the combination of a good Bordeaux with cocaine sold extremely well.[16] Not only did the drink have the attractive effects of both of its ingredients going for it but Mariani was also an excellent publicist, obtaining affidavits from all kinds of famous people. These included, believe it or not, both the pope and the chief rabbi of France. Eventually Mariani marketed a large number of cocaine products in addition to his wine, including tea, lozenges, and cigarettes.[16]

Inspired by success of Vin Mariani, John Permberton, a drugstore owner in Columbus, Georgia, formulated his own version known as "Pemberton's French Wine Coca." However, when Fulton County where he

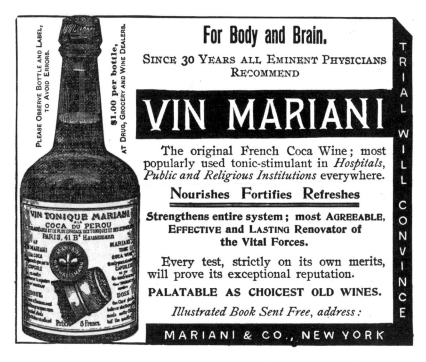

Figure 8.7:
Vin Mariani, a mixture of cocaine and claret, was one of the typical cocaine-containing "nerve tonics" widely available in the mid nineteenth century. The pope, Queen Victoria, and Thomas Edison were all fans.
(© Associated Press)

lived prohibited the sale of alcohol, he had to change his drink and came up with a nonalcoholic version based on kola nut extracts and other ingredients in addition to coca. Kola nuts are another natural source of significant amounts of caffeine. Thus the original Coca Cola, as the drink was eventually named, contained both cocaine and caffeine. Coca Cola was originally sold as a "nerve tonic" and was claimed to have numerous health-giving and restorative powers. The cocaine content was radically reduced in 1903, but to this day coca leaves are still used to flavor the drink once most of their normal content of cocaine has been removed.

COCAINE HITS THE STREETS

For serious cocaine consumers, other products were also available in the late nineteenth century. Large drug companies such as Parke-Davis in Detroit also got into the cocaine game. They developed processes for the mass production of easily crystallizable and soluble salts like cocaine hydrochloride, which could be accurately measured and dispensed. Finely powdered "lines" of cocaine could easily be "snorted" through a cut straw or rolled up banknote and would enter the well-vascularized mucous membranes in the nose and move from there into the blood and then the brain relatively quickly. Naturally, the most efficient way of taking cocaine, just like morphine, was to inject it intravenously. To satisfy this portion of the cocaine market, drug companies like Parke-Davis also came up with drug-taking paraphernalia such as nifty little boxes that contained syringes, needles, and supplies of cocaine all packaged together as a fashion accessory for the smart set. According to Parke-Davis' own ads, cocaine "could make the coward brave, the silent eloquent, and render the sufferer insensitive to pain." As we have seen with other powerful and potentially dangerous drugs, the end of the nineteenth and the beginning of the twentieth century was a time when these things were generally available and not illegal. In fact, cocaine could be purchased over the counter in the United States until 1916.

In recent years the consumption of cocaine has also been associated with innovations in how the drug is prepared, marketed, and used. Freebase or "crack" cocaine, which started to appear in urban areas in the 1980s, is often the method of choice today. Making crack is very simple and can be achieved with a few basic ingredients heated together in something like a spoon. The products can be collected and dried to form large crystalline "rocks."

Crack cocaine vaporizes very easily—the sound of the heated rocks crackling being responsible for its name. These vapors can be inhaled and blood levels rapidly approach those produced by intravenous injection because of the extensive surface area allowing absorption into the pulmonary circulation, and the drug reaches the brain within a few seconds. On the other hand, cocaine salts such as the hydrochloride do not vaporize in this way and so cannot be used in this manner. A similar technique to the use of crack is known as "freebasing" in which the cocaine base is first precipitated out from its aqueous salt using alkali and then extracted into an organic solvent like ether and dried. However, as such preparations may still contain appreciable amounts of organic solvents they are likely to flare up when heated and this can be very dangerous, as might be imagined. Overall, there are numerous ways in which cocaine can be utilized today and these result in somewhat different drug experiences.

Unfortunately, cocaine is certainly very addictive and even today its use constitutes an enormous drug abuse problem throughout the world. The story has often been told of how many of the people who pioneered the use of cocaine, including Freud and Halsted, ended up as addicts.[15] Today, cocaine addiction is still with us in a major way and it is not restricted to any particular part of society.

EPHEDRINE AND AMPHETAMINE

As we have seen, the consumption of cocaine is an ancient habit. However, there are other psychostimulant drugs that produce similar effects that were developed much more recently. Amphetamine and the related molecule methamphetamine are the best known of these substances.[17] However, even the development of amphetamine started with research on another ancient substance. As we have seen, the Chinese had a very sophisticated understanding of the therapeutic properties of many plants. Another example of this was the preparation known as *Ma Huang* which was made from the plant *Ephedra vulgaris*. One traditional use for this preparation was in the treatment of asthma because of its powerful bronchodilator effects. However, our modern experience with the drug has shown that it also has a number of effects that are suspiciously like those of cocaine, including the ability to counter fatigue and hunger and to act as a stimulant. The active principle of Ma Huang was actually isolated in Japan in 1885, but it didn't really come to the attention of Western scientists until it was rediscovered and synthesized in 1923 and named *ephedrine* (Figure 8.8).

Some years prior to this, there had been considerable interest in the fact that glands could secrete biologically active molecules which became known as *hormones*. One of the first of these to be characterized was the active principle of the adrenal gland. This had been isolated and named *adrenaline* or *epinephrine*. Adrenaline was marketed by Parke-Davis in 1901, as it mimicked the effects of stimulation of the adrenal gland. In particular, adrenaline had a powerful "pressor" effect; that is, it constricted blood vessels and raised blood pressure. It also acted as a bronchodilator. These properties meant that adrenaline was useful for counteracting "anaphylactic shock," which is associated with a profound fall in blood pressure. Generally

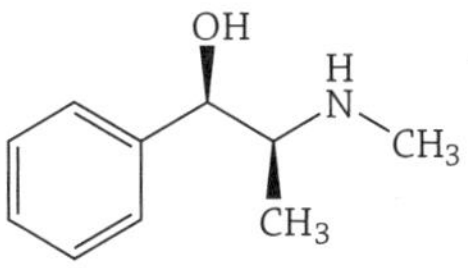

Ephedrine

Figure 8.8:
The structure of ephedrine isolated from the Chinese herb, Ma Huang.

speaking, these and other effects of adrenaline were noted to mimic many of the effects of stimulating the sympathetic branch of the autonomic nervous system, and so drugs like adrenaline became known as *sympathomimetics*. The sympathetic nervous system is responsible for what is known as the "fight or flight" response. This is a basic physiological mechanism for mobilizing all the resources of your body simultaneously in order to be able to either engage with or avoid danger from a predator or similarly acute life-threatening situation. Indeed, the introduction of adrenaline alerted people's attention to the fact that drugs that mimicked or suppressed the activity of the sympathetic nervous system were a real possibility, something that could potentially be very useful for numerous reasons.

The success of adrenaline prompted a search for drugs with a similar profile of effects, and indeed ephedrine fits this description rather well. However, as we have mentioned, ephedrine also has effects on the brain because it can penetrate the central nervous system much more easily than adrenaline, whose effects are really restricted to the periphery. One particular advantage of ephedrine over adrenaline proved to be the fact that it was found to be very effective at constricting blood vessels in the nasal mucosa, and this could be achieved by taking it as a nasal spray or as a pill. Thus, when Eli Lilly and Co. marketed ephedrine in 1926 it had enormous success as a decongestant, something for which it was successfully marketed as an over-the-counter drug until the FDA put restrictions on its use in the early years of the twenty-first century.

Originally, supplies of ephedrine were limited and Eli Lilly basically had the market to itself. This naturally prompted other companies to try to come up with something similar. They were particularly interested in drugs which, like ephedrine and unlike adrenaline, were orally effective. With this in mind Gordon Alles synthesized phenylisopropylamine sulfate in 1927, a structure closely related to ephedrine and adrenaline, which he tested orally on himself. He noted a "feeling of well being," "palpitation," and eventually a "sleepless night" in which his "mind seemed to race from one subject to another."[17] The drug later became known as "amphetamine," derived from *alpha-methyl-phenethylamine,* an alternative chemical name for this molecule (Figure 8.9). Subsequent tests demonstrated that the drug was not particularly effective in asthma patients, although it was a fairly good decongestant, and it was also noted that many patients felt "exhilarated" after taking it.

Alles gave some public talks about amphetamine, and soon afterward the drug was put on the market by the Smith, Kline and French (SKF) company. SKF had apparently come up with the compound independently, although it is very likely that they had heard one of Alles' presentations. Actually, the

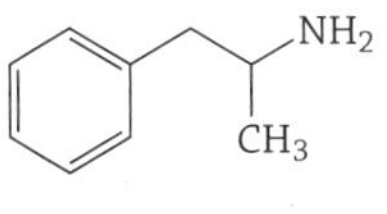

Amphetamine

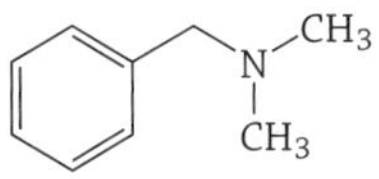

Methamphetamine

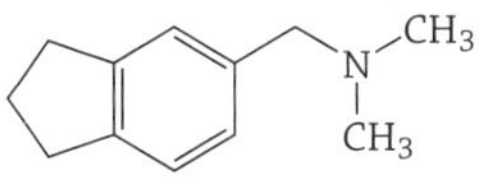

Methylenedioxymethamphetamine (MDMA)

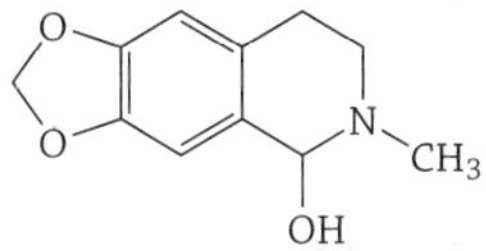

Hydrastinine

Figure 8.9:
The structure of the stimulant amphetamine, and related structures including MDMA ("XTC").

first synthesis of amphetamine occurred in Germany in 1887, and of the closely related molecule methamphetamine (Figure 8.9) in Japan in 1920, but their psychoactive properties were not generally recognized until later. SKF's original marketing ploy was to sell amphetamine as a volatile free-base dispensed from an inhaler as a decongestant, under the trade name Benzedrine. However, it was clear from the earliest times that however effective amphetamine and the closely related substance methamphetamine were as sympathomimetics, they also had very marked psychostimulant effects that were extremely similar to those of cocaine.

These psychostimulant properties were so widely recognized, that during the Second World War, Allied and Axis soldiers were all supplied with amphetamine-like drugs to ward off fatigue. Since that time many a student has used the drug as a study aid late at night, amphetamines have been widely employed as appetite suppressants in diet pills of one sort or another and, of course, amphetamines are widely abused as psychostimulants.

ECSTATIC AMPHETAMINES

However, the story of amphetamines had yet another interesting twist.[18] In 1912 the Merck pharmaceutical company in Germany was trying to synthesize compounds similar to the molecule hydrastinine, which had been patented by the Bayer company as a "styptic" or hemostatic agent (i.e., one that stops bleeding). Indeed, hydrastinine itself was a semisynthetic derivative of the alkaloid hydrastine, which the company had previously isolated from the plant *Hydrastis canadensis,* also known as the goldenseal, a relative of the buttercup (Figure 8.9). As an intermediate in this process, the Merck chemists prepared the compound MDMA, or methylenedioxymethamphetamine (Figure 8.9). The chemical similarity of MDMA to amphetamine will be clear to us now, but at the time the psychostimulant properties of amphetamine had not been identified and Merck had no real interest in MDMA except as a synthetic chemical intermediate.

Of course we have seen that the amphetamines not only act as psychostimulants, but many amphetamine-related molecules with simple substitutions, such as DOI or DOM, also act as powerful hallucinogens (Chapter 2). In fact, in the first investigations of the psychological effects of MDMA, it was used as an analogue of the hallucinogen mescaline rather than as a psychostimulant. As we have discussed (Chapter 2), the chemist Alexander Shulgin synthesized a large number of amphetamine derivatives and determined that many of them, such as DOI, acted as mescaline-like hallucinogens. During his extensive investigations, he resynthesized MDMA and performed some of his personal brand of "human" studies with it, concluding that it produced a unique spectrum of psychological effects—something akin to an amphetamine-like psychostimulant and something akin to a mescaline-like hallucinogen.[19] Initially MDMA was taken up by several psychiatrists, who tried to use it as an adjunct to therapy and, like LSD before it, the drug was very popular in this context for a brief time. However, such attempts quickly waned. At any rate the psychological effects of MDMA were well appreciated by the 1970s, and it became widely used as a street drug. Starting in the 1980s the drug became very popular under the name Ecstasy (XTC) and is the prototype of a class of compounds which the pioneering medicinal chemist David Nichols has named "entactogens" (Chapter 2). Entactogens seem to have effects that place them somewhere in between the hallucinogenic amphetamines like DOM and DOI, and the psychostimulants such as amphetamine and methamphetamine. Thus, some people report that Ecstasy produces hallucinations, and it also seems to produce its own type of psychostimulant effects. To repeat a point raised in a previous chapter (Chapter 2), it is quite amazing just how many interesting psychologically active molecules can be produced from the simple phenethylamine nucleus, including many different types of drugs and biogenic amine neurotransmitters (see Figure 2.13).

Although today amphetamines are widely used and abused for their psychostimulant effects, they do have some bona fide therapeutic uses. A mixture of amphetamine salts sold under the trade name Adderall is used for narcolepsy, which seems reasonable enough, but is also one of the leading treatments for attention deficit hyperactivity disorder (ADHD) in children.

Additionally, other amphetamine-like stimulants, such as the drug methylphenidate, an analogue of amphetamine sold under the trade name Ritalin, are used for the same purpose. Methylphenidate certainly produces similar effects to amphetamine and cocaine and can be abused just like these other psychostimulants. It may seem completely counterintuitive to use drugs like this for a disorder characterized by hyperactivity. Nevertheless, Adderall and Ritalin seem to be effective, although the reasons for their beneficial effects in this context are not well understood.

PSYCHOSTIMULANTS AND BIOGENIC AMINES

Considering the fact that the biological effects of the amphetamine psychostimulants and cocaine are very similar, one might suspect that they have common mechanisms of action and this is certainly the case. The primary target for both types of drugs is neurotransmission mediated by biogenic amines.[20] Of course, this has been a common theme in this book and we have already seen how the actions of hallucinogens, antidepressants, and antipsychotic drugs involve these same important neurotransmitters. We have discussed how, following their release as neurotransmitters, biogenic amines are taken up again into nerve terminals using specific reuptake transporter molecules, each with their own unique expression pattern and substrate specificity (Chapter 4). We have seen, for example, that many widely used antidepressants are active at blocking both norepinephrine and 5-HT reuptake into nerve terminals. Cocaine also blocks both norepinephrine and 5-HT uptake and, in addition, blocks dopamine uptake. This means that cocaine is able to increase the synaptic concentration of all three of these neurotransmitters, enhancing their neurotransmitter effects both in the peripheral and central nervous systems.

The reuptake transporter proteins for the three biogenic amine transmitters are also the site of action for amphetamine. However, amphetamine's mechanism of action is somewhat different from that of cocaine when we consider it closely at the molecular level. Rather than blocking these transporter proteins, amphetamine is actually a substrate for them. It binds to them and is transported into the nerve terminal just as if it were dopamine, norepinephrine, or 5-HT.[21] Exactly what happens after that is not completely clear, and there are several competing hypotheses that try to explain the consequences of amphetamine's transport. Nevertheless, the ultimate result is quite clear. Following the uptake of amphetamine, it causes the release of biogenic amines from their storage vesicles into the cytoplasm. They now bind to the uptake transporter protein and move in the reverse direction, outward from the nerve terminal into the synaptic space. Thus, even though their mechanisms are different, the net result of the actions of both cocaine and amphetamine is increased synaptic concentrations of norepinephrine, 5-HT, and dopamine, both in the brain and in the peripheral nervous system.

THE INDIANS GO UP IN SMOKE

The diverse family of psychostimulant drugs includes one other very important member that also comes to us from the New World. When Columbus and his followers arrived in the Americas in 1492 they found many things to amaze them. Among these things was the observation of the local Taino Indians apparently "drinking" smoke (Figure 8.10).[16] The smoke came from a roll of dried leaves, to which the Indians set fire. Sometimes instead of drinking smoke from the dried leaves the Indians would grind them up

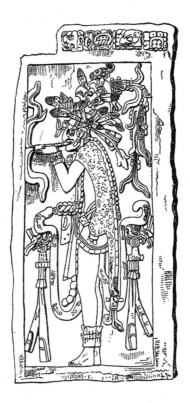

Figure 8.10:
Engraving of a Mayan priest "smoking."
(INTERFOTO / Alamy)

and use them as snuff. The name of the leaf used by the Indians was *tobaco,* which later became "tobacco" in Europe. It appeared that the Indians used tobacco for several purposes. It was said that the plant was originally a gift from the gods, and so it was used by Indian shamans during religious ceremonies. Additionally, it was used in various forms as a medicine or for recreational purposes. Tobacco produced a sense of relaxation and mild euphoria, together with a sharpening of intellect, alertness, and memory— something along the same lines as caffeine, cocaine, or amphetamine.

During early voyages to the New World, several of the crew members tried tobacco and, finding it to their liking, adopted the habit. When Rodrigo de Jerez brought tobacco back to Spain from an early voyage to the New World, he was immediately imprisoned by the Inquisition who assumed, reasonably enough, that someone who exhaled smoke from their mouth and nose was in league with the devil. However, tobacco "smoking" caught on quickly. It is said[16] that by the time Rodrigo was released from jail, lots of folks in Madrid could be seen doing precisely the same thing. As with many other new drugs arriving in Europe, tobacco was first acclaimed for its medicinal properties, which were said to be numerous. In terms of the Galenic humoral theory, tobacco was "hot and moist" and could act as a corrective for conditions that were characterized as "cold and dry." On the other hand, the use of tobacco by the Indians as a mild stimulant in order to help them "go out of their wittes" was not necessarily met with immediate approval. From the earliest times when the Spanish Inquisition had taken exception to the habit, there has always been a debate about its desirability. Not everybody liked it. In particular, in 1604 King James I of England published his "Counterblaste to Tobacco" in which he described smoking as unhygienic.[22,23]

In 1559 Jean Nicot, a French diplomat, was sent to Lisbon where he encountered tobacco and became deeply impressed with its medicinal virtues. Taking tobacco back to Paris, it is said that he used it successfully to cure the French queen from migraine and the tobacco habit quickly caught on. So did Nicot's name, as in 1753 the great Linnaeus named the tobacco plant after him. In fact there are numerous members of the genus *Nicotiana.* The plant first encountered by Columbus in North America is known as *Nicotiana rustica.* The Spaniards later encountered another variety in South America which is known as *Nicotiana tobacum.* This was found to be a better source of tobacco and was later imported into Virginia and the Carolinas by the British, and is what is normally used to produce tobacco today.

The practice of smoking tobacco spread rapidly throughout Europe. One of the important things to realize about tobacco was that smoking not only introduced a new drug to the public, but also a whole new way of using drugs. Prior to its introduction, drugs were not used in this way. However, as the tobacco habit moved from Europe to the Middle East and then to India and China, smoking opened up a new way of using many drugs that has been widely adopted ever since. In modern times the invention of the cigarette, an adaptation of the ancient Indian practice of putting a wrapper around tobacco in order to smoke it, together with powerful advertising and mass marketing campaigns, catapulted tobacco cultivation and use to being one of the largest industries in the world. Health considerations have now curtailed the use of tobacco extensively in America and Europe, but not in the rest of the world where its use continues unabated.

NICOTINE: PLEASURE AND POISON

The active principle from tobacco, the alkaloid nicotine, was first isolated in 1843 and its structure was determined in 1893 (Figure 8.11).[24]

Nicotine taken in small amounts (tobacco contains between 0.5% and 3.0% alkaloid per dry weight) in a cigarette or snuff obviously has pleasant effects as far as many people are concerned. However, pure nicotine is another matter. Concentrated nicotine is highly toxic to most animals including humans, and has been used as an insecticide for many years. To illustrate the point, in Agatha Christie's story entitled "Three Act Tragedy," the villain carries out his murders by getting people to drink cocktails laced with pure nicotine. Nevertheless, with his unparalleled knowledge of neuropharmacology, Inspector Poirot figures everything out and the baddies get what's coming to them in the end.

In addition to its use as a drug or poison, nicotine played a vital role in the development of our entire concept of neurotransmission. At the start of the twentieth century John Langley, a professor at Cambridge University and the editor of the *Journal of Physiology,* was examining how different drugs including nicotine affected the activity of the autonomic nervous system. The results of his experiments led him to propose that

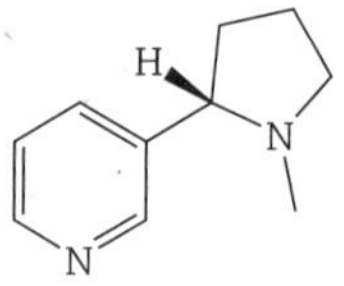

Nicotine

Figure 8.11:
The structure of nicotine.

the drugs produced their effects by activating "receptor substances."[25] He imagined these substances as being inactive until a drug actually bound to them, after which the activated receptor substance would carry out the observed effect of the drug on the tissue. At the same time, Paul Ehrlich in Germany was developing similar concepts (Chapter 3). In 1904 Langley's student Henry Dale spent some time working with Ehrlich. He acted as a conduit for the transmission of scientific information between the two laboratories, and after a while Ehrlich was also using Langley's term "receptor substance." Gradually the concept of a drug "receptor" as the site of action of a drug developed from these ideas.

Henry Dale continued to make fundamental discoveries in neuropharmacology for many years to come and eventually won the Nobel Prize for his efforts. One of Dale's most important contributions was his identification of acetylcholine, which he subsequently predicted would act as a neurotransmitter in the peripheral nervous system, something that would be actually proved some years later by his fellow Nobel Laureate Otto Loewi. In one series of experiments Dale compared the effects of acetylcholine on several tissues with those of the drugs nicotine and muscarine. He found that in some cases nicotine produced the same effects as acetylcholine and that in others, muscarine mimicked acetylcholine. From these studies he concluded that there were two different types of acetylcholine receptors, which he named *nicotinic* and *muscarinic*. Subsequent studies by many other scientists demonstrated that nicotinic receptors were highly localized to the area of the synapse. This included cholinergic synapses in autonomic ganglia and synapses at the junctions between motor neurons and skeletal muscle. In fact, the nicotinic acetylcholine receptor was the very first receptor to be identified from the biochemical point of view, and provided the initial breakthroughs in understanding the molecular properties of receptors in general (e.g., see Chapter 1).

The nicotinic receptor proved to be a ligand gated ion channel (Chapter 1). Electrophysiological studies demonstrated that activation of nicotinic receptors produced an electrical current resulting from the flow of cations, mainly Na and K. Further studies demonstrated that the complete receptor protein complex had a molecular mass of around 250,000 and consisted of four different, but closely related, protein subunits—two α chains, one β chain, one γ chain and one δ chain arranged as a pentamer.[26] Modern cloning techniques have determined the amino acid sequences of each subunit. We now know that there are several types of α and β subunits that can arrange themselves in different combinations, producing some variations in the properties of nicotinic receptors found at different synapses. This is reminiscent of the same type of heterogeneity observed in the composition of GABA-A receptors in different parts of the brain (Chapters 1 and 6). In fact the nicotinic receptor is the archetype for the entire family of ligand gated ion channels. Its structure was the first to be understood at a molecular level and has since been seen to be repeated by other ligand gated ion channel receptors of this type.

As we have seen, nicotine produces numerous effects on the central and peripheral nervous systems. Some of these, such as the effects of the drug on cognitive functions including memory, concentration, arousal, and alertness, are highly desirable and potentially therapeutically useful. On the other hand, effects such as those on the cardiovascular system, the gut, the vomiting center, are not at all desirable. Additionally, of course, there is the fact that like the other psychostimulants we have discussed, nicotine is highly addictive. The question therefore is whether the same subtypes of nicotinic receptors produce the desirable and undesirable effects of the drug. If they could be separated from one another along these lines, then drugs that only stimulate certain nicotinic receptor subtypes might be produced and might produce very useful and selective effects. Under what circumstances might they be useful?

Here one should consider the fact that there are several important neurodegenerative diseases in which deficits in cognitive function are a major symptom. This is certainly true for Alzheimer's disease (AD).[27,28] In AD one finds that certain proteins accumulate into large aggregates in the brain and this results in the death of neurons. Neurons in the cortex and hippocampus are particularly badly affected. In particular, cholinergic neurons in the nucleus basalis of Meynert that innervate the cortex degenerate in AD. Thus at least some of the symptoms of Alzheimer's disease are caused by a lack of cholinergic function in the brain. We might therefore suppose that a drug like nicotine that could increase cholinergic function in the brain might be helpful in diseases like AD. In fact, this idea has been discussed and several drug companies are trying to produce drugs of this type. Indeed, there are now good indications that it may be possible to produce a "useful" nicotinic agonist drug. It turns out that many of the undesirable effects of nicotine are due to the fact that it activates receptors in autonomic ganglia, thereby stimulating or inhibiting various functions of the autonomic nervous system. Thus, nicotinic agonists that avoid these receptors should be free of the undesirable autonomic effects produced by nicotine. Indeed, a large number of novel molecules that activate these subtypes of nicotinic receptors have been produced and have demonstrated encouraging therapeutic profiles.[27-29]

One should note that it is not only drugs that activate nicotinic receptors that might be theoretically employed as "cognition enhancers" in conditions such as AD. As we have seen, drugs like caffeine that act as antagonists at adenosine receptors also produce some highly desirable effects. Generally speaking, the effects of adenosine antagonists are modest compared to those of the other psychostimulants. This includes both its stimulant effects as well as its addictive potential. So, there are also attempts at this time to develop novel adenosine antagonists for use in AD. Perhaps they will produce some beneficial effects and have a reasonable safety profile. Time will tell, but excuse me... the kettle is on the boil and the Darjeeling is waiting!

NOTES

1. Robert Fortune. *A Journey to the Tea Countries of China* (2005 ed.). Elibron Classics.
2. Sarah Rose. *For All the Tea in China: How England Stole the World's Favorite Drink and Changed the World*. Viking Press. 2009.
   Beatrice Hohenegger. *Liquid Jade: The Story of Tea for East to West*. St. Martin's Press. 2006.
3. David Mitchell. *The Thousand Autumns of Jacob De Zoet*. Sceptre Press. 2010.
4. Amitav Ghosh. *River of Smoke*. Farrar, Straus and Giroux. 2011.
5. Bennett Alan Weinberg, Bonnie K. Bealer. *The World of Caffeine: The Science and Culture of the World's Most Popular Drug*. Routledge. 2002.
6. Fredholm BB. Notes on the history of caffeine use. *Handb Exp Pharmacol*. 2011, (200):1–9.
7. Ribeiro JA, Sebastião AM. Caffeine and adenosine. *J Alzheimers Dis*. 2010, 20 Suppl 1:S3–15.
8. Burnstock G. Physiology and pathophysiology of purinergic neurotransmission. *Physiol Rev*. 2007, 87(2):659–797.
9. Fredholm BB, Jacobson KA. Adenosine Receptors: the contributions of John W Daly. *Heterocycles*. 2009, 79:73–83.
10. Daly JW. Caffeine analogs: biomedical impact. *Cell Mol Life Sci*. 2007, 64(16):2153–2169.
11. Chen JF, Yu L, Shen HY, He JC, Wang X, Zheng R. What knock-out animals tell us about the effects of caffeine. *J Alzheimers Dis*. 2010, 20 Suppl 1:S17–24.
12. Calatayud J, González A. History of the development and evolution of local anesthesia since the coca leaf. *Anesthesiology*. 2003, 98(6):1503–1508.
13. Goldstein RA, DesLauriers C, Burda AM. Cocaine: history, social implications, and toxicity—a review. *Dis Mon*. 2009, 55(1):6–38.
14. Ruetsch YA, Böni T, Borgeat A. From cocaine to ropivacaine: the history of local anesthetic drugs. *Curr Top Med Chem*. 2001, 1(3):175–182.
15. Howard Markel. *An Anatomy of Addiction. Sigmund Freud, William Halsted and the Miracle Drug Cocaine*. Pantheon. 2011.
16. Mike Jay. *High Society: The Central Role of Mind-Altering Drugs in History, Science and Culture*. Park Street Press. 2010.
17. Rasmussen N. Making the first antidepressant: amphetamine in American medicine 1929-1950. *J Hist Med*. 2006, 61:288–323.
18. Freudenmann RW, Oxler F, Bernschneider-Reif S. The origin of MDMA (ecstasy) revisited: the true story reconstructed from the original documents. *Addiction*. 2006, 101(9):1241–1245.

19. Anne and Alexander Shulgin. *PIHKAL: A chemical love story.* Transform Press. 1991.

20. Elliott JM, Beveridge TJ. Psychostimulants and monoamine transporters: upsetting the balance. *Curr Opin Pharmacol.* 2005, 5(1):94–100.

21. Fleckenstein AE, Volz TJ, Riddle EL, Gibb JW, Hanson GR. New insights into the mechanism of action of amphetamines. *Annu Rev Pharmacol Toxicol.* 2007, 47:681–698.

22. http://en.wikipedia.org/wiki/History_of_smoking

23. http://en.wikipedia.org/wiki/Tobacco_smoking

24. http://en.wikipedia.org/wiki/Nicotine

25. Elliot S. Valenstein. *The War of the Soups and the Sparks. The Discovery of Neurotransmitters and the Dispute Over How Nerves Communicate.* Columbia University Press. 2005.

26. Steinlein OK, Bertrand D. Neuronal nicotinic acetylcholine receptors: from the genetic analysis to neurological diseases. *Biochem Pharmacol.* 2008, 76(10):1175–1183.

27. Haydar SN, Dunlop J. Neuronal nicotinic acetylcholine receptors—targets for the development of drugs to treat cognitive impairment associated with schizophrenia and Alzheimer's disease. *Curr Top Med Chem.* 2010, 10(2):144–152.

28. Poorthuis RB, Goriounova NA, Couey JJ, Mansvelder HD. Nicotinic actions on neuronal networks for cognition: general principles and long-term consequences. *Biochem Pharmacol.* 2009, 78(7):668–676.

29. Dolder CR, Davis LN, McKinsey J. Use of psychostimulants in patients with dementia. *Ann Pharmacother.* 2010, 44(10):1624–1632.

30. Fields DR. Non synaptic and non vesicular ATP release from neurons and relevance to neuron-glia signaling. *Seminars in Cell and Developmental Biology.* 2011,22(2):214–219.

CHAPTER 9

Papillons

"Every sickness is a musical problem, its healing a harmonic resolution."
Novalis (1772–1801)

By the latter part of the twentieth century the great psychopharmaco-logical revolution that had produced antipsychotic, antidepressant, and anxiolytic drugs had started to lose its momentum. As we have discussed, it is getting harder to come up with novel strategies for producing new drugs for the treatment of mental illness. So, where do we go next? One possibility has its origins in the idea that the brain doesn't function in isolation but is always in contact with regulatory elements such as the endocrine and immune systems. Typically we think of the immune system as something that fights infection or produces inflammation. It turns out that many of the pathological processes that produce mental illness are accompanied by increased activity of the immune system in the brain—a phenomenon which is known as *neuroinflammation*. Neuroinflammation operates through the actions of molecules known as *cytokines*. Although these are not neurotransmitters in the conventional sense of the word, they do have the capacity to regulate the activity of neurons and so we may be able to manipulate them to produce novel types of drugs. Sometimes the neuroinflammatory response can be extremely strong, such as in the disease multiple sclerosis. The neuroinflammation that accompanies mental illness is probably much more subtle, but it is there nevertheless. There is now a great deal of interest in the connection between neuroinflammation and mental illness, and how cytokines might contribute to the genesis and progression of numerous brain disorders. As with many other things, the signs of neuroinflammation and its effects on the brain have been known for many years. Let us start with a good example of how neuroinflammation can be associated with "insanity."

THE TRAGIC STORY OF ROBERT SCHUMANN

Just before 11am on the morning of September 30, 1853, a handsome young man named Johannes Brahms sat on a bench on the Bilkerstrasse in Dusseldorf. It was raining and Johannes, who had been sitting there for a considerable time, was wet through. In spite of this fact he felt completely unable to move. What he really wanted to do was to walk across the road and knock on the door of number 1032. But somehow he couldn't. He was in a state of high anxiety, with feelings of "butterflies" in his stomach that had produced total mental and physical paralysis.

Johannes had spent the previous week hiking along the river Rhine. Now he had arrived in Dusseldorf and was ready to fulfill the ultimate goal of his trip, which was to speak to the resident of number 1032 Bilkerstrasse: the composer Robert Schumann.[1] Johannes was himself a composer, just setting out on his chosen career, and he desperately wanted to show Schumann some of his music and receive his criticisms and, hopefully, his endorsement.

Robert Schumann was an influential figure in contemporary music for numerous reasons. To begin with, Schumann was one of the most important composers of the time. In his earliest works, particularly his piano pieces such as "Papillons," he had introduced new musical forms and had forged a major friendship with Felix Mendelssohn, another of the great composers of the mid nineteenth century. He also had the respect of the musical avant garde, composers such as Liszt, Wagner, and Berlioz, who were composing the "music of the future"—music that was supposed to embrace all forms of art and politics. Schumann was the editor of the *Neue Zeitschrift fur Musik,* the leading publication for music criticism. As editor of the journal, Schumann had a position of great intellectual leadership and was known for fostering the careers of many young composers. For example, he had famously declared—"Hats off, gentleman, a genius!" when speaking of Chopin. Most people, including Johannes Brahms, agreed with that sentiment. All in all, getting Schumann's opinion about his music was of the greatest importance to Johannes.

Johannes Brahms was from the city of Hamburg. His musical talents had been obvious from an early age, and his parents had regularly sent him to play the piano in one of the *animierlokale,*[2] the brothels that lined the waterfront of the Hamburg docks. Johannes was a beautiful child with golden curls and bright blue eyes, and apparently was routinely abused by the whores in the *animierlokale* as well as their clients. It was not surprising that Johannes had grown up with a somewhat ambivalent attitude toward the opposite sex. He consorted with women out of necessity, but was suspicious of them in general and rarely formed relationships of a meaningful nature.

Nevertheless, there were exceptions. For example, there was Schumann's wife, the formidable Clara Wieck, one of the world's most gifted pianists.[3] Johannes had heard her play when she and Robert had visited Hamburg, and been truly impressed with the sensitivity of her performance. He had sent the Schumanns a package of his music to their hotel, but it had been returned unopened. He was not surprised. After all, they had no idea who he was. But now things were different, and the reason for this was his friendship with Joseph Joachim.[4]

Joachim was a young Hungarian violinist who was the toast of Europe. His ability was legendary, and he was actively sought out and befriended by all of the most important composers of the day. Joachim had become particularly close to Robert Schumann and his wife, and regularly visited to play chamber music with them. He had been introduced to Johannes Brahms by another Hungarian violinist, and Joseph and Johannes had become fast friends. They traveled together, and Joachim was enthusiastic about the music that Brahms had shown to him. He said he would write to the Schumanns telling them to receive Brahms, and so they would certainly do so. Nevertheless, Johannes continued to harbor nagging doubts about his abilities; so there he was, still sitting on a bench, getting wetter and wetter.

But then he did decide—it was now or never! He got up, walked across the road and knocked. Within seconds Robert Schumann himself, in his dressing gown, pajamas and slippers answered the door.

"Oh yes, Johannes Brahms, of course, of course! We had a letter about you from Joachim, please do come in, come into the parlor and make yourself at home."

Johannes sat down and he and Schumann talked for a while. One thing led to another, and soon Brahms was invited to play his music, and Clara Schumann joined to listen. Brahms launched into his Opus 1, a sonata.

After a few seconds the Schumanns caught each other's glances. What a bold and virtuosic introduction! Incredibly difficult and exuberantly Romantic. The opening, with its thick chords and decisive rhythm—the likeness to the opening of Beethoven's great Hammerklavier sonata was unmistakable! They were frankly amazed at what they heard. Indeed, as they discussed afterwards, perhaps this was the man who would take up Beethoven's mantle?

The Schumanns invited Brahms to stay. And he did. He stayed for a very long time, and set the path of music in a new direction. He also formed the one relationship with a woman that would last a lifetime.

London Feb 26th 1861. 17 Half Moon Street, Piccadilly (⁵).

How glad I am to be able at last to find a quiet hour this evening for you, dearest Johannes, all the more so because I am able to inform you that your Sextet was produced with great success at the Popular Concert yesterday. Joachim had, of course, practiced it well and played magnificently. The reception was most enthusiastic, particularly after the first three movements. The Scherzo was encored, but Joachim wanted to keep the audience fresh for the last movement and so did not respond to the call. I enjoyed it thoroughly, and should have loved to have been the first violin. I really wanted to play the A Major Quartet, but Joachim insisted on the Sextet, which he thought more suitable for the first performance of one of your works in England. I gave way, but most unwillingly. After all it went splendidly and that is the chief thing.

In my opinion the most beautiful thing in England is the countryside. How it invigorates and refreshes one! I could contemplate the sort of tree one sees here and which spreads its branches on all sides down to the earth for hours at a time and find a world of poetry in it—such varied and luxuriant vegetation is really wonderful. And now imagine whole parks of such trees about which one can wander for hours. I saw the most beautiful of all these parks for the first time yesterday at Windsor and also the most beautiful of all castles. I cannot attempt to describe it, but when you see it you live through the whole of Shakespeare.

Of course there is another side to England as well. Its great industrial cities like Manchester. Here you will find factories, great temples for worshipping the machine. I played a recital there this week and was given a tour by Mr. Behrens, a rich Manchester man with whom Joachim always stays. You would be surprised how many young Germans there are working in Manchester. Mr. Behrens took me to the factory of Roberts, Dale and Co. Here they make great varieties of dyestuffs. You have never seen anything like it. Great vats containing every colour of the rainbow. The smell I did not like, but the place was fascinating. My guide was a young German named Heinrich Caro who has been working here for some time. We spoke in German and so he could say exactly what was on his mind. He told me that many Germans come here to gain experience in the dye making trade. However, he also told me that most of them hope to return to Germany and start a chemical industry there. Indeed, Mr. Caro is hoping to return this year. He told me that he had an offer of a job in Mannheim. He says that they make a kind of tar when they are producing gas for lighting the streets and that this tar is the raw material for making dyes and other chemicals. Imagine that! So, it is his goal to help to set up a chemical company there that would be like the ones they have here in England. Mr. Caro's enthusiasm and intelligence impressed me greatly. I will look forward to seeing how things progress! He is a music lover and I have invited him to hear my recital in Mannheim next year.

Now let me come to the main reason for writing you this letter. It is now 5 years since the death of my dear Robert, and I have had time to think about the events leading up to his death. In particular, I have tried to understand what happened at the end. How was it that this terrible insanity descended upon my dear Robert? Where did it come from and could anything have been done to prevent it? Now here I am in London a long way from home and perhaps I can organize my thoughts properly.

First of all let me recall some of the things that happened. It was in 1854 when the final act of the tragedy began. But things had been going that way for some time. From the time we moved to Dusseldorf, Robert's behavior had become increasingly bizarre. I mean stranger than normal. The first thing to consider is Robert's personality. He was truly an artist and everybody understands what that means. A creative genius never has a personality like other men. He was unique. So what does normal mean? Ever since I first met Robert, when he was a student of my father's, he was somewhat eccentric. He was very sensitive, as is any great artist. He frequently believed himself to be ill. No, not "believed"—he really was ill. There were all sorts of complaints that tormented him. First of all he had trouble with his hand, a peculiar weakness in the third and fourth fingers of his right hand that certainly affected his playing. He tried to correct it with all kinds of mechanical devices—something of which my father vehemently disapproved. Then there were a whole variety of other symptoms which he suffered from to a greater or lesser degree over the years. Aches in his limbs, cramps, problems with his bowels, headaches, dizziness, insomnia and such things. For example, when we toured Russia together he had such a bad attack of dizziness that he was incapacitated for several days.

Another aspect of Robert's personality was the extensive variations in his mood. Sometimes he would be full of energy and incredibly productive. I actually went so far as to calculate how many songs he wrote every year of his life; in 1840 he composed more than 150 songs. A few years later in 1844 he was completely depressed and composed virtually nothing. Then again in the years 1849–1850, more than 100 songs were produced and yet in a couple of years he went into a terminal decline that lead to his death.

I have heard it said that some people have changes in their moods that are so extreme that they are practically insane. Perhaps something like that was a part of Robert's family? His sister Emilie died when she was only 29—I think she drowned herself, she was so depressed. And so it is quite possible that Robert was afflicted by something like that. Nevertheless, I should point out that people do not die from such things, unless of course it is by their own hand. Because of

Robert's attempt to end his life, the picture is somewhat confusing. However, I cannot believe that whatever was responsible for Robert's changeable moods was also responsible for his other symptoms and ultimately for his death. The quality of the insanity that accompanied his end was of a totally different type. Therefore, I have repeatedly asked myself where this could have originated?

I have concluded that Robert was the recipient of bad blood. And where could the bad blood have come from? Here I have a suspicion. There is something I should tell you, in the strictest confidence, and of course I have no doubt at all that you will treat it in this manner. I knew Robert from my childhood when he was a frequent visitor to our house in Leipzig where he was a student of my father's. Early on in 1831 when I was just 11 years old and Robert was 20, something happened. I do not blame Robert for this. He was a young man and as such had his natural needs. He had his friends. He liked to drink—we both know that was sometimes to excess. And of course he was certainly aware of women.

There was a servant girl that lived in our house. Her name was Christel. I have come to believe that there was a relationship between her and Robert. Moreover, I believe it lasted a long time and that it was as serious as such things can be between people of such different classes. Indeed, I have every reason to believe that he may have fathered her child. And what did she give to him? Bad blood. Yes, I believe it came from her. I have heard things and read things in his diaries that lead me to this conclusion. In his diaries he often calls Christel by the name "Charitas," but I know they were one and the same.

Here is what happened—I even have the date from his diary—May 11th, 1831. Robert went to see his doctor, Christian Glock. Whatever it was Robert showed Dr. Glock, the latter was not pleased. Next day Dr. Glock came to our house and examined Christel herself. Again he was not pleased. Dr. Glock reprimanded Robert commenting on his loose and licentious life style, which he considered potentially dangerous. So, perhaps this is when Robert was infected with bad blood. Perhaps this is why he was ill so often over the years? I know Dr. Glock treated him and considered him to be cured. But how about the catastrophe that occurred so many years later? Was he truly cured, or had the medicine just made the bad blood hide somewhere in his body to rise up again many years later and take his life? Perhaps such things are possible?

At any rate, Robert was up and down with his health and his moods for many years. However, once we moved to Dusseldorf in 1850 things took a turn for the worse. To begin with I didn't really understand what was going on. When people complained about his direction of the choir and the orchestra, I assumed that these were just the opinions of a group of badly trained amateur musicians. I defended him and was indignant on his behalf. What else should I have thought and done? Indeed, I am quite sure that it was true that the musicians did resent him in some way and wanted to make his life difficult. But then it became increasingly apparent that perhaps Robert himself was to blame for some of what was going on.

In 1852 all his old illnesses returned in a very serious manner. His dizziness, headaches and insomnia seemed to be getting worse. He had an attack of intense nervous agitation. Then there was an incident when he found it difficult to speak for some days as if he had suffered a fit of apoplexy. Reports started to reach me about the state of things with the choir and orchestra. It seemed that Robert was conducting the music at unnaturally slow tempi. At that time they told him that in future the choir would be conducted by his assistant Herr Tausch. Then in 1853 I was told that when conducting a performance of Moritz Hauptmann's Mass, Robert continued to conduct after the piece was finished! It seemed at that point he was hearing the music in his head rather than with his ears. He was constantly dropping the baton and resorted to tying it to his wrist. Indeed, he seemed less and less in control of both his body and his mind. It was at this point that the committee instructed him that all of the choir and orchestral concerts were to be conducted by Tausch, with the exception of performances of his own music.

But Robert also had many days when he appeared entirely normal. It was about this time that you made your appearance at our door—a day I shall never forget. Hearing you play in our parlor that day was a revelation to both Robert and I. We realized that you were a fresh and individual voice whose music would take us along new paths. Since that time your friendship and support for me, both during that difficult time and subsequently, have been one of the great mainstays of my life. But you would surely admit that the first day you met us, nothing seemed amiss. You remained with us for several weeks, and when Joachim also joined us, the music making was some of the most exhilarating I have ever experienced.

However, it was only the lull before the storm. Strange things began to happen. First, you will recall when the painter Herr Laurens visited us and made sketches of all three of us. He told me something which made no sense to me at the time—"Frau Schumann—have you noticed that one of your husband's pupils is much larger than the other?" I looked and saw that this was certainly the case, but I didn't know what it meant. Now I think this was an effect of the bad blood that was finally starting to fatally degrade his body.

In the subsequent months other strange things began to happen. Around the time we toured Holland in late 1853, he started to repeatedly hear a single tone in his head. This was an odd affliction indeed and produced several nights of insomnia. However, the effect waned only to return with terrifying force the next February. He started hearing the tone again on Feb 11th and the next day started to hear complete music. He said "that it is so glorious and with instruments sounding more wonderful than ever one hears on earth." He became convinced that angels hovered about him, and he would lie awake all night staring at the heavens. At one point he got up and wrote down one of the themes that a particular angel, a manifestation of the spirit of Schubert, dictated to him. Eventually he composed a series of variations on this theme, as you yourself did following Robert's death.

But over the next few days the voices changed from being angels to being demons. They said he was a sinner and wanted to throw him into Hell. Their music was terrifying. They came to him in the shapes of tigers and hyenas threatening to rip him limb from limb. He lived in a paroxysm of terror. I was 5 months pregnant but stayed with him night after night until he was able to find some rest. For some weeks after that he was alternately afflicted with demons or angels shouting at him, so that he was in a state of unnatural terror or bliss—but to me all was torture.

Eventually he instructed me to keep him away from knives because he was afraid he would do me harm, and then, worst of all, that he should be taken to an asylum! This from a man whose greatest fear had always been that he would someday lose his sanity! Then on Mon Feb 27th the crisis came to a head and it was the beginning of the end. I had gone to stay with my friend Elise so as not to be too near Robert, as it was my presence that seemed to upset him the most. Our daughter Marie was upstairs looking after him. But at some point he eluded her and he left the house, running into the pouring rain wearing nothing but his dressing gown and slippers. He made his way to the Rhine, climbed down to the boats below the bridge, and slid into the freezing waters!

There is no doubt that he intended to take his life. However, soon after, he was seen by some fishermen in a boat and they rescued him—although apparently he resisted them. Then they brought him home through the streets on an open cart, dripping wet and for everybody to see! Can you imagine what people must have thought? When he arrived home his rescuers brought him into the house, and he was hiding his face with his hands. His doctors made a rapid decision that he should indeed be sent to the asylum. As you know I never saw him again until the day he died. He went to the asylum at Endenich just outside Bonn. It was recommended to us because it was run by Dr. Franz Richarz, a man who was renowned for being up to date with modern developments and for the humane care of his patients. Before he left I sent him a bouquet of flowers. I was told that before he got into the carriage he handed a flower to everybody—like the mad Ophelia.

It was there, Johannes, that you visited him in August and told me that he seemed relatively well—but that he never asked about me. Indeed, once he had left he rarely inquired about my health or that of his family. It was as if he had now entered a new universe where we no longer existed. I had frequent reports from Dr. Richarz over the next two years. Robert continued to have delusions, spasms, convulsions and other symptoms. Some days he would be better and some days worse. However, there was a clear downward trend. Occasionally he became violent and had to be put into a straightjacket. At other times he seemed fine and he would go for a stroll, even as far away as Bonn.

However, when I returned from my concert tour of England in July of 1856, you were visiting Robert. You told me not to come to see him—presumably because you thought it would upset me. But now his behavior was becoming increasingly erratic and lewd, and his physical symptoms had worsened. He would not eat and was starving himself. I received this news and was resolved to visit. When I arrived in Endenich on the evening of July 27th what I encountered distressed me more than I can possibly say. Robert was in bed, completely emaciated, he could hardly speak or move. I think he recognized me. I believe he tried to embrace me and to say my name—but perhaps I am imagining all of this? You will recall that the next morning you and I went to the station to meet Joachim, and by the time we returned my dear Robert was no more.

Afterwards Dr. Richarz told me that his diagnosis was that Robert suffered from a "General Paralysis of the Insane."[6] I have his postmortem report which he believes is consistent with this diagnosis, and with the symptoms Robert displayed such as delusions, dementia and eventual loss of his bodily functions. Nevertheless, my question has always been—"Where did this come from?" As I have now told you I believe it was bad blood, and I believe that he was infected with this many years before when he had his relationship with Christel. But in truth I do not know this or really what it means—it is just a feeling that I have. I know that Dr. Richarz also suspected something along these lines, as he questioned Robert about his previous relationships with women and their consequences. I am sure that as long as I live I will never stop pondering this question.

So there it is. I shall remain here until Easter week and then I shall have earned sufficient to be able to look forward calmly to next year. But I shall hardly be able to put anything aside. I have nothing but good news from my family. Ferdinand is turning out very well and Ludwig's master is also pleased with him. Felix often gives us great amusement with his letters, in which his vigorous nature stands revealed. Julie is being well looked after, and is studying diligently with Lachner; and Elise is doing a lot of music apart from her lessons. On the 26th of March Joachim is going to France again, and this time to the provinces. He has earned a lot of money this winter, for which I am very glad. I only hope he has laid a good deal aside. He is seriously considering moving to Berlin....

I am longing for news from you. I hope you are quite well, dearest Johannes, and may sometime remember—Your Clara.

May 5th 2011. 9am Northwestern University, Chicago. A lecture theatre.

Good morning everybody! Has everyone got their coffee or whatever else they need to stay awake? OK—that's good. So we should begin.

Over the last few weeks we have discussed different problems that can afflict the nervous system, their manifestation as psychiatric and neurodegenerative diseases, and their potential treatment. Today I want to turn to something slightly different, and that is the influence of the immune system on the development of brain pathology and disease. Yes, I know you are not immunologists! Don't worry I'm not going to drown you in a lot of immunological vernacular—but really some of these things are very important, and so we should be acquainted with at least the basic concepts. It turns out that interactions between the immune and nervous systems probably play an important role in many neurodegenerative and psychiatric diseases, and targeting these interactions may be an important therapeutic approach that is just starting to be appreciated.

I thought it might be interesting to introduce the subject by considering a particular case—the composer Robert Schumann. How many of you have heard of Robert Schumann or anything he composed?

Ah, that's a good try Ms. Cook, but that's Schubert, not Schumann. Yes, it's true they do sound similar. And indeed you are not the first to make a mistake like that. I am reminded of a story. In 1956 the German Democratic Republic issued a stamp to commemorate the anniversary of Schumann's death. Unfortunately the music depicted in the background of the stamp was from the song "Wanderers Nachtlied" written by Johann Wolfgang von Goethe, with music composed by Franz Schubert. What a scandal! Due to this error, it was decided to issue a new stamp with corrected music in the background. The new set now showed a song composed by Robert Schumann, his "Mondnacht" to poetry written by Joseph von Eichendorff. Collectors value the incorrect version of the stamps very highly. So Ms. Cook you are in good company—that is, if you consider the GDR good company.

Anyway, Robert Schumann was one of the great figures in nineteenth-century Romantic music (Figure 9.1). He was extremely influential and I encourage all of you to listen to his music. His life was that of the archetypal Romantic artist. There are various things that happened to him which have made him famous—I mean apart from his music. First of all there is the story of his courtship and eventual marriage to Clara Wieck (Figure 9.1). Clara was a child prodigy and grew up to be one of the most celebrated pianists in Europe. When she was 11 years old, and Robert Schumann was 20, he started coming to her house to take lessons with her father Friedrich Wieck, a celebrated pedagogue. He was always attentive to the little girl. Gradually, as she grew into her teenage years, their feelings for each other deepened into something much more complicated.

However, Friedrich Wieck was vehemently against any kind of relationship between the two of them. He had groomed Clara to be a great pianist and didn't want anything to get in the way of her career and also, I dare say, her potential income. In the end Clara and Robert had to bring a court case against her father, which they won and so they were able to marry.

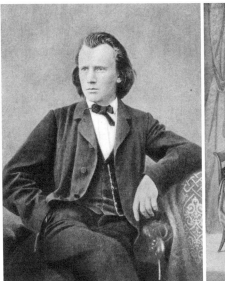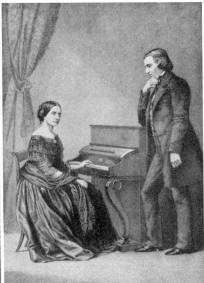

Figure 9.1:
Johannes Brahms, Robert Schumann, and Clara Wieck in their youth.
(Photoscom)

Another thing that Schumann is famous for is the manner in which he died. The last few years of his life in particular were characterized by increasingly bizarre behavior, finally resulting in dementia and attempted suicide by throwing himself into the Rhine. However, he was rescued and then sent to an insane asylum where he died two years later. There has been a good deal of speculation as to the nature of Schumann's final illness. He was certainly a man of shifting moods and probably suffered from something along the lines of bipolar disorder. However, it is unlikely that this was the cause of his ultimate demise. A far more likely scenario is that he suffered from syphilis and, in the end, from the manifestations of the effect of this disease on the brain.[6]

Syphilis was the bête noir of nineteenth-century diseases,[7] although since the introduction of penicillin it has been virtually eradicated, at least in Western countries. There is one major exception, and that is in the HIV-1 infected population, where syphilis is once again making its mark. However, such patients are routinely screened for the disease and treated with antibiotics. The first case of syphilis that we know about occurred in Naples in 1494.[7] As this is just a couple of years after Columbus' voyage to the Americas, it has been hypothesized that it must have originated in the New World, although this is still widely debated.

Syphilis is easily spread by sexual contact. Following its introduction into Europe in the fifteenth century, it was probably initially spread by soldiers during the numerous wars that were always going on somewhere on the continent, and especially by prostitutes and other camp followers who were associated with armies at that time. During the industrial revolution of the nineteenth century there was a vast overall movement of the population from the countryside to the rapidly growing cities. This resulted in overcrowding, poor living conditions, and the growth of activities such as prostitution. Such an urban environment was also ideal for the spread of sexually transmitted diseases like syphilis, and it became a very widespread problem.

Moreover, because it was known to be spread by sexual contact, the diagnosis of syphilis often brought with it a degree of shame and social rejection of the patient. It is also possible to transmit syphilis between a pregnant mother and a fetus during birth. This results in what is known as *congenital syphilis*. This is the subject of Henryk Ibsen's 1861 play "Ghosts." The public and critics at the time found the play unacceptably disgusting and immoral, which tells us something about what they thought about the subject in general. The course of both sexually transmitted and congenital syphilis is well described and consists of numerous stages which may extend over a period of many years following the initial infection. Ultimately, severe disruption of the nervous system is one commonly observed outcome. Such a manifestation is generally known as *neurosyphilis*.

The organism which causes syphilis is a bacterium called *Treponema pallidum subspecies pallidum*, and it is what is called a *spirochete*; that is, a member of the order Spirochaetales, family Spirochaetaceae, and genus Treponema.[8] There are also three other members of the same genus which can infect humans, and which produce three different diseases. *T. pallidum subsp. pertenue* causes a disease called "yaws"; *T. pallidum subsp. endemicum* causes a disease called "bejel"; and *T. carateum* causes a disease called "pinta."

T. pallidum is a unicellular organism with a coiled helical shape. It is about 10 μm long and 0.15 μm wide (Figure 9.2). It has long been known that *T. pallidum* can cause dementia and associated neurodegenerative and demyelinating disease in the late phases of neurosyphilis. The occurrence of dementia has also been reported in association with Lyme disease caused by another spirochete, *Borrelia burgdorferi*. Both spirochetes are neurotropic; that is to say, they can productively infect the nervous system. In particular, they can both persist in the infected host tissues and play a role in chronic neuropsychiatric disorders, including dementia. Let's discuss the course of the disease and examine how this might be related to the fate of Robert Schumann.

Traditionally syphilis follows a chronic course that is divided into primary, secondary, and tertiary phases, which may last for many years. The primary phase of the infection is typified by the appearance of a blister, known as a *chancre*. This usually forms after about 3 weeks at the original site of inoculation. It is very likely that this was the case with Schumann. He probably initially became

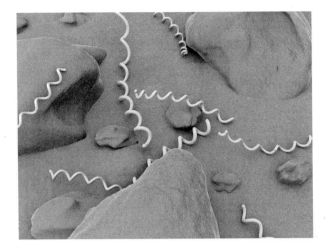

Figure 9.2:
The spirochete *Treponema Pallidum* the infectious agent responsible for syphilis.
(Sebastian Kaulitzki © Shutterstock)

infected because of a relationship he had in his early twenties with a servant girl living in his future wife's house. We know from his diaries that he went to see his doctor, who was somewhat shocked by what he observed—likely a primary chancre on Schumann's penis.

In those days, when the basis of the disease was not understood, patients were usually treated with metals such as mercury and arsenic—ideas that went back to medieval times.[7] As you can imagine these treatments were extremely toxic and people feared them almost as much as contracting the disease itself. It is likely that Schumann received treatment of this type. Eventually, in 1910, the great pharmacologist Paul Ehrlich developed organic derivatives of arsenic that were actually quite effective as antiluetics (that is, for treating syphilis) and certainly much less toxic than arsenic itself. Drugs he developed, such as arsphenamine (Salvarsan) became the first really effective treatment for the disease, only to be eventually displaced by antibiotics such as penicillin.[9]

Even when it isn't treated, the chancre that is associated with primary *T. pallidum* infection usually resolves completely. Although the chancre is a highly localized lesion, it is believed that during this initial period of infection *T. pallidum* invades the bloodstream and becomes widely disseminated around the body, including the central nervous system. Approximately two months later, the spread of the organism shows itself again by the appearance of a rash that can occur virtually anywhere. This rash also usually goes away completely, leaving the victim without any apparent symptoms.

However, the organism has not actually disappeared and is still present in a "latent" form. In some patients, many years or even decades later, *T. pallidum* can reappear and produce "tertiary" disease. This can take many forms including cardiovascular disease, neurosyphilis, or "gummas," the latter being large bulbous lesions of the skin, bones, or organs. When patients are untreated with antibiotics, around 15%–40% eventually develop some form of tertiary disease.[7-9]

As I have said, it is thought that *T. pallidum* invades the CNS early in the course of the infection and seeds the meninges during the primary and secondary phases of the disease. Indeed, testing cerebrospinal fluid (CSF) samples from patients with primary or secondary syphilis has revealed signs of CNS disease in up to 50% of patients. It is thought that most patients clear the CNS infection spontaneously, leaving only a small percentage who will ultimately exhibit the signs of late stage neurosyphilis.

Interestingly, "early" neurosyphilis, which might occur some 2–5 years following the primary infection, involves infection of the meninges and central blood vessels. This results in symptoms such as headaches, dizziness, and fever, which are precisely the kinds of things that plagued Robert Schumann throughout his life. He may well have eventually transitioned to "late" neurosyphilis which, in addition to the cerebral vasculature, also involves infection of the parenchyma (that is the general tissue) of the brain or spinal cord. Typically this occurs many years following the primary infection, so 20 years would not be uncommon. Inflammation of the meninges and blood vessels may lead to strokes in these patients, whereas it is infection of the parenchyma of the brain that is associated with "General Paralysis of the Insane (GPI)," a syndrome associated with progressive personality changes and dementia.

It is interesting to note that during the last years of his life, Robert Schumann was subject to symptoms such as transitory loss of speech, which may have been the manifestation of a stroke. Moreover, the psychiatrist at the asylum where he finally died diagnosed him as suffering from GPI, although in those days its connection with tertiary syphilis was not understood. Another manifestation of tertiary syphilis, in some patients, is a syndrome known as *tabes dorsalis,* which is the result of infection of the spinal cord. This may be manifest as bowel problems, and again Schumann certainly was plagued with these, as well as proprioceptive problems and pain.

Interestingly, another symptom of tertiary syphilis is a syndrome known as Argyll-Robertson pupils.[10] In this case the patient may have a pupil that does not contract when exposed to bright light, resulting in pupils of different sizes. We know that prior to his attempted suicide, such a phenomenon was noted in Robert Schumann by an artist who came to paint his picture. He pointed this out to Schumann's wife, who confirmed its existence and mentions this in her diaries. Although it is unlikely that we will ever know exactly what was wrong with Robert Schumann, I think that it is likely, as commented on by many writers, that he suffered from syphilis and the manifestations of tertiary neurosyphilis. It was certainly not unique for young men at the time to contract this disease and indeed, other famous artists at the time such as the composers Hugo Wolf and Franz Schubert may have suffered similar fates. The question that should concern us is, how the infectious organism leads to the eventual symptom of dementia.

In 1913 *T. pallidum* was first identified in the brain of patients suffering from GPI, and so finally established a direct link between infection of the parenchyma of the brain and the observed dementia. Classic late neurosyphilis, which is associated with GPI or tabes dorsalis, is the result of extensive damage to the brain or spinal cord respectively. These days the use of antibiotics has made such manifestations very rare in Western countries. When GPI does occur, it usually appears initially as a form of dementia associated with impaired cognitive function, changes in mood and, frequently, psychotic symptoms such as hallucinations and speech impediments. The severity of these symptoms becomes worse with time, together with the appearance of other types of symptoms associated with a general lack of control of numerous normal bodily functions. When one examines the brains of patients with advanced GPI and observes the widespread evidence of neuronal death and demyelination, it is hardly surprising that severe psychological problems are associated with this condition. Huge numbers of spirochetes may accumulate in the cerebral cortex in association with the disease. The death of neurons and demyelination of axons can be so severe that the characteristic layering pattern of neurons in the cerebral cortex is no longer apparent. Spirochetes may also occur in other parts of the brain, such as the basal ganglia. Look at this picture, which shows a brain section from a patient with neurosyphilis. Can you imagine having that lot crawling around in your brain?

There is another thing that can be observed in the brains of patients with GPI—and this is certainly one of the keys to understanding what is going on— and that is the occurrence of widespread inflammation. By this I mean the observation that numerous white blood cells that are part of the immune system have entered the brain from the blood. A further aspect of this inflammatory response is that certain brain cells called microglia become "activated." This state of activation is associated with the synthesis of numerous molecules called *inflammatory cytokines*. These are the important molecules that orchestrate the inflammatory response. Although the inflammatory response may initially play a role in the body's attempt to clear infection, when it becomes chronic it is probably the major factor in producing damage to the nervous system.[11]

The appearance of neuroinflammation is a manifestation of the immune and nervous systems interacting with one another. Every tissue contains resident cells of the immune system, which are known as *tissue macrophages*. These cells are constantly sampling their environment for signs of trouble; that is, anything that might upset normal tissue homeostasis.[11] When they detect a problem they mount a response and try to correct it. Tissue macrophages are part of the front line in regulating what is known as the *innate immune response*. Tissue macrophages express a large group of receptors that can recognize "pathogen associated molecular patterns" or PAMPs.[12] These are general molecular patterns associated with damaged cells or infectious pathogens. PAMPs could be things like bacterial cell wall lipopolysaccharide, proteins from bacterial flagella, viral DNA, or RNA or molecules like stress or heat shock proteins that cells synthesize when they are confronted with damage of some kind: basically, anything that signals that cells are in trouble.

For example, following a period of ischemia in association with a stroke, cells will make heat shock proteins as part of their protective response to the situation. If these proteins leak from damaged cells, they will activate PAMP receptors expressed by tissue macrophages. When innate immune receptors expressed by tissue macrophages recognize PAMPs, they activate biochemical signaling pathways that direct the synthesis of inflammatory cytokines. As I have indicated, these molecules then help to organize the subsequent inflammatory response and instigate the synthesis of molecules such as nitric oxide (NO) and reactive oxygen species (ROS) that are designed to destroy pathogens.

When we speak of "inflammatory cytokines" we know that this is a very large family of molecules including members of the interleukin and tissue necrosis factor (TNF) families, such as interleukin -1 and TNF-α, as well as different kinds of growth factors and chemotactic cytokines (chemokines). The idea is that as a result of activation of the innate immune response, inflammatory cytokines elicit local cellular responses that are designed to help solve the prevailing problem, and indeed that may certainly happen. However, if things do not work out and the problem persists, reinforcements are called in. These reinforcements are the white blood cells of the immune system that enter the tissue to help with its protective response.[12]

As opposed to the innate immune response, which is a general response to a variety of potential problems, the *adaptive immune response* constitutes the body's specific response to individual pathogens. It includes the production of antigen-specific populations of immune system cells including T lymphocytes, B lymphocytes that make specific antibodies, as well as phenomena such as immunological memory that ensure a rapid response to subsequent infections by the same pathogens. Once the innate and adaptive immune responses have been triggered, a battle takes place in which these immune responses go head to head with the prevailing problem, and perhaps it is ultimately successfully resolved. However, if it is not, the presence of chronic inflammation will itself become problematic and produce extensive collateral damage leading to the general destruction of intrinsic tissue cells.

So, how do these events play out in the brain in particular? The brain certainly does contain numerous tissue macrophages, which are the microglial cells. In fact in some parts of the neuraxis they may constitute around 20% of the resident cells in the brain.[13] As opposed to cells such as neurons and glia, which are derived from neural stem cells, the microglia are derived from precursor cells from the yolk sac which enter the brain during embryogenesis. So, really, the name *microglia* is a misnomer because these cells are more related to immune cells than to the real glial cells of the nervous system—the astrocytes and oligodendrocytes.

The microglia enter the brain during embryogenesis and take up permanent residence there. In other words, microglia represent a part of the immune system that is normally resident in the brain. Under normal conditions, when no problems need to be addressed, microglia are often described as being in their "resting" state—but nothing could be further from the truth. Recent real-time imaging studies of live brain tissue have demonstrated that under resting conditions microglia display a highly branched morphology with many extensions or "processes" extending from these cells like arms. These microglial processes continually waggle about in what appears to be an attempt to explore and sample the local environment, as might be expected of a tissue macrophage with a surveillance function. In addition we now also suspect that microglia have an important role in the shaping of synaptic connections and regulating the strength of synaptic transmission between nerve cells.

Microglia are highly plastic cells that can adopt a large number of cellular and molecular identities depending on what is going on in the cellular microenvironment they are surveying. When microglia adopt these phenotypes, we refer to them as "activated." The activation of microglia was a phenomenon that was actually first described by the famous neuroanatomist Nissl, a friend and colleague of Alois Alzheimer, who originally described the neurological disease which now bears his name. Nissl observed what he described as "strung-out, often infinitely long, extremely slim glial cells" that "may cross the entire layer of the large pyramidal neurons." He also observed that these microglial "rod cells" typically aligned themselves with the apical dendrites of neurons, often extending to adjacent neuronal surfaces and even wrapping around somatic membranes (Figure 9.3). Rod cells are only one manifestation of the activation of microglia. At the molecular level, states of microglial activation are associated with the synthesis of PAMP receptors, inflammatory cytokines, and elements of the complement system. So, as you can see, microglia in the brain are really the key cells that communicate between what is going on in the brain and the immune system.

The expression of different PAMP receptors by microglia is a key element in understanding the inflammatory response of the brain to pathogens like *T. pallidum*, because this is the way problems are first detected and how the local immune response is first activated. There are several types of receptors of this type. They are quite different from the ligand gated ion channels and GPCRs we have discussed previously. One class are the Toll-like receptors (TLRs). There are

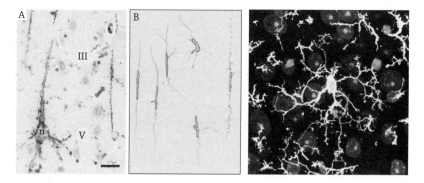

Figure 9.3:
Microglial cells. Right panel illustrates a contemporary image. Panels A and B are images from 1922 illustrating microglial cells in a "rod like" conformation as typically seen in General Paralysis of the Insane (arrow), sometimes associated with the dendrites of nerve cells (n).

Micrograph reproduced courtesy of Dr. Jaime Grutzendler, Yale University, and Panels A and B reproduced courtesy of *Science* magazine.

also "NOD"-like and "RIG1"-like receptors. Some of these receptors—like the TLRs, which can recognize bacterial components such as lipopolysaccharide and flagellin—are located in the plasma membrane, while other receptors, such as some of the TLRs as well as the NODs and RIGs, are intracellular. When these PAMP receptors recognize a molecule that signals the presence of a pathogen or some type of cell damage, they activate a signaling pathway that leads to the increased synthesis of numerous inflammatory cytokines. The microglia may also behave like cells called *phagocytes* and migrate to the area of infection or tissue damage, where they attempt to ingest and destroy cellular detritus or produce bacteriocidal molecules such as nitric oxide (NO) and reactive oxygen species (ROS) in an effort to kill invading pathogens. Such responses are designed to take care of the recognized problem. If this does not occur, a full scale neuroinflammatory response may also involve the participation of an adaptive immune response, and the influx of different classes of white blood cells into the brain.[14]

But why does all of this take up to 20 years to happen in response to *T. pallidum* infection of the brain? There is no definite answer to this question. It is clear that during the primary phase of *T. pallidum* infection, the body mounts an adaptive immune response. That is to say that *T. pallidum*–associated antigens are picked up at their points of tissue entry by antigen-presenting cells called *dendritic cells*, which then migrate to lymphoid organs and present these molecules to populations of immature T lymphocytes (T cells).[14] These cells are stimulated to develop into various subclasses of activated T cells, while other cells develop into antibody secreting cells. At any rate, the combination of an innate and adaptive immune response to a pathogen constitutes the body's defense against an organism and is normally expected to be able to wipe it out and get rid of the problem. In some people infected with *T. pallidum,* however, that does not seem to happen. Somehow the spirochete manages to hide out in tissues such as the parenchyma of the brain for many years. What probably happens is that when *T. pallidum* is threatened by the immune response, it forms cysts or "granular" forms of the organism which can persist within infected cells and where it can live in a quasidormant state protected from its environment, including the surveillance of the immune system. We know this is the case both for *T. pallidum* and also for *B. burgdorferi.* So, it appears that *T. pallidum* lives in this form in the brains of some patients for many years and then, for some reason that we don't fully understand, it awakens once more and begins to actively replicate. When this happens the PAMPS derived from the organism will activate microglia.[14]

Of course the infected individual will also mount an adaptive immune response based on the original infection many years previously. Clearly, however, in some people the combined immune response is not capable of restraining the ever growing threat of rapidly dividing *T. pallidum.* As it tries to defend the brain more and more desperately, reinforcements in the form of immune cells from the bloodstream enter the brain in greater and greater numbers. The potentially bacteriocidal molecules produced during this chronic, full blown neuroinflammation now start to kill more and more oligodendrocytes and neurons in a destructive dance of death, until the brain is no longer a viable organ and that is that. Not a pretty picture!

This kind of scenario fits very well with what was observed with Robert Schumann. His doctor is on record as probably observing the primary chancre following his initial infection. Perhaps many of the diverse symptoms he exhibited over the years were the result of low-grade inflammation of the meninges of the brain? The symptoms reported for the last few years of his life, including increasing dementia, possible strokes, and Argyll-Robertson pupils, clearly support the ongoing effects of tertiary neurosyphilis and eventual death.

Owing to the introduction of antibiotics, neurosyphilis is not a major problem in Western countries these days, although it is still found quite extensively in the third world. On the other hand, inflammatory diseases of the brain do constitute widespread problems for other reasons.[15] Consider the following scenario. Suppose at some point in your life you are infected with a pathogen. As we have discussed, normally your immune system takes care of the problem. There will be both an innate and an adaptive immune response mounted against the invader. Now consider this. The adaptive immune response is based on the presentation of antigens derived from the organism, and activated T cells or antibody-expressing cells develop to specifically attack the organism based on the presence of the particular antigens which it expresses. Our immune system knows that these antigens are associated with the invading organism and are not normally part of ourselves, and so attacks the invader in a specific manner. In other words, it is critically important that the immune system knows how to recognize antigens that represent "non-self" from those that represent "self"; otherwise, it would spend its time attacking our normal tissues.

However, what happens if the immune system makes a mistake? What happens if a particular antigen presented by an invading organism closely resembles something that is normally expressed by our own cells? Then it is possible that the immune system will erroneously start to attack our own organs. This is what happens in the case of what is known as "autoimmune disease." Autoimmunity as the mechanistic basis for different diseases is something we are increasingly aware of these days. For example, rheumatoid arthritis is an autoimmune response against joint synovium. In the case of systemic lupus erythematosus, circulating anti-DNA anti-nucleoprotein antibodies produce damage to the kidneys and blood vessels due to deposition of immune complexes and subsequent activation of the complement cascade and neutrophils. T cell mediated autoimmune diseases are almost universally due to the activity of self-reactive or "autoreactive" T cells with the cooperation of inflammatory cytokine activated macrophages that are the major effector cells producing tissue damage.[15]

The major autoimmune disease that affects the nervous system is multiple sclerosis (MS), which affects more than a million people worldwide. Although the cause of the disease is unknown, it is thought to be triggered by something such as a virus or other pathogen that mistakenly activates T cells that recognize antigens associated with myelin, a layer of insulating material derived from oligodendrocytes that surrounds many nerve cell axons.[16] Once activated in lymph nodes, these "autoreactive" T cells enter the circulation. However, the parenchyma of the brain and spinal cord is not a friendly environment for T cells, which do not survive there unless restimulated by the same antigen that they were initially stimulated by in the peripheral lymphoid organs. This process probably occurs in the choroid plexus, meninges, and perivascular spaces that surround the brain. Once restimulated in this fashion, autoreactive T cells and activated microglia can elicit an inflammatory cytokine response that allows white blood cells to efficiently invade the brain. It is these cells that are primarily responsible for producing the effects like demyelination and axonal degeneration that are observed in multiple sclerosis.

Indeed, the major pathological signs of the disease include infiltrates of immune cells associated with areas of demyelination known as *plaques*. The clinical presentation of multiple sclerosis can include a wide range of symptoms, including problems with movement and coordination, spasticity, fatigue, pain, and sensory impairments. Examination of the brains and spinal cords from multiple sclerosis patients reveals multiple demyelinating lesions. Damage to axons and neuronal death can also be observed, as well as areas of inflammation.

Lesions containing inflammatory cells such as T cells are usually observed in both the brain and the spinal cord.

Investigations into the causes and treatment of multiple sclerosis have been aided by the development of several good animal models of the disease. The most sophisticated of these is called "experimental autoimmune encephalomyelitis" (EAE).[16] In this case rodents are usually injected with myelin-derived antigens so that they mount an immune response against them. Alternatively, T cells from a mouse with EAE can be isolated and transfused into a normal mouse, which will then develop the disease—a technique known as "adoptive transfer." The inflammatory cells that enter the brain, as well as the pathological signs of demyelination seen in EAE, are clearly similar to those that have been observed in human multiple sclerosis. The fact that EAE can be induced by the adoptive transfer of myelin-specific T cells also clearly supports the notion that these cells are the key to understanding the mechanisms underlying the disease. The EAE model allows investigations into the mechanisms which give rise to the disease, as well as the development of new drugs for combating it. Overall, it is currently believed that the pathogenesis of EAE is triggered exclusively within the peripheral immune system. However, the influx of autoreactive T lymphocytes into the central nervous system is clearly associated with the subsequent activation of microglia, which may then be of central importance in the progression of the disease. Indeed, inhibition of microglial function in mice using genetic methods leads to a strong suppression of the symptoms of EAE.[16]

How can we treat neuroinflammation? Current treatment of multiple sclerosis is primarily based on drugs with "immunomodulatory" properties that inhibit the ability of reactive T cells to exit the lymphoid organs or enter the brain.[16,17] Steroids, which are effective treatments for inflammatory diseases in general, can be used to treat acute attacks. However, many patients with relapsing remitting disease are treated with either the cytokine molecule interferon-β or glatiramer acetate, marketed under the trade name Copaxone. The use of interferon-β in multiple sclerosis was originally based on the fact that this cytokine has well known antiviral properties, and it was thought that the disease might well be caused by a virus. However, it is not at all clear if this is the basis of its beneficial effects. Interferon-β reduces the relapse rate in multiple sclerosis by about 30%, and new lesion activity by about 65%. As far as its molecular mechanism is concerned, however, it has been shown that interferon-β regulates the expression of literally hundreds of genes in immune cells and it is not clear which of these effects are the most relevant. Copaxone is a random polymer of the four amino acids: glutamate, lysine, alanine, and tyrosine. It is approximately as effective as interferon-β. However, again, it is not entirely clear how it works. It appears to mimic the structure of myelin basic protein to some extent, and to shift the population of T cells from those that are proinflammatory to other populations that have anti-inflammatory actions, and this has a beneficial effect on the course of the disease. How this is achieved is not at all clear.

Aside from these treatments, there are now more recent therapies that have a clearer mechanism of action. For example, there is a monoclonal antibody called *natalizumab,* marketed under the name Tysabri. Tysabri is an antibody against the α4 integrin molecule and was specifically designed to inhibit the entry of T cells into the brain and spinal cord. The idea here is that passage across the blood-brain barrier by inflammatory cells such as autoreactive T lymphocytes requires that they first need to interact with receptors on the endothelial cells within blood vessels which form part of the blood-brain barrier. Tysabri works by inhibiting the influx of immune cells into the brain by binding to and blocking α4β1-integrin receptors. These are molecules on the surfaces of endothelial cells that are essential for this influx. Tysabri is basically used to treat patients who are resistant to the effects of interferon-β or Copaxone and is at least as effective as these other agents.

However, as we are continually learning, unpredictable events can intervene in the smooth course of drug development. It is clear that normally there is a degree of immune surveillance of the central nervous system by circulating T lymphocytes; that is to say, there are always some of these cells that do traverse the brain on the lookout for infection and damage. This is part of the normal function of our immune system. Consequently, totally blocking the access of immune cells to the brain could have unfortunate consequences. In the case of Tysabri, this is precisely what happened. While the drug was being successfully used to treat many patients with multiple sclerosis, it was observed that a few people developed a serious and potentially fatal side effect, particularly when the drug was combined with other drugs with immunosuppressant actions. These patients developed progressive multifocal leukoencephalopathy (PML), an inflammatory disease of the white matter caused by the JC virus. It is assumed that the effects of this virus are normally kept at bay by the immune response, but that under immunosuppressed conditions, which might produce a deficit in the basic immune surveillance of the brain, this can fail, leading to the observed syndrome. When the first few patients developed PML, Tysabri was withdrawn from the market, only to be allowed back some time later with the appropriate usage warnings.

Are there any new possible therapeutic strategies for treating neuroinflammation? As I have said, it is likely that the activation of microglia is an important factor in this phenomenon.[18] Indeed, it is likely that a microglial response is present in association with many types of neuropathology, including neurodegenerative diseases such as Alzheimer's, Parkinson's, Lou Gehrig's, and Huntington's diseases, and even psychiatric disorders as well, where signs of neuroinflammation are also observed. An active area of research at the moment is to determine how these activated microglia contribute to the course of each disease.[19] For example, if it is the case that microglia activated to assume their phagocytic role are important in the body's attempts to clear amyloid plaques in Alzheimer's disease, or the debris of dying neurons in other neurodegenerative diseases, then disturbing this function would not seem like a good idea. On the other hand, the chronic nature of these diseases and the ultimate inability of the brain's innate immune and other defense systems to keep up with them may mean that ultimately the collateral damage caused by the products of activated microglia are more trouble than they are worth. Thus, it may be the case that inhibiting microglial function and local inflammation in the brain is a good therapeutic strategy, and it may well be that agents designed to regulate microglial functions will find a therapeutic niche in treating a variety of brain disorders. Indeed, new research has started to show that a neuroinflammatory response probably accompanies diseases like schizophrenia and depression. This is not as strong as the response in a disease like multiple sclerosis. However, it appears that cytokines produced by the response may influence the activity of neurons that are involved in these diseases. Hence, manipulating the immune responses of the brain, such as the activation of microglia or the production and action of cytokines, is a new direction for psychopharmacology that may be of great importance in the future treatment of mental disorders as well as diseases like multiple sclerosis.

Let us propose that our goal is to inhibit the activation of microglia associated with a neuroinflammatory response Are there any likely mechanisms that might be able to produce effects such as these? How about the cannabinoid receptors (Chapter 7)? We know that CB1 receptors are widely expressed in the nervous system, and that CB2 receptors are widely expressed by white blood cells. Interestingly it appears that under "resting" conditions microglia don't express either of these receptors to any great extent. However, when activated, both CB1 and CB2 seem to be expressed by microglia.[20] Moreover, the activated phenotypes of microglia can be effectively inhibited by stimulation of such receptors.[20] Thus, endocannabinoid signaling may normally constitute a negative feedback regulatory system for controlling microglial activation. We know that activation of CB1 receptors in the brain produces the psychotropic effects associated with cannabis, so a drug that activates CB1 receptors in the brain, even if it has profound anti-inflammatory effects, is unlikely to be acceptable. On the other hand, activation of CB2 receptors is not associated with any psychotropic effects that we know about. Hence a drug that activates CB2 in the brain might represent a reasonable drug for treating microglial activation in the context of brain disease. But, of course, this is just one possibility.

OK, that ends our brief survey of neuroinflammation and how it might be important in the context of brain disease. Now here's what I would like you to do for your homework assignment for next time: invent a new treatment for multiple sclerosis based on the actions of a new drug that regulates the properties of microglia. It should be no more than one page. Explain the mechanism of action of your new drug based on what you can glean from the literature and our discussion today. Email me your answers. I will read them and announce a winner next time. As you may know, we are supposed to be encouraging you to think about the translational potential of your research these days. This is the directive that has come down from the NIH. I look forward to hearing your ideas!

The near future . . . . .

PRESS RELEASE FROM MONARCH PHARMACEUTICALS[21]
MON-52 for Multiple Sclerosis
MON-52

MON-52 and MON-52D are the lead compounds synthesized by our medicinal pharmacology team under the direction of Dr. Bob Schumann. This series was designed to produce agonists at the CB2 cannibinoid receptor. Importantly, owing to significant pharmacological differences between CB2 receptors in humans and rodents, the members of this series were all screened against human CB2 as expressed in tissue culture cells and using our proprietary "HOTmouse" lines of mice, which express human microglia in their nervous systems. MON-52 is an effective agonist at human CB2 receptors. MON-52D is a prodrug derivative of MON-52, which is only active when it enters the brain, and is enzymatically modified to produce MON-52, a conversion process that takes place very easily and which we have shown to occur with high efficiency. The use of MON-52D ensures that the drug will only act as an effective agonist at CB2 receptors when they are expressed within the central nervous system, such as by microglia under neuroinflammatory conditions. This also means that activation of CB2 receptors on immune cells in the periphery does not occur, and so the use of MON-52D is predicted to be free of any immunosuppressive effects that would result from such an action. Our studies have clearly demonstrated that MON52/52D suppressed the production of proinflammatory cytokines (IL-1ß, TNF-α) and enhanced the production of the anti-inflammatory cytokines (IL-4, IL-10) in mice with experimental autoimmune encephalomyelitis.

Based on the potential mechanisms of action of MON52/52D, our preclinical data, and the issuance of a U.S. patent covering the method of using MON2/52D to treat the disease, we have decided to pursue development of MON-52D as a novel, oral agent for the treatment of multiple sclerosis (MS). Clinical trials are being planned both in the United States and Europe in collaboration with our partners Schmetterling & Co. (Germany) and Skurefugal (Denmark). We will make further announcements about the progress of this novel drug development in the near future.

NOTES

1. Robert Schumann (1810–1856) was one of the key figures in the Romantic era. Born in Zwickau, Saxony, he started out training to become a pianist but was unable to continue owing to a hand injury. He established himself as one of the most important composers of the Romantic era, as well as an important music critic. His works for the piano and his lieder are particularly well known, although he composed many different types of chamber, orchestral, and choral music. He became the mentor for many younger composers, particularly Johannes Brahms. He married the pianist/composer Clara Wieck over the opposition of her father, who was also his piano teacher. He died at the age of 46 in a mental asylum following a suicide attempt while he was living in Dusseldorf.

2. *Animierlokale*. These were bar/brothels situated at the dockside in Hamburg where Brahms was born. As a child piano prodigy Brahms played in these brothels to make money for his family. There is good evidence that he was sexually abused by both men and women at this time.

3. Clara Wieck Schumann (1819–1887). Born in Leipzig, Clara was a child piano prodigy groomed carefully by her father Friedrich Wieck to have a career as a concert pianist. She became one of the leading pianists of her generation and also composed for the piano. When she was a young teenager she met Robert Schumann, who was studying piano with her father. Following a long romance they were married when she was 21 years old, but first had to overcome the opposition of Clara's father. In the end they had to bring a lawsuit against Friedrich Wieck to obtain permission to marry. Clara and Robert Schumann had 8 children. Following a move to Dusseldorf, Clara and Robert Schumann met Johannes Brahms and encouraged him. Following Schumann's death, Clara and Brahms had a relationship over many decades which resulted in a long correspondence. The precise nature of their relationship has remained unclear but it was probably platonic.

4. Joseph Joachim (1831–1903) was a famous Hungarian/Jewish violinist and composer and a close friend of both Johannes Brahms and Robert Schumann.

5. The first two paragraphs of this letter are adapted from Berthold Litzman (ed.). The letters of Clara Schumann and Johannes Brahms (1853–1896). Hyperion Press. 1979.
   Letter p. 206 from 1867 and letter p. 268 from 1873.

6. Jänisch W, Nauhaus G. Autopsy report of the corpse of the composer Robert Schumann—publication and interpretation of a rediscovered document. *Zentralbl. Allg Pathol.* 1986, 132(2):129–136.
   Lederman RJ. Robert Schumann. *Semin Neurol.* 1999, 19 (Suppl 1):17–24.
   Bazner H, Hennerici MG. Syphilis in German speaking composers—"Examination results are confidential." 2010. *Frontiers Neurol Neurosci.* 2010, 27:61–83.

7. Kaplan RM. Syphilis, sex and psychiatry, 1789–1925: Part 1. *Australas Psychiatry.* 2010, 18(1):17–21.
   Kaplan RM. Syphilis, sex and psychiatry, 1789–1925: Part 2. *Australas Psychiatry.* 2010, 18(1):22–27.
   Chahine LM, Khoriaty RN, Tomford WJ, Hussain MS. The changing face of neurosyphilis. *Int J Stroke.* 2011, 6(2):136–143.
   Ghanem KG. Neurosyphilis: A historical perspective and review. *CNS Neurosci Ther.* 2010, 16(5):e157–168.

8. Miklossy J. Biology and neuropathology of dementia in syphilis and Lyme disease. *Handb Clin Neurol.* 2008, 89:825–844.

   Marra CM. Neurosyphilis. *Curr Neurol Neurosci Rep.* 2004, 4(6):435–440.

   Kent ME, Romanelli F. Reexamining syphilis: an update on epidemiology, clinical manifestations, and management. *Ann Pharmacother.* 2008, 42(2):226–236.

9. Peeling RW, Hook EW 3rd. The pathogenesis of syphilis: the Great Mimicker, revisited. *J Pathol.* 2006, 208(2):224–232.

   Burke ET. The arseno-therapy of Syphilis; Stovarsol, and Tryparsamide. *Br J Vener Dis.* 1925, 1(4):321–338.

10. http://en.wikipedia.org/wiki/Argyll_Robertson_pupil

11. Medzhitov R. Origin and physiological roles of inflammation. *Nature.* 2008, 454(7203):428–435.

   Infante-Duarte C, Waiczies S, Wuerfel J, Zipp F. New developments in understanding and treating neuroinflammation. *J Mol Med (Berl).* 2008, 86(9):975–985.

   Wee Yong V. Inflammation in neurological disorders: a help or a hindrance? *Neuroscientist.* 2010, 16(4):408–420.

12. Baccala R, Gonzalez-Quintial R, Lawson BR, Stern ME, Kono DH, Beutler B, Theofilopoulos AN. Sensors of the innate immune system: their mode of action. *Nat Rev Rheumatol.* 2009, 5(8):448–456.

   Man SM, Kaakoush NO, Mitchell HM. The role of bacteria and pattern-recognition receptors in Crohn's disease. *Nat Rev Gastroenterol Hepatol.* 2011, 8(3):152–168.

   Rivest S. Regulation of innate immune responses in the brain. *Nat Rev Immunol.* 2009, 9(6):429–439.

13. Perry VH, Nicoll JA, Holmes C. Microglia in neurodegenerative disease. *Nat Rev Neurol.* 2010, 6(4):193–201.

   Graeber MB. Changing face of microglia. *Science.* 2010, 330(6005):783–788.

   Graeber MB, Streit WJ. Microglia: biology and pathology. *Acta Neuropathol.* 2010, 119(1):89–105.

   Ransohoff RM, Cardona AE. The myeloid cells of the central nervous system parenchyma. *Nature.* 2010, 468(7321):253–262.

   Prinz M, Mildner A. Microglia in the CNS: immigrants from another world. *Glia.* 2011, 59(2):177–187.

14. Shin JL, Chung KY, Kang JM, Lee TH, Lee MG. The effects of Treponema pallidum on human dendritic cells. *Yonsei Med J.* 2004, 45(3):515–522.

   Miklossy J, Kasas S, Zurn AD, McCall S, Yu S, McGeer PL. Persisting atypical and cystic forms of Borrelia burgdorferi and local inflammation in Lyme neuroborreliosis. *J Neuroinflammation.* 2008, 5:40.

   Myers TA, Kaushal D, Philipp MT. Microglia are mediators of Borrelia burgdorferi-induced apoptosis in SH-SY5Y neuronal cells. *PLoS Pathog.* 2009, 5(11):e1000659.

   Ramesh G, Borda JT, Gill A, Ribka EP, Morici LA, Mottram P, Martin DS, Jacobs MB, Didier PJ, Philipp MT. Possible role of glial cells in the onset and progression of Lyme neuroborreliosis. *J Neuroinflammation.* 2009, 6:23.

   Chauhan VS, Sterka DG Jr, Furr SR, Young AB, Marriott I. NOD2 plays an important role in the inflammatory responses of microglia and astrocytes to bacterial CNS pathogens. *Glia.* 2009, 57(4):414–423.

   Chauhan VS, Sterka DG Jr, Gray DL, Bost KL, Marriott I. Neurogenic exacerbation of microglial and astrocyte responses to Neisseria meningitidis and Borrelia burgdorferi. *J Immunol.* 2008, 180(12):8241–8249.

15. Goverman J. Autoimmune T cell responses in the central nervous system. *Nat Rev Immunol.* 2009, 9(6):393–407.
16. Steinman L. A molecular trio in relapse and remission in multiple sclerosis. *Nat Rev Immunol.* 2009, 9(6):440–447.
    Baker D, Gerritsen W, Rundle J, Amor S. Critical appraisal of animal models of multiple sclerosis. *Mult Scler.* 2011, 17(6):647–657.
17. Palmer AM. Pharmacotherapy for multiple sclerosis: progress and prospects. *Curr Opin Investig Drugs.* 2009, 10(5):407–417.
    Rudick RA, Goelz SE. Beta-interferon for multiple sclerosis. *Exp Cell Res.* 2011, 317(9):1301–1311.
18. Heppner FL, Greter M, Marino D, Falsig J, Raivich G, Hövelmeyer N, Waisman A, Rülicke T, Prinz M, Priller J, Becher B, Aguzzi A. Experimental autoimmune encephalomyelitis repressed by microglial paralysis. *Nat Med.* 2005, 11(2):146–152.
19. Long-Smith CM, Sullivan AM, Nolan YM. The influence of microglia on the pathogenesis of Parkinson's disease. *Prog Neurobiol.* 2009, 89(3):277–287.
    Naert G, Rivest S. The role of microglial cell subsets in Alzheimer's disease. *Curr Alzheimer Res.* 2011, 8(2):151–155.
20. Stella N. Endocannabinoid signaling in microglial cells. *Neuropharmacology.* 2009, 56 Suppl 1:244–253.
    Stella N. Cannabinoid and cannabinoid-like receptors in microglia, astrocytes, and astrocytomas. *Glia.* 2010, 58(9):1017–1030.
    Bisogno T, Di Marzo V. Cannabinoid receptors and endocannabinoids: role in neuroinflammatory and neurodegenerative disorders. *CNS Neurol Disord Drug Targets.* 2010, 9(5):564–573.
    Atwood BK, Mackie K. CB2: a cannabinoid receptor with an identity crisis. *Br J Pharmacol.* 2010, 160(3):467–479.
21. This "press release" is based on an actual report from a drug company: http://www.medicinova.com/html/research_multiplesclerosis.html.

BIBLIOGRAPHY

John M. Allegro (2009) *The sacred mushroom and the cross.* (40th anniversary edition) (Gnostic Media Research and Publishing)

Charles Baudelaire (1998) *Artificial Paradises*, trans. Stacy Diamond (Citadel Press)

Alex Baenninger, Jorge Alberto Costa e Silva, Ian Hindmarch, Hans-Juergen Moeller, and Karl Rickels (2004) *Good Chemistry. The life and legacy of valium inventor Leo Sternbach.* (McGraw-Hill)

J. Bernath (ed.) (1999) *Poppy: The genus Papaver.* (Harwood Academic Publishers)

Martin Booth (1996) *Opium: A history.* (St. Martins Press)

Martin Booth (2005) *Cannabis: A history.* (Picador)

Sir Thomas Browne (1977 ed.) *The major works.* (Penguin Press)

J. Bogousslavsky, F. Boller (eds.) (2005) *Neurological disorders in famous artists.* Frontiers of Neurology and Neuroscience. Vol. 19 (S. Karger AG)

J. Bogousslavsky, M. G. Hennerici, H. Bazner, C. Bassetti (eds.) (2010) *Neurological disorders in famous artists Part 3. Frontiers of Neurology and Neuroscience*, Vol. 27 (S. Karger AG)

Harry Bruinius (2006) *Better for all the world. The secret history of forced sterilization and America's quest for racial purity.* (Knopf)

Stephen Calloway and Lynn Federle Orr (2011) *The cult of beauty: The Aesthetic movement 1860–1900.* (Victoria and Albert Publishing)

Alan F. Casy and Robert T. Parfitt (1986) *Opioid analgesics: Chemistry and receptors.* (Plenum Press)

Frank H. Clarke (ed.) (1973) *How modern medicines are discovered.* (Futura Publishing Co)

Doris H. Clouet (1971) *Narcotic drugs. Biochemical Pharmacology.* (Plenum Press)

Sidney Cohen (1970) *The beyond within. The LSD story.* (Antheum)

Colin Cruise (2005) *Love Revealed. Simeon Solomon and the Pre-Raphaelites.* (Merrell)

Thomas De Quincy (1998) *Confessions of an English Opium Eater.* (Oxford World's Classics)

N. N. Dikov (1971) *Mysteries in the rocks of ancient Chukotka*, trans. Richard L. Bland. (Nauka, Moscow)

William Emboden (1972) *Narcotic Plants. Hallucinogens, stimulants, inebriants and hypnotics, their origins and uses.* (Studio Vista)

Robert Fortune (2005) *A journey to the tea countries of China.* (Elibron Classics)

Simon Garfield (2002) Mauve. *How one man invented a color that changed the world.* (Norton)

E. Gerlach and B. F. Becker (eds.) (1987) *Topics and Perspectives in adenosine research.* (Springer-Verlag)

Amitav Ghosh (2011) *River of smoke.* (Farrar, Straus and Giroux)

Jonathon Green (2002) *Cannabis.* (Thunder's Mouth Press)

Clark Heinrich (2002) *Magic mushrooms in religion and alchemy.* (Park Street Press)

Diarmuid Jeffreys (2004) *Aspirin. The remarkable story of a wonder drug.* (Bloomsbury)

Diarmuid Jeffreys (2008) *Hell's cartel. IG Farben and the making of Hitler's war machine.* (Metropolitan Books)

Joel G. Hardman, Lee L. Limbird, Perry B. Molinoff, Raymond W. Ruddon, and Alfred Goodman Gilman (1996) *Goodman and Gilman's The pharmacological basis of therapeutics.* (McGraw-Hill)

Alethea Hayter (1968) *Opium and the romantic imagination.* (University of California Press)

Lucinda Hawksley (2004) *Lizzie Siddal. Face of the Pre-Raphaelites.* (Walker and Co)

David Healy (2008) *Mania. A short history of bipolar disorder.* (Johns Hopkins University Press)

David Healy (2004) *The creation of psychopharmacology.* (Harvard University Press)

Gwynneth Hemmings and W. A. Hemmings (eds.) (1978) *The biological basis of schizophrenia.* (University Park Press)

Barbara Hodgson (1999) *Opium. A portrait of the heavenly demon.* (Chronicle Books)

Albert Hofmann (2005) *LSD, my problem child.* (MAPS, multidisciplinary association for psychedelic studies)

Beatrice Hohenegger (2006) *Liquid jade: The story of tea from east to west.* (St. Martins Press)

Aldous Huxley (2009) *Island.* (Harper Perennial Modern Classics)

Aldous Huxley (2010) *Brave New World.* (Harper Perennial Modern Classics)

Aldous Huxley (2011) *The Doors of Perception: Heaven and Hell.* (Frontal Lobe Publishing)

Leslie L. Iversen (2007) *The science of marijuana.* (Oxford University Press)

Mike Jay (2010) *High Society: The central role of mind-altering drugs in history, society and culture.* (Park Street Press)

Kathleen Jones (1991) *Learning not to be first: The life of Christina Rossetti.* (St. Martins Press)

E. J. Kahn (1975) *All in a century: The first 100 years of Eli Lilly and Company* (Eli Lilly and Co.)

H. W. Kosterlitz, H. O. J. Collier, and J. E. Villarreal (1973) *Agonist and antagonist actions of narcotic analgesic drugs.* (University Park Press)

Andy Lechter (2007) *Shroom: A cultural history of the magic mushroom.* (Harper Collins)

Martin A. Lee and Bruce Shlain (1992) *Acid Dreams: The complete social history of LSD. The CIA, the sixties and beyond.* (Grove Press)

Louis Lewin (1998) *Phantastica.* (Park Street Press)

Jie Jack Li (2006) *Laughing Gas, Viagra, and Lipitor: The human stories behind the drugs we use.* (Oxford University Press)

B. Litzmann (1979) *Letters of Clara Schumann and Johannes Brahms (1853–1896).* (Hyperion, pp. 103, 206)

Fitzhugh Ludlow (1903 ed.) *The Hasheesh Eater.* (S G Rains and Co, New York)

James H. Madison (2006) *Eli Lilly: A life, 1885–1977.* (Indiana Historical Society Press)

Howard Markel (2011) *An anatomy of addiction: Sigmund Freud, William Halsted, and the miracle drug cocaine.* (Pantheon)

Jan Marsh (1985) *Pre-Raphaelite sisterhood.* (Quartet Books)

Jane Martineau (ed.) (1997) *Victorian Fairy Painting.* (Merrell Holberton)

Raphael Mechoulam (1973) *Marijuana: Chemistry, pharmacology, metabolism and clinical effects.* (Academic Press)

Yutaka Mino and James Robinson (1983) *Beauty and Tranquility: The Eli Lilly Collection of Chinese Art*. (Indianapolis Museum of Art)

David Mitchell (2010) *The thousand autumns of Jacob De Zoet* (Sceptre)

Eric J. Nestler, Steven E. Hyman, and Robert C. Malenka (2001) *Molecular Neuropharmacology. A foundation for clinical neuroscience*. (McGraw-Hill)

Jonathan Ott (1996) *Pharmacotheon: Entheogenic drugs, their plant sources and history*. (Natural Products Co)

D. M. Perrine (1996) *The Chemistry of mind altering drugs: History, pharmacology, and cultural context*. (American Chemical Society, Washington DC)

R. Pertwee (2007) *Cannabinoids*. Handbook of Experimental Pharmacology, Vol. 168. (Springer)

H. C. Peyer (1996) *Roche—a company history 1896–1996*. (Editiones Roche, Basel)

Sadie Plant (1999) *Writing on drugs*. (Faber and Faber)

Roy Porter (2002) *Madness. A brief history*. (Oxford University Press)

Roy Porter and Mikulas Teich (eds.) (1995) *Drugs and narcotics in history*. (Cambridge University Press)

Claire Preston (2005) *Thomas Browne and the writing of early modern science*. (Cambridge University Press)

Oakley Ray and Charles Ksir (1996) *Drugs, society and human behavior*. (WCB McGraw-Hill)

Nancy B. Reich (2001) *Clara Schumann: The artist and the woman*. (Cornell University Press)

Simon Reynolds (1984) *The Vision of Simeon Solomon*. (Catalpa Press)

Sarah Rose (2009) *For all the tea in China. How England stole the world's favorite drink and changed history*. (Viking Press)

Christina Rossetti, ed. Jan Marsh (*1995)* Poems and Prose (Orion Publishing Group)

Mark Sedgwick (2004) *Against the modern world: Traditionalism and the secret intellectual history of the twentieth century*. (Oxford University Press)

Alexander and Ann Shulgin (1991) *PIHKAL: A chemical love story*. (Transform Press)

Alexander and Ann Shulgin (1997) *TIHKAL: The continuation*. (Transform Press)

W Snaeder (2005) *Drug discovery: A history*. (Wiley-Interscience)

Jan Swafford (1999) *Johannes Brahms: A biography*. (Vintage Books)

Alan Staley (2011) *The new painting of the 1860s: between the Preraphaelites and the Aesthetic movement*. (Yale University Press)

Paul Stamets (1996) *Psilocybin mushrooms of the world: An identification guide*. (Ten Speed Press)

Leo H. Sternbach (1980) *The benzodiazepine story*. (Editiones Roche, Basle, Switzerland)

Melanie Thernstrom (2010) *The pain chronicles: Cures, myths, mysteries, prayers, diaries, brain scans, healing and the science of suffering*. (Farrar, Straus and Giroux)

Andrea Tone (2009) *The age of anxiety: A history of America's turbulent affair with tranquilizers*. (Basic Books)

Elliot S. Valenstein (2005) *The war of the soups and the sparks: The discovery of neurotransmitters and the dispute over nerve communication*. (Columbia University Press)

Douglas Valentine (2004) *The strength of the wolf: The secret history of America's war on drugs*. (Verso)

Jessica Warner (2002) *Craze: Gin and debauchery in an age of reason*. (Random House)

R. G. Wasson (1971) *Soma: Divine Mushroom of Immortality*. (Harcourt, Brace, Jovanovich)

R. Gordon Wasson, Stella Kramrisch, Jonathan Ott and Carl P. Ruck (1986) *Persephone's Quest: Entheogens and the origins of religion*. (Yale University Press)

R. G. Wasson, A. A. Hofmann and C. A. P. Ruck (2008) *The road to Eleusis: Unveiling the secrets of the mysteries.* (North Atlantic Books)

Bennett Alan Weinberg and Bonnie K. Bealer (2002) *The world of caffeine. The science and culture of the world's most popular drug.* (Routledge)

Sasha Su-Ling Welland (2007) *A thousand miles of dreams: The journeys of two Chinese sisters.* (Rowman and Littlefield)

John Worthen (2007) *Robert Schumann: Life and death of a musician.* (Yale University Press)

INDEX

2C-B (4-bromo-2,
5-dimethoxyphenethylamine), 64

Abbaye de Plaincourault, France, 16f
Abilify (aripiprazole), 109
Accomplia (rimonabant), 267–268
acetaminophen (Tylenol), 183
acetanilide, 90f
acetylcholine, 18–19, 21, 189
acolytes, 5
Adam and Eve, 16
Adams, John Bodkin, 216
adaptive immune response, 326
Adderall, 302–303
addiction
    barbiturates, 214–215
    Veronal, 214–215
adenosine triphosphate (ATP)
    energetic neurotransmitter, 289–293
    structure, 290f
adrenaline, 299–300
Aesthetic Movement, 256
Afghanistan, poppies, 165–166
agent provocateur, 62, 68, 154
Age of Anxiety, 210–211, 232n.9
Agfa (Aktiengesellschaft fur
    Anilinfabrikation), 88
agonists, 23
agranulocytosis, 108
AIDS patients, 261, 266
alchemy, opium and, 167–168
alcohol, 23, 66, 230–232
Alcott, Louisa May, 247
aldehyde dehydrogenase, 135
Alice in Wonderland, Carroll, 11
alizarin, red dye, 88, 89f
Allegro, John Marco, 15–17, 164
Alles, Gordon, 300

Allom, Thomas, 278f
Alpert, Richard, 5, 67
alphaxalone, 229
Alston, Charles, 170
Alzheimer, Alois, 327
Alzheimer's disease (AD), 111, 289,
    308–309, 332–333
Amanita muscaria, 6, 8–13, 15, 17, 18,
    25, 32, 40, 52
    photograph, 8f
    religious fertility sacrament, 15
    role in brain, 22
Amanita pantherina, 9, 17, 18
Amanita strobiliformis, 19
Ambien, 28, 227
American Indians, peyote, 56–59
American Pharmaceopeia, 242
American Psychiatric Association, 133
amitriptyline (Elavil), 140
amobarbital (Amytal), 213
amphetamines, 62, 114, 299–301
    ecstatic, 301–303
    hallucinations, 111–112, 302
    structure, 301f
amyloid precursor protein (APP), 111
Amytal, 127, 213
ananda, 263
anandamide, 263
anesthesiology, thiopental, 213
Angel Dust, 77, 112
anhalonium, mescaline, 5, 58
Anhalonium Lewinii, 4, 54
aniline, 82, 82f, 84
animal model, psychosis, 110–113
anorexia nervosa, 145
Anslinger, Harry, 235–238, 240–244,
    251, 269–271
antagonists, 23